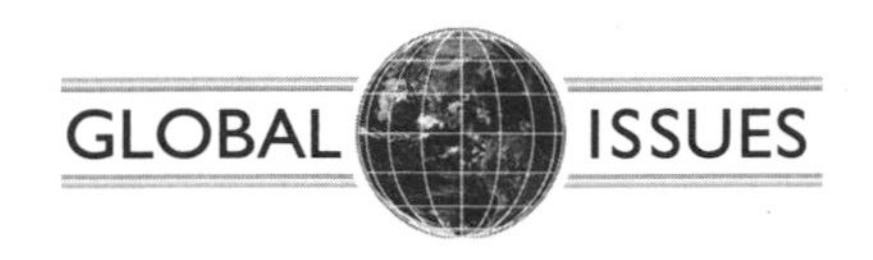

PANDEMICS AND GLOBAL HEALTH

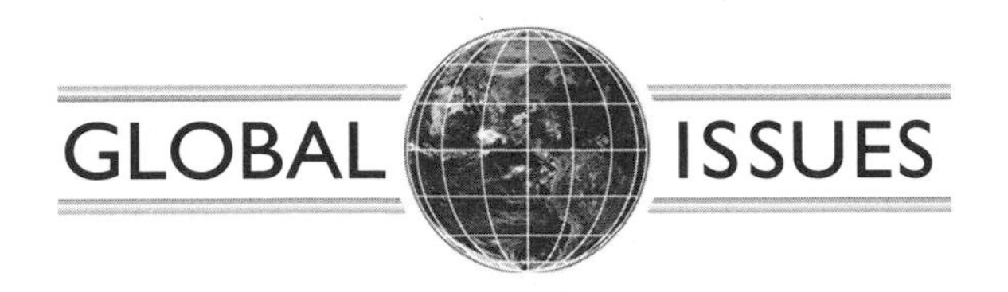

PANDEMICS AND GLOBAL HEALTH

Barry Youngerman

Foreword by Susan Foster
Professor, Department of International Health, Boston University

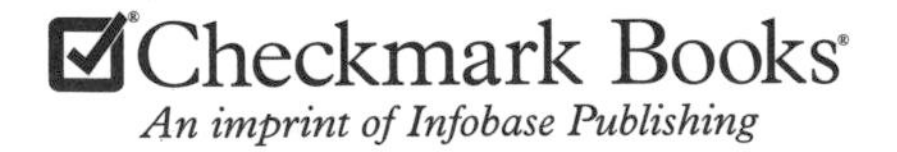

GLOBAL ISSUES: PANDEMICS AND GLOBAL HEALTH

Checkmark Books
An imprint of Infobase Publishing
132 West 31st Street
New York NY 10001

Library of Congress Cataloging-in-Publication Data
Youngerman, Barry.
Pandemics and global health / Barry Youngerman ; foreword by Susan Foster.
p. cm. — (Global issues)
Includes bibliographical references and index.
ISBN-13: 978-0-8160-7740-3
ISBN-10: 0-8160-7440-1
1. Epidemics—History. 2. Communicable diseases—History. 3. World health—Diseases—History. I. Title.
RA649.Y65 2008
614.4'9—dc22 2007021749

Checkmark Books are available at special discounts when purchased in bulk quantities for businesses, associations, institutions, or sales promotions. Please call our Special Sales Department in New York at (212) 967-8800 or (800) 322-8755.

You can find Facts On File on the World Wide Web at http://www.factsonfile.com

Text design by Erika K. Arroyo
Cover design by Salvatore Luongo
Illustrations by Dale Williams

Printed in the United States of America

Bang BVC 10 9 8 7 6 5 4 3 2 1

This book is printed on acid-free paper.

CONTENTS

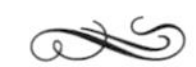

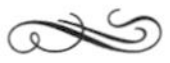

Foreword

With newspapers full of international health news and headlines declaring, "Airplane Trips by Resistant-TB Patient Trigger Alert," "Air Canada Grounds Planes As 'Ruinous' SARS War Hits Home," and "Vietnam on Alert after Latest Human Bird Flu Death," we have increased our awareness of how much we have in common with people in other countries—and how interdependent we are. HIV/AIDS, a disease that started to spread in small remote villages in rural Central Africa probably some 50 or 60 years ago, has now extended worldwide and claimed more than 25 million lives, leaving behind millions of orphaned children, and devastated communities.

Given the high profile of global health issues, it is not surprising that young people (and many older ones too) are eager to become involved. Although advances in biology and medicine are important for global health, it would be unattainable without the public health workers who implement solutions. They must be able to manage, analyze, and evaluate the situation and also communicate with the at-risk population. Without consideration of sociology and anthropology, economics, epidemiology and statistics, and even history and law, the complex health problems facing the world today cannot be solved.

The cases presented in *Pandemics and Global Health* show that these problems truly are multifaceted, and that their solutions are rarely technical in nature. There may be an improved technology at the core, such as the development of ivermectin or Mectizan® for river blindness, but the real challenge comes in distributing the ivermectin to the remote rural populations who need it most. Smallpox eradication could not have been achieved without an effective vaccine, but the real difficulties arose in getting the vaccine to the last few people who were still susceptible to the disease. The solution to SARS was not in the drugs used but, rather, in using proper infection-control practices and isolating the few patients until the disease had died down. The role of public health workers and authorities in these successes is crucial.

Barry Youngerman has done an excellent job of bringing together, in one engaging volume, key information on many of the major contemporary international public health issues, and he has situated each of the major diseases and events in their socioeconomic, historical, and political contexts. Youngerman is also careful not to slight the importance of major historic events, such as the 1918 influenza epidemic, and he has highlighted the elements of that experience that are relevant to the possibility of another pandemic flu outbreak in the next few years. This book will both intrigue and inspire readers to know more and to become involved, and those readers will find a good starting point for their own investigations in the sections on resources for further study.

Part I sets the scene by defining the issues and the challenges involved and provides a brief history of international health. Chapter 1 begins with a review of the major types of infectious agents—bacteria, viruses, parasites, worms, fungi, prions, and so on—and gives useful background for a reader with limited, or outdated, knowledge of biology. It continues with an explanation of the major modes of transmission of disease, a fascinating history of infectious disease from ancient times to the present, and the development of our understanding of causation and attempts to control epidemics, which includes our recent and ongoing efforts to eradicate smallpox, polio, and measles.

The reader is offered a review of the history of epidemics and infectious disease in the United States in chapter 2, which begins with the colonial period and continues to the present. The chapter ends with an examination of the major U.S. agencies involved in public health: the Centers for Disease Control (CDC), the Food and Drug Administration (FDA), the National Institutes of Health (NIH), the Department of Health and Human Services, and the U.S. Public Health Service.

Chapter 3, in some senses the heart of this book, goes beyond U.S. borders and addresses global health issues. It makes the case for governments being open about the presence and scope of infectious disease within their borders and to be willing to take required action. It begins with a riveting account of the SARS outbreak and the response of China and the World Health Organization. The history of SARS demonstrated the need for openness, government commitment, and adequate finance in the fight against major diseases. As Youngerman states in the conclusion to the section on SARS, "It is to be hoped that the world's governments have learned the lesson that transparency and cooperation are essential to protect their populations from infectious disease." The chapter then continues with an account of the discovery and rapid spread of HIV/AIDS, with a focus on the very different responses of Uganda and of South Africa. In Uganda President Yoweri Kaguta

Museveni became personally involved in the effort to increase awareness and change behavior, while in South Africa, President Thabo Mbeki, who succeeded Nelson Mandela as president, came under the influence of "AIDS denialists" who say there is no proof that HIV causes AIDS. Many crucial years were lost during which the epidemic continued to spread unchecked among the South African population, to the extent that now more than 5 million South Africans—11 percent of the total population—are infected with HIV. Three hundred and fifty thousand of those infected are children, many of whom could have been protected by a single-dose treatment given to their mothers at the time of their birth. The Mbeki government's misconception of the disease has led to millions of unnecessary HIV infections.

Next comes an account of the decades-long and successful campaign against onchocerciasis, or river blindness, in West Africa. Youngerman notes that this success required "three decades of persistent hard work by a coalition of governments and international agencies," which has yielded a remarkable if little-known success story. In former times, nearly all the adults above 35 years of age in remote African villages affected by river blindness would be showing signs of incipient blindness. Following a remarkably successful intervention program, hundreds of thousands of African villagers have escaped blindness, and millions of fertile acres of land have been returned to cultivation as a result. The story is not over, however, as this success will continue to require funds, medications, human resources, and a major effort if it is to be sustained. Complacency is the enemy of continued success in public health.

The severe penalty that may be paid for relaxing the level of public health effort is clearly described in the following section. Malaria was under control and nearly eradicated in India, but pressure to stop using DDT brought about a major resurgence of malaria in that country and elsewhere around the world. Youngerman reports that "the total malaria caseload for the entire country fell to below 50,000 by 1961; in 1965, not a single malaria death was reported in India." But that victory was short-lived due to a combination of complacency, slackening of government effort, rise in the price of DDT due to the oil embargo of 1973, and, finally, the appearance of resistance to DDT in the mosquito that spreads the disease. Approximately 20,000 people are now thought to die of malaria each year in India.

Part I ends with a consideration of influenza—past, present, and possible (some would say likely) future. This section includes both a historical review of past flu epidemics, particularly the Spanish flu of 1918, and considerations regarding a possible impending avian flu epidemic. Those interested in the possible avian flu pandemic will find very useful background information here to enhance their understanding of the pandemic flu issues.

Part II provides original source documents, both historical and contemporary and domestic and international. These give readers a starting point for their own investigations into how public health works. The reader will find here a rich selection of documents, including heart-rending accounts of yellow fever in Philadelphia in 1793 and the 1918 flu pandemic in Indian pueblos in New Mexico, discussion of quarantine plans to keep cholera from being brought into the United States by immigrants and the latest U.S. plan for dealing with pandemic flu. It also provides documents on the controversy about the treatment of Lyme disease, showing the diverging opinions offered by two different U.S. scientific bodies. Even top scientists are not always in agreement on the best ways to proceed.

Finally, Part III provides resources for people wanting to further explore public health issues. The student is given practical tips for finding and using a wide variety of sources on public health, from encyclopedias to blogs. The advice on using historical sources is particularly useful and not often found in public health texts. In chapter 8 there is a "who's who" of public health that includes many—but certainly not all—of the greats of public health. Students wanting to know, for example, who Jonathan Mann was and why they hear his name so often will find the answer here. And chapter 9 presents a listing and description of some key organizations in international health, including some important nongovernmental organizations such as Doctors without Borders and the Bill and Melinda Gates Foundation.

One of the best features of *Pandemics and Global Health* is that it completely engages the reader. It provides not so much the "end of the story" but, rather, a point of departure for the reader wanting to begin his or her own investigation of global and international health issues. It will be a valuable resource to anyone wanting to become more informed on global health issues, whether or not he or she hopes one day to make a career in international health.

—Susan Foster

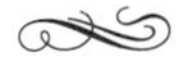

Preface: 1918

My aunt Rose was not sure if her husband was still breathing. After hours of tossing and turning beside her under the sweat-soaked coverlet, his hacking cough keeping her from any hope of sleep, he had suddenly sunk into a stupor. He lay immobile on his back, his eyes blindly focused on the gas lamp hanging from the ceiling.

"Sam?" she whispered. No answer. "God, don't let him die," she prayed over and over. And then: If he goes, how will I feed two kids, and a third one on the way? That is, if any of them survived. He stirred, still alive. Rose looked through the open window toward the street. It was a bright autumn afternoon, but there wasn't a sound outside. No children playing on the stoop or in the gutter, no streetcars lumbering past; only the slow clip-clop this morning on the cobblestones, as the horse cart came to pick up the dead from the overcrowded tenements on St. Mark's Place in New York. It had stopped in front of four buildings today, according to Joey, her five-year-old.

"Joey, listen to me," she called to him in heavily accented English.

"When are we eating, Ma?" he asked from the door. "I'm hungry."

"Joey, take the baby." She summoned all her strength to lift herself a few inches on her elbow. "Go. Go knock on Mrs. Shechter upstairs. Ask her to feed you. I can't. I can't, Joey." She sank back on the bed, her burning lungs exhausted by the effort to talk. The Shechters on the top floor had all gotten sick when the epidemic first hit last month—it killed their 19-year-old. But they say, once you survive you're safe. "Stay there, Joey, at Shechter's" she whispered. The frightened child had started to cry. "I'll get you later. I promise, little lamb." I should never have come to America, Rose thought. At least at home they don't leave you to die. And there was fresh air in the mountains; you could breathe.

But the mountain air had failed to check the plague in Sinowodska, a village 5,000 miles away. Rose couldn't know, as there had been no contact since the outbreak of war, but the "Spanka"—the "Spanish flu"—had swept into the villages of the eastern Carpathians just as the second wave hit New York City.

There Rose's brother, Hersh, had taken sick together with half the village. The only doctor had run away to the Black Sea as soon as the first cases turned up in the province. "Nothing keeps you healthy like the salt air," he had said.

"Salt air? Fairy tales!" Hersh's mother, Sarah, said with a dismissive wave. "Can you run away from the Angel of Death? God is punishing the whole world, like the generation of the Flood." She dipped a rag in a pan of water and wiped Hersh's face before forcing a bit of soup between his peeling lips. For a week she had been nursing him—and most of her neighbors. She would wash down the feverish patients, make them drink water, and talk to them.

It was starting to lift, thank God. Yesterday only four bodies were taken out from the village. God willing, in a few days Sarah could rest. That evening, she felt an ache in her back, so she slipped into bed at nightfall. Two days later Hersh was back on his feet, helping to carry his mother's body to the waiting cart. He insisted on following the corpse to the edge of the forest, where it was slid into a mass grave, in which Poles, Ukrainians, and Jews lay next to one another promiscuously, united in death as they had never been in life. As Hersh chanted a psalm, fresh lime was shoveled over the bodies, by orders of the progressive new mayor, schooled in sanitation.

The news reached Rose in New York a few months later, just after she gave birth to her second son. By then the scourge had cut a swathe through the entire world, striking hundreds of millions in its fury.

—Barry Youngerman

PART I

At Issue

1

Introduction

THE PAST—AND THE FUTURE

The 1918 influenza took a higher toll than any previous epidemic. The precise numbers can never be known, but by the time it ended in 1920, it had killed tens of millions of people, hitting every race and nation, taking the rich and powerful along with the helpless poor, reaching the most remote habitations. Perhaps a third of humanity had fallen ill,[1] and as many as one person out of 20 alive in 1917 was dead by 1919. Among young adults, the flu's special targets, the proportion may have been a good deal higher. Millions of others had been physically and psychologically damaged by the virus,[2] which left its mark on an entire generation.

Although the total number of people who died was exceptional, the suffering caused by this epidemic was unfortunately far from unique. The Black Death of the 14th century probably killed a higher percentage of the population in Asia and Europe. In the Americas, smallpox and other diseases unintentionally introduced after 1492 by European conquerors and settlers may have wiped out as many as 95 percent of the native population over a period of 130 years.[3]

But that was ancient history for the citizens of the industrial world of the early 20th century. Proud of their technical and scientific prowess, they had even begun to "conquer" disease, facing down such age-old enemies as smallpox, yellow fever, and cholera through scientific breakthroughs as well as advances in public health. The world's most advanced countries had just been successfully mobilized for an unprecedented war effort. How could such people be so vulnerable, so helpless before an influenza bug? The shock left its imprint on the memories of a generation.

First-person stories gradually fade. Most young people today would regard 1918 as the distant past. But has the world really changed that much? True, medical science has continued to advance, aided by a larger degree of international cooperation. The mass media have also helped raise awareness.

Today, the first clear sign of a serious pandemic threat would trigger an immediate worldwide deployment of resources undreamed of by the overwhelmed doctors of 1918.

Would it be enough? If a dangerous new human disease were to appear, the scientific and medical establishments might still need precious months (or years) to understand the threat, and to develop new vaccines or treatments. In the meantime, there would not be nearly enough hospital beds or trained nurses to care for the victims. In 1918 the majority of the deaths occurred in just a few months.

If the wealthy countries would be in trouble, what would happen to the poor ones? As it is, in the early 21st century, millions in Asia and Africa are suffering and dying from diseases like malaria that could be much better controlled, if not eradicated, if only enough resources were allocated for preventive measures. Millions of others are dying of AIDS (acquired immunodeficiency syndrome) because they live in countries too poor to maintain adequate health care delivery systems, and because the richer countries have been slow to respond with cheap or subsidized drug treatments.

If anything, our species may be more susceptible than ever to pandemics. Improvements in transportation have brought the entire world into one network of trade, mass migration, and tourism. Today, if a new or newly dangerous pathogen (disease-causing microbe) emerges anywhere, no matter how remote from population centers, it can quickly find its way around the world, as infected individuals drive or fly across countries and continents. In fact, such a pathogen may not even have to seek out human society. According to some observers, as our civilization penetrates previously isolated ecological areas such as rain forests (or other planets[4]), it almost invites attack from pathogens that rarely if ever before infected humans.[5] Climate change, according to other scientists, could also allow some diseases to expand beyond their current geographic limits.[6] Moreover, many experts believe we face a real danger that criminals or terrorists may release specially enhanced infectious agents into our environment, causing human-made pandemics.[7]

Nevertheless, there is no reason to despair. We have more and better tools to deal with deadly organisms: Scientists can quickly isolate and analyze new microbes; laboratories are developing new techniques for rapid production of vaccines; and antiviral drugs are being developed that have at least some effectiveness. Doctors have also learned how to keep more patients alive while infectious diseases run their course, by techniques such as rehydration (to maintain adequate fluids) and treatment of secondary infections. Instant communication via 2 billion mobile phones and over 1 billion Internet accounts means that new threats should be recognized and dealt with faster than ever. International campaigns against smallpox, AIDS, SARS, polio, and measles have brought governments, nongovernmental organizations, and the private sector together to learn habits and skills that will be invaluable in facing new threats.

Knowledge—including more and better information in the hands of the public—is ultimately the best weapon against pandemics. Toward that end, this book will provide an updated survey of pandemic diseases, their history, and the various strategies being used to fight them today. Also included is a selection of source materials that can be used for students in their own research, as well as a survey of many of the available books and other resources in the field. Knowledgeable readers will be better equipped as individuals and members of the human community to resist any pandemics the future may have in store.

THE SCIENCE

What Are Infectious Diseases, Endemic Diseases, Epidemics, and Pandemics?

INFECTIOUS DISEASE AND ENDEMIC DISEASE

An *infectious* disease is any illness caused by an external organism (usually microscopically small) that enters (*infects*) the body. An infectious disease is considered *endemic* to a particular region if it afflicts a more or less steady number of people at any one time. For example, malaria is endemic in much of sub-Saharan Africa. Some 1 to 3 million Africans, mostly small children, die of the disease over the course of the year, with little variation from year to year. The majority of the population escapes: Some people will take ill and recover; others acquire a "subclinical infection"—they are infected without showing symptoms; and some fortunate people are *immune*—their bodies know how to resist the disease. An endemic disease will usually persist in an area if the current victims go untreated, and if the natural conditions that encourage it remain unchanged (in the case of malaria, the presence of mosquitoes).

EPIDEMIC

An *epidemic* is a sudden outbreak of a disease that is new to an area, or a sudden increase in the number of new cases of a previously endemic disease. Childhood diseases like chickenpox can break out in local epidemics; in the past, measles and polio also spread through local or national epidemics. An endemic disease can become epidemic when the pathogen (the organism that causes the disease) mutates to a more dangerous form or when there is a change in the social or natural environment (for example, a long wet spell that increases the mosquito population).

PANDEMIC

The difference between epidemic and pandemic is a matter of degree. When an epidemic rapidly spreads around the world, or over a large part of the world, and strikes a large part of the population, it is called a pandemic.

What Causes Infectious Diseases, Endemics, Epidemics, and Pandemics?

In the past, pandemics usually occurred only in times of political, social, or economic change. For example, the 13th-century conquest by the Mongols of a vast empire, which brought Asia, the Middle East, and Europe closer together, may have facilitated the spread of the Black Death in every direction in the next century.[8] Human immunodeficiency virus (HIV), the virus that causes AIDS, probably first crossed over from an animal to humans in Africa in the 1940s, but did not spread widely there until the independence era of the 1960s and 1970s, when civil wars, boundary changes, and rapid urbanization drove millions of people to move, often far from their homes.[9] In today's shrunken and interconnected world, however, we must assume that conditions are *always* ripe for new pandemics.

Of course, these events and changes would not cause pandemics if the disease organisms did not exist. These pathogens, nearly all invisible to the naked eye, fall into a number of classes: viruses, bacteria, parasites (protozoa), worms, and other epidemic causes.

VIRUSES

Until the recent discovery of prions (see the prion section on pg. 11), viruses were the smallest known infectious agents. A virus is a tiny organism composed of a small amount of genetic material (DNA or RNA) packed into an envelope that can attach to and enter a cell. Once inside, the virus takes over the cell's reproductive machinery in order to produce copies of itself. A virus often kills or weakens the host cell (the cell it has infected); it can also cause damage by overstimulating a person's immune system, which can sometimes harm and kill the body's own cells while attacking the invaders.

Viruses need a host cell to reproduce, but many varieties can survive in the air, in water, and on surfaces for varying amounts of time, which makes them difficult to eradicate. Most of them infect only particular species of animals or plants; unfortunately for humans, a few of the most lethal have been able to jump from animals to humans. Each virus can come in different strains or varieties, which can be more or less harmful to people.

Contagious viruses cause many human diseases, ranging from the common cold and herpes sores to influenza, smallpox, polio, measles, and AIDS.

They can cause at least some cancers (e.g., the human papilloma virus causes most cervical cancers), and are even suspected by some researchers of being involved in multiple sclerosis[10] and other neurological diseases as a complicating factor. From time to time the medical community learns about new viruses. The terrifying Ebola virus first surfaced in Central Africa in 1976, and HIV was first identified in 1983, two years after the first cases of AIDS came to the attention of doctors. Virologist Scott Weaver wrote, "There are undoubtedly a huge number of viruses that infect people all the time that go unnoticed;"[11] he was commenting on an epidemic of crippling chikungunya virus disease that struck the islands of the Indian Ocean in 2005–06. The virus is endemic in most of Africa and Southern Asia.

Antibiotic drugs are useless to combat viruses. Viral diseases sometimes respond to new antiviral drugs like ribavirin or oseltamivir, but they are most often fought with vaccination—injection by a piece of the virus itself, which primes the body's immune system to fight any future infection. Global vaccination programs finally vanquished smallpox, which had killed hundreds of millions of victims over the centuries. The last natural case was recorded in 1977.[12] Polio and measles have also been nearly eliminated, and the world community hopes to declare complete victory over these two diseases in the near future. On the other hand, AIDS still rages unchecked in many countries, although new antiviral medicines can maintain most patients in reasonable health for years.

Certain strains of influenza virus may have the potential to cause a human pandemic, a repeat of the 1918 experience. In the early 21st century a deadly strain of avian flu caused an epidemic among domestic fowl and wild birds, especially in Southeast Asia, and spread to small numbers of people who lived or worked closely with infected birds. In 2007 a few suspected cases of people-to-people transmission had been reported, and health authorities around the world were closely monitoring the situation.

Apart from these global threats, certain viral diseases remain endemic in some countries, with the potential to become epidemic. Several epidemics of dengue fever, transmitted to humans via mosquito bites, have occurred in recent decades; some 24,000 victims died in 1995 in Latin America.[13] Tens of thousands are infected with the severe hemorrhagic (blood loss) dengue strain every year, mostly in Southeast Asia, but most victims survive. Yellow fever, another viral disease spread by mosquitoes, once caused massive epidemics even in northern climates; 10 percent of the people of Philadelphia died in the 1793 epidemic. Yellow fever vaccination has been available for 100 years, and treatment is effective (large volumes of fluids, and at times blood transfusions). Nevertheless, some 30,000 unvaccinated and untreated people in South America and Africa continue to die of yellow fever every year.[14]

BACTERIA

Bacteria are tiny organisms, each comprising a single cell; they are sometimes classified as plants, but they move around like animals. They can live in earth, rocks, or water, on decaying plant and animal matter, and within living things.

The first bacteria emerged at the dawn of life on Earth a few billion years ago. They are so abundant that their biomass (the weight of all individual bacteria added together) may well exceed that of all other plants and animals combined.[15] Many types of bacteria perform vital tasks necessary for the cycle of life. Billions of them live in each of our bodies—mostly on our skin and in our body openings and digestive tract. They help their hosts (the people they live in), fight harmful microbes, and digest food.

Their ability to break down organic (plant or animal) materials makes them useful in environmental cleanups, but it also can make them deadly to human hosts. Disease-causing bacteria damage the body's tissues and organs "both directly through chemical substances that they emit, and indirectly" when the host's immune system overreacts.[16]

These bacteria cause debilitating, crippling, and even fatal diseases. They have caused many of the deadliest epidemics and pandemics in history, including bubonic plague and cholera. Epidemics of tuberculosis, typhoid fever, typhus, and food poisoning (such as from *Salmonella* or *E. coli*) used to be common in America, and they still cause great suffering under certain conditions, often in poorer countries. Chronic (long-lasting) bacterial illnesses such as leprosy and syphilis may take years to kill their hosts. Lyme disease, which is transmitted by deer and mouse ticks, has become endemic in large parts of the United States in recent decades, as dense forests have taken over abandoned farms across much of the country, and suburban development has extended adjacent to these forests.

Much deadly pneumonia is caused by bacteria, often among people who have been weakened by other diseases or old age. Common bacteria such as *Streptococcus* or *Staphylococcus* can cause severe localized infection or can become systemic (infecting the entire body), causing sepsis (blood poisoning) and death. The highly contagious *Chlamydia* bacteria, if untreated, can lead to trachoma, a leading cause of blindness. As a sexually transmitted infection, affecting some 4 million Americans a year, chlamydia can cause infertility in both men and women.

Bacterial illnesses are often highly contagious. Paths of infection can include the air, food, water, insect bites, and physical contact. Some of these organisms can live in host animal populations. For example, the bubonic plague bacteria lives in rats and wild rodents; fleas that feed on these rodents ingest the bacteria, and then pass it along to human hosts.

Fortunately, most harmful bacteria are vulnerable to the many antibiotic drugs that have been developed since the introduction of penicillin in the mid-20th century. These drugs either kill off the bacteria or limit their growth. Other measures that have reduced bacterial disease are: improved garbage removal and pest control, clean water supplies, sanitary regulations for restaurants and food processing plants, and antiseptic practices in doctors' offices and hospitals.

Unfortunately, many disease-causing bacteria have developed resistance to antibiotics, partly due to overuse of the drugs. Public health authorities worry that this growing resistance might one day expose us to renewed pandemics of diseases that we thought were under control.

PARASITES (PROTOZOA)

Protozoa are microscopic one-celled creatures that have some of the characteristics of animals. They live in a variety of habitats. Some of them are capable of infecting people; they become parasites, taking their nutrition from the food their victims eat or from the victim's own cells. They can cause severe symptoms, sometimes leading to death.

These parasitic diseases tend to be endemic, and these days they are generally confined to tropical and poorer regions. While they lack the dramatic impact of sudden pandemics, they affect hundreds of millions of people around the world, who are periodically or chronically unable to work or study. As such, they are a severe drain on developing economies and cause much individual suffering.

Malaria has been the most widespread and the most devastating of the parasitic diseases, with a few hundred million new infections and 1–3 million deaths each year,[17] mostly in Africa and mostly among young children. Although preventive measures and drugs are available to fight this plague, and promising vaccines are being developed, neither have been sufficiently deployed, due to lack of resources and lack of a sense of urgency in the world. Controversies have complicated the matter as well. DDT, a cheap, effective killer of mosquitoes, was banned in rich countries because it was toxic to some wildlife; most malaria experts want it used more extensively in poor countries, where, they say, suffering from malaria far outweighs the possible ill effects of DDT on people or wildlife when used carefully and appropriately.[18] In another issue, anti-malaria groups differ about how widely to use the drug artemisinin—it kills the parasite, but overuse may encourage the microbe to develop drug resistance, which would leave victims without any recourse.[19]

One group of protozoa, the trypanosomes, is responsible for several deadly parasitic diseases, all transmitted to their human hosts via insects. The famous tsetse fly passes along sleeping sickness, the aptly named assassin bug spreads Chagas disease (which infects 20 million victims and kills 20,000 of them each years in various parts of Latin America),[20] and certain sand fly species spread Leishmaniasis in Africa, Asia, and Latin America, causing disfiguring skin sores, organ failure, and sometimes death.

Sleeping sickness in still endemic in parts of sub-Saharan Africa; it infects a few hundred thousand people each year. Many of them develop chronic and repeated episodes of illness and many of them die. Major, long-lasting epidemics have been recorded, the worst in 1896–1906.

"Elephantiasis," a severe form of filariasis, is transmitted by a mosquito. It affects some 120 million people in tropical countries, one-third of them seriously.[21] Symptoms include leatherlike skin and crippling enlargement of the legs and genitals due to blockage of lymph vessels.

Many protozoa enter the body through contaminated food and water. The victims in turn pass on the organisms—and the disease—in their body wastes (urine or fecal matter) Where sanitation is inadequate, the parasites can reenter the water supply, or be passed along in foods handled by infected people. Parasitic diseases like giardiasis, amoebiasis, and a host of others can cause severe, debilitating intestinal distress; if untreated by antibiotics they can become chronic or cyclical. They are endemic to many regions, and migration and tourism have helped spread them to new areas, causing unexpected local epidemics.

WORMS

The majority of the many thousands of roundworm and flatworms species are parasitic (they live off a plant or animal host) but only a small number infect humans. The diseases they cause, like the protozoan diseases, tend to be endemic in poorer tropical countries.

Some 200 million people in Latin America, Africa, and Asia are infected with schistosomiasis, some 10 percent of them severely.[22] The larva (immature form) of the schistosoma flatworm develops in freshwater snails and attaches itself to humans swimming in infested waters; the eggs develop within the human host, and return to the water through body wastes. The disease has spread in certain regions when new dams create artificial lakes, ideal homes for the larvae.[23] The disease is rarely fatal, but it is chronically debilitating. A cheap, readily available drug can safely eliminate the parasite, but reinfection is common.

The less dangerous tapeworm, another parasitic flatworm, can be found in all climates, and can cause malnutrition and serious complications. It is often transmitted via infected and improperly cooked food, especially meat. It rarely reaches epidemic proportions.

Nematodes (roundworms) are responsible for two harrowing illnesses that, thankfully, have been largely suppressed: onchocerciasis (river blindness) and Guinea worm disease. The onchocerca parasite is transmitted to people by black flies living along rivers; it can cause severe inflammation and often leads to blindness. A World Health Organization (WHO) program launched in 1974 eliminated most transmission of the disease in West Africa, through aerial spraying with insecticides and treatment of patients with donated medicine. The agency estimates that over 60 million acres of infested riverfront land was freed for safe farming and resettlement.[24]

Guinea worms (dracuncula, or "little dragons") infected some 3 million people in Africa as recently as 1986. They incapacitate their victims through severe pain, as the long, thin worm slowly burns away a path out of the victim's body. An international eradication campaign has eliminated the pests in most locations in Africa, with only 12,000 cases reported in 2005.[25]

OTHER EPIDEMIC CAUSES

Fungus

Many common types of fungus that are found everywhere in the environment can infect people. Some are harmless; others cause only relatively minor problems (athlete's foot, yeast infections)—except when individuals are weakened by other conditions, such as AIDS.

Prion

A new type of infectious disease agent has come to the attention of scientists and a frightened public in recent decades—the prion. A prion is a protein molecule that has become misfolded; it can convert normal protein molecules into its own misshapen and harmful form. One type of prion is the probable cause of "mad cow disease" (bovine spongiform encephalopathy), a fatal affliction of the brain and nervous system.

Mad cow disease became epidemic in cattle herds in the United Kingdom in the 1980s. It was apparently transmitted to some 180 Europeans, who became ill in the 1990s after eating meat or meat products. Some epidemiologists feared that large numbers of Britons would eventually succumb, and that the global trade in meat might already have laid the basis for a pandemic. Massive cattle culls, strict import controls in other countries, and a change in animal feeds seem to have contained the epidemic. Isolated cases have continued to emerge among cattle in several countries around the world.

Multiple causes

Finally, some deadly conditions, such as severe diarrhea (responsible for close to 2 million deaths each year among children under five[26]), can be caused by a variety of different viruses, bacteria, or parasites, which are endemic in the food or water supply in many regions. The treatment is often the same whatever the cause: It is based largely on oral rehydration (replacing lost liquids). Prevention depends largely on clean supplies of drinking water. Early in 2007, the WHO approved an affordable vaccine for rotavirus, which causes fatal diarrhea in 600,000 young children a year in poor countries.[27]

How Do They Get Us?: Modes of Transmission

If the huge variety of infectious disease agents does not frighten you, think about all the different pathways these agents use to infect humans. But also bear in mind, we can use each of these pathways to prevent and fight epidemics.

HUMAN-TO-HUMAN

Probably the most common way to get sick is to have contact with another person who is sick. Many diseases, such as influenza, tuberculosis, and smallpox, are typically "airborne"; they are acquired by breathing air into which patients have coughed or sneezed. People may catch smallpox, for example, by being within six or seven feet of a patient for two or three hours. The microbes can also survive for a while on clothing, dishes, doorknobs, or any surface, waiting for a new victim to touch them and then touch their face or mouth. Other human-to-human pathogens such as HIV and chlamydia are much less contagious. For these diseases transmission generally requires more direct physical contact, such as sex or sharing needles.

INSECT-TO-HUMAN

Mosquitoes, flies, lice, ticks, fleas, and other bloodsucking insects constitute another major disease vector (transmitter). Some insects pass the microbe from one person to other, such as in malaria, yellow fever, and typhus. Other insects serve as middlemen in this process; the pathogens live in animal "reservoirs"—such as cattle in sleeping sickness and rats in bubonic plague—until transmitted by the insect to humans.

ANIMAL-TO-HUMAN

Some diseases are transmitted to people only or primarily through direct infection from animals. Such is the case with rabies, and with the deadly H5N1 strain of avian flu. Nearly all recorded human cases of this avian flu were clearly passed to people after close contact with infected birds, as of mid-2007. However, many pathogens that originated in animals have mutated over time to become contagious between humans. Such was apparently the case with the SARS virus, which killed some 800 people in 2002–03 before it was stopped by relentless case-tracking and stringent quarantine procedures.

FOOD AND WATER

Many diseases are contracted primarily by eating contaminated food or drinking (or bathing in) water contaminated by fecal matter and other waste. Typhoid fever, guinea worms, polio, mad cow disease, and hepatitis A are among the afflictions often transmitted in this fashion.

MOTHER-TO-BABY

Tragically, some infectious diseases can be transmitted from mother to fetus during pregnancy, childbirth, or breast-feeding, including hepatitis B (endemic in Southeast Asia) and HIV infection. This mode is called "vertical transmission."

MEDICAL PROCEDURES

A large number of unrelated ailments can be passed along during blood transfusions and organ transplants, or by the use of unsterilized medical and dental equipment. Increased vigilance by medical professionals and more accurate testing of blood and organs have limited this mode of transmission in most of the industrialized world, although it may still be an important mode of transmission in other areas, such as China or India.

HISTORY OF EPIDEMICS

An Overview

Infectious disease has been with the human race since prehistoric times. In fact, such diseases are a fact of life for all animal and plant species. From the perspective of evolution, infectious diseases are major engines of evolutionary change. They eliminate vulnerable populations and encourage diversity as a survival tactic.[28]

Many of the familiar pathogens that caused major historic epidemics were already present among primitive hunter-gatherers tens of thousands of years ago. The diseases are evident in ancient remains. Scientists called paleopathologists have examined samples of human and animal bones and other remains (including preserved mummies) at sites all over the globe, dating from prehistoric to recent eras. The bones and teeth found in these sites often show the characteristic marks of tuberculosis, syphilis, leprosy, and other infections. In addition, these scientists have found traces of DNA from deadly bacteria in ancient human bones.[29]

Scientists have tried to estimate when certain viruses or bacteria first began to infect humans by tracing the genetic variations between different strains of these pathogens in current patients. If the strains vary widely, the pathogen has probably lived in human hosts for thousands of years, giving it time to mutate and evolve.[30]

Historians have used this and other evidence to trace a rough history of human health and disease. The results can be surprising. The earliest humans, who ate only what they could hunt or gather in the wild, were relatively tall and vigorous. When people learned to cultivate grains and domesticate animals some 10,000 years ago, the total number of humans soared; however, the health of the average individual seems to have declined. Their skeletons are shorter and they show more evidence of malnutrition and chronic disease than the "cavemen" who came before.

Epidemic disease may have been the main cause of this deterioration. Agriculture required permanent settlements. These settlements eventually grew into crowded villages and towns, where everyone lived close to human waste and garbage. The hunter bands of the past had developed immunity to the pathogens endemic to their communities. In the new towns people encountered unrelated individuals, each one carrying his or her own collection of microbes. Manageable infections turned into "crowd diseases" or epidemics; with so many more hosts, some microbes were able to mutate into deadlier forms.

Domesticated animals, living in close quarters with their human masters, were another source of microbes; no one was immune to these new diseases. Smallpox, influenza, bubonic plague, tuberculosis, and other deadly diseases spread like wildfire. Eventually, the surviving population developed a degree of immunity to the more common diseases, which became endemic. The reprieve would last only until one of the microbes mutated, or environmental conditions changed, or war, migration, or trade brought formerly isolated populations together.

All the early civilizations of the Old World, including Mesopotamia, Egypt, India, and China, left written records of the ravages of epidemic disease. In a lament dating from the 14th century B.C.E., a Hittite priest (from modern-day Turkey) wrote of a terrible plague that had decimated his nation for 20 years. The disease had apparently been brought to the country by Egyptian prisoners of war; nevertheless, the priest attributed it to the wrath of a river god, angry that a wartime pledge had not been fulfilled.[31]

Such explanations were common in ancient times. The book of Exodus in the Hebrew bible reports that Egypt was struck with a devastating livestock epidemic, followed by a human plague of unbearable skin boils. The book explains the plagues as God's punishment for the wickedness of

Pharaoh and the Egyptians; the plagues also served to convince Israel and the world that the sacred Egyptian idols were worthless. In the biblical narrative, the two epidemics are preceded by plagues of lice and flies, both of which are known transmitters of human and animal disease.

As with the Hittite epidemic, international war often helped diseases to disperse over long distances; large numbers of soldiers and refugees living under ad hoc conditions are perfect incubators for epidemics. The great historian Thucydides wrote a terrifying description of such an epidemic, which decimated Athens in the late fifth century B.C.E. during the Peloponnesian War. The disease (whose symptoms do not exactly correspond to any known modern disease) wiped out one-third of the population, including much of the army and political leadership, leading to the defeat of Athens and thus changing the course of Western history. According to the author, the plague began in Ethiopia, spread to Egypt, and thence to Piraeus, the port city of Athens.[32]

The First Pandemics

The merging of widely dispersed countries into vast, integrated empires like that of Rome (which covered parts of three continents) allowed genuine pandemics to take hold. One such catastrophe (generally believed to have been smallpox and/or measles) ravaged the entire Roman Empire in 164–180 C.E.; it was brought to the capital by soldiers returning from the eastern provinces. Some historians believe it triggered a long-term population decline, which accelerated during a repeat pandemic in the following century (251–270).[33]

By this time, the different civilized regions of the Old World (in the Mediterranean Basin, the Middle East, northern India, and China) had grown more interconnected, through expanding settlements, migration, trade, and unfortunately, disease. The outbreak of bubonic plague that began in Constantinople in 541 C.E., known in the West as "Justinian's Plague," struck Europe (as far as Denmark and Ireland), North Africa, the Middle East, and Central and South Asia; by the end of the century it hit China as well. Millions died in the first wave; even worse, the disease did not completely disappear—Europe saw new outbreaks (often localized) every few decades for 200 years. Some historians claim that the total European population declined 50 percent over this period; if so, the plague can take major credit for the final decline of the Roman Empire and the beginning of the "Dark Ages" of European history.[34]

Bubonic plague entered a 600-year period of dormancy, only to reemerge with greater force in the epidemic known in Europe as the Black Death (1347–51); the plague killed about one-third of the continent's population and had profound effects on economic, religious, and cultural life.[35] Including Europe, the Middle East, India, and China, about 75 million people died. The Black Plague, much like its Justinian predecessor, ushered in an era of intermittent local plagues, like the one that devastated London in 1665–66.

These pandemics were confined to the Old World. The peoples of the Americas, safe behind two oceans, were spared, but as a consequence, their populations had no immunity to these microbes. In Europe and Africa, measles and even smallpox had become largely nonfatal childhood diseases, which conferred immunity on the survivors.

The very first contacts between the Old and New Worlds had terrible results. The Spanish conquests of the Aztec Empire in Mexico in 1519 and the Inca Empire in Peru in 1532 were aided by smallpox epidemics, which wiped out much of the local population and left the survivors demoralized. In Peru, typhus came in 1546, influenza in 1558, diphtheria in 1614, and measles in 1618. In each case, the first outbreak was followed by periodic returns. In New England, early European explorers reported that the coast was settled with thriving American Indian villages. In 1616 a French ship was shipwrecked on Cape Cod; its crew was captured and divided among neighboring tribes. Apparently the crew carried a disease, possibly viral hepatitis. Within three years as many as 90 percent of the American Indians in coastal New England had died, leaving large stretches of unsettled land for the first colonists from England to claim and settle. By 1650 the pre-1492 population of the Americas had been reduced by as much as 95 percent, in the opinion of some scholars.[36]

Nor did the Europeans come away unscathed. Along with maize, tomatoes, potatoes, chocolate, and tobacco, they apparently brought back venereal syphilis (although the claim is still controversial[37]) and possibly typhus as well. The Old World was ravaged by a ferocious syphilis epidemic at the start of the 16th century, appearing first in Italy in 1494, reaching the Middle East by 1499, and arriving in China a few years later.[38] The disease subsided to endemic levels by the end of the 15th century, but it remained widespread until the advent of 20th-century antibiotics.

How Did People Cope?

Despite the attempts of brilliant and dedicated physicians, premodern cultures around the world proved largely helpless in the face of epidemics. In fact, they were not too successful in treating ordinary illness. The prevailing medical theories in the West, China, and India ascribed most disease to an imbalance of basic substances within the body. Such imbalance was supposedly caused by diet, poisons, climate, the movements of the stars and planets, behavioral excesses, and other factors. The Greek philosopher Aristotle posited four "humors": blood, phlegm, black bile, and yellow bile; the Chinese wrote about yin and yang; Indian Ayurveda posited five basic elements.

Diets and treatments based on such views, combined with knowledge of medicinal herbs, often helped people maintain general health, and a healthy person is somewhat more likely to resist epidemics. Some religious practices designed to ensure ritual and moral purity also helped prevent physical illness. Egyptians stressed frequent ritual washing and shaving; the Hebrews would not eat animals that died on their own, or any slaughtered animal whose entrails appeared damaged or diseased. Both cultures practiced male circumcision, which gives some protection against sexually transmitted diseases, at least under premodern sanitary conditions.[39]

Since ancient times people have known that deadly diseases can spread from person to person and from place to place, and they have responded with measures designed to isolate the sick. In September 1793, during a yellow fever epidemic in Philadelphia, the state legislature declared a quarantine against ships arriving from the West Indies, preventing their crews from landing; one such ship may have brought the first cases to the city a month before.[40] The practice derived from the European Middle Ages, when ships would often be required to wait offshore 40 days (*une quarantaine de jours,* in French) in times of plague, to see if any cases turned up on board. Rich people would flee crowded cities for the country at the first sign of an epidemic.

But the method of transmission remained a frightening mystery. Often, foreigners or feared minority groups were blamed for spreading epidemics. During the Black Death of the 14th century, thousands of Jews were murdered in various European countries on suspicion of having spread the plague by poisoning wells. When venereal syphilis spread across Europe in the 16th century, the English called it "the French disease," the French called it "the English disease," and Arabs called it the "disease of the Christians."

Without support from medical theories, certain folk practices around the world reflected at least a practical intuition of how diseases spread. Historians have uncovered many examples from Europe, India, China, the Middle East, and Africa in which people introduced pus from smallpox sores into healthy individuals, giving them a mild form of the disease but protecting them against the more serious epidemic form.[41] The successful vaccination experiments of British doctor Edward Jenner in the 1790s, in which subjects were protected from smallpox infections after being injected with pus taken from cowpox victims, provided scientific support for such practices, made them acceptable around the world, and eventually led to the discovery of viruses as a disease agent.

Many European doctors and public officials, from ancient times to the late 19th century, blamed epidemics on "miasmas"—unhealthy fogs made up of particles of decomposed or toxic material. They were wrong, but the theory proved useful nevertheless. While the bad odors that often come from swamps are not in fact harmful, such swamps encourage the growth of mosquitoes, the vector that passes yellow fever and malaria (the Italian word for "bad air") from victim to victim. Similarly, foul-smelling garbage attracts rats, which can bear contagious diseases, and the water from undrained sewage can seep into wells, spreading cholera and other diseases.

The London physician John Snow proved, at least to a wide public if not to all scientists, that the agent that caused cholera was passed in drinking water and not air. His careful observations during the epidemic of 1854 traced many cases of the disease to drinking water from a pump in Broad Street. Those who lived near the pump but obtained their water from other sources were spared, evidence that the disease did not pass through the air. Parliamentary legislation mandating cleaner water supplies and an efficient sewer system soon eliminated cholera from the city.[42]

Breakthrough: The Germ Theory

In the second half of the 19th century, all earlier theories of disease transmission were overturned by the triumph of the germ theory, which captured the imagination of both scientists and the wider public across the world. It became a key foundation of modern medicine and public health. According to this theory, all infectious diseases are caused by invisible microscopic living organisms that enter the body through direct or indirect contact with other diseased individuals, animals, or insects.

Some ancient philosophers had similar ideas, but the theory became plausible only after Dutch scientist Antoni van Leeuwenhoek used his powerful hand-made microscopes in the late 17th century to discover a vast invisible world of single-celled microorganisms all around us. In the course of the 19th century, scientists like Agostino Bassi of Italy, Louis Pasteur of France, and Robert Koch of Germany were able to isolate and observe some of the actual microscopic fungus and bacteria that were killing both animals and humans. By 1876 Koch had discovered the bacterium that causes anthrax; in 1882 he announced his discovery of another, even smaller bacterium that causes tuberculosis,[43] a far more widespread disease. In 1894, during a plague epidemic in Hong Kong, the Swiss doctor Alexandre Yersin and the Japanese bacteriologist Kitasato Shibasaburo discovered the bacterium that causes bubonic plague.[44]

The germ theory was a great advance—but it was only the first step in fighting epidemics. Biologists still had to identify most of the microbes (viruses were first seen only in the 1940s, using electron microscopes). Then they had to develop vaccines, antitoxins (blood products taken from mildly infected animals), and antibiotics to fight them. Doctors and hospitals had to discover the best ways of preventing the spread of disease and treating the victims. They were helped by the new field of epidemiology (the study of how disease spreads). The first university department of epidemiology was set up at Johns Hopkins University in Baltimore in 1919. But even before then, epidemiologists had begun careful studies of past epidemics and pandemics to see what preventive measures and what treatments really worked.

At least by the 18th century governments around the world began to assume responsibility for enforcing healthier conditions in housing and the workplace, and to ensure a safer food and water supply. Bavaria passed a law requiring vaccination of infants against smallpox in 1804;[45] similar laws were passed in many other countries and in most American states over the next hundred years. As new vaccines were developed, including "booster" doses for older children to reinforce immunity, the laws were generally expanded to cover these vaccines as well.

By the end of the 19th century, public health authorities were granted legal powers to incarcerate uncooperative disease carriers (those who harbored disease-causing microbes without getting sick themselves). The notorious "Typhoid Mary" of New York City was an asymptomatic carrier of the typhoid virus—she carried the bacteria that lived within her without causing illness. She had infected 22 people over seven years working as a domestic cook, until she was apprehended in 1907 and put into isolation, where she was kept for 30 years.[46] Physicians were required to report any cases of deadly contagious disease to public authorities, and contract tracing was enforced to locate others who might have been exposed. When New York authorities discovered in 1943 that penicillin was a highly effective drug against syphilis, they instituted a contract tracing policy for the disease, backed up by the police; similar policies around the country helped reduce the incidence of the disease by 90 percent.[47] Such mandatory health measures have often attracted opposition on grounds of civil liberties; the laws have sometimes been modified to offer more leeway when possible.

A Shrinking World Learns to Cooperate

Epidemics pay little attention to boundaries of nation, race, or even economic status. In ages past, geographical barriers—oceans, deserts, and mountains—could provide some protection. By the 15th century, however, nearly all of Asia, Europe, and North Africa had been knit together by trade, conquest, and travel. In the next century the Americas and the entire coastline of Africa were brought into the fold. For the last 400 years human beings have constituted one large, integrated "herd," from the viewpoint of disease microbes. Infectious disease anywhere is a threat—at least potentially—to people everywhere. This is true of existing diseases like AIDS, malaria, and plague as well as any new disease that may appear.

To put the matter in a more positive light, any advance in knowledge and practice anywhere can help people everywhere. However, such help is not automatic. As the 21st century begins, millions of people in Africa and parts of Asia are still suffering and dying from preventable and treatable endemic and pandemic diseases that have largely been eliminated from Europe, the Americas, and East Asia. However, persistent, well-funded cooperation by governments, international bodies, professional and charitable groups, and the private sector can surely spread the benefits of medical advances to the entire world.

Fortunately, the foundation for such work already exists, laid down over the past 150 years, at first largely on the initiative of the European powers (including the Ottoman Empire of Turkey). In the 1830s a Sanitary, Medicine, and Quarantine Board was established in Alexandria, Egypt, to keep track of any disease outbreak in the Middle East that could affect Mediterranean trade, or that could spread to Europe (as had happened, it was believed, several times in the past). Eventually the board assumed responsibility for inspecting the health of the many Muslim pilgrims traveling to and from Mecca, whose numbers were soaring thanks to modern means of transportation. Similar boards were soon set up at Constantinople and Tangier, with European representation.

In 1851 the first International Sanitary Conference was held at Paris, largely to combat the persistent cholera epidemics that plagued Europe. Later meetings were held at Constantinople, Vienna, Venice, and Washington, D.C., leading up to the International Sanitary Convention or treaty in 1882, which was strengthened in 1903, 1913, and 1926. Under the convention the signatory governments agreed to observe rules of hygiene, inspection, quarantine, and public reporting that could prevent the spread of cholera, plague, and other epidemic diseases. Such measures (including inspections, rat extermination, and reporting of contagious disease) were largely confined to ports and border crossings, although wider reporting requirements were added during later revisions.

The sanitary conferences were stimulated in part by European fears of "Asiatic diseases," and reflected a degree of racism. However, they helped erect a structure of international health law and create global awareness of health interdependence. Unfortunately, the measures were enforced only in part. Also, from the 19th century to the present many international disputes have arisen concerning "excessive measures" by individual countries that restricted trade and the free movement of people using the threat of disease as a convenient excuse.

In parallel to the governmental efforts, international medical conferences were held, starting in Paris in 1867. They helped spread new medical discoveries and methods to the Americas and Asia, which eventually became centers of medical research in their own right. In 1894, when an outbreak of bubonic plague from southern China hit Hong Kong, its governor appealed for help to France, whose government sent one of the top researchers from the Pasteur Institute, Alexandre Yersin, and to Japan, where the noted expert in infectious diseases Shibasaburo Kitasato assembled a team to investigate the problem. They eventually isolated the plague bacteria (later named *Yersinia pestis*) in both humans and rodents.[48]

The century also saw a substantial growth in organized nongovernmental activity in the field of global health. Starting in the 1830s, European and American Protestant and Catholic missionaries began developing an infrastructure of doctors and hospitals in non-Christian countries in Asia and Africa, starting with the Medical Missionary Society of China, founded in 1838,[49] continuing in India in the 1860s, sub-Saharan Africa in the 1870s, and Korea in the 1880s. This work, eventually staffed by locally trained professionals, helped lay the groundwork for modern medicine throughout the non-European world. It also established lines of communication that facilitated the spread of modern medicine and medical science.

The first permanent international health organization was founded in 1902, in the Western Hemisphere—the International Sanitary Bureau, later renamed the Pan American Health Organization (PAHO). PAHO serves simultaneously as the Americas Regional Office of the UN World Health Organization (WHO). In 1909 L'Office Internationale d'Hygiène Publique (the "Paris Office") was founded with a mission to gather and spread information on infectious diseases and epidemics around the world. World War I brought an upsurge of typhus and malaria in Europe; these threats, together with the influenza pandemic of 1918, led the new League of Nations to set up a Health Organization, which continued to function alongside the Paris Office until World War II. In 1924 the organization created a Malaria Commission, which organized visits through Italy, the Balkans, and the Soviet Union to investigate the problem and work with local authorities to eradicate the disease.

The Modern Era

The World Health Organization, founded by the new United Nations in 1946 during the brief era of good feeling and international cooperation following World War II, was the culmination of these global efforts. On its inception in 1948 it took over the responsibilities of the Paris Office and the League of Nations Health Organization, with an even more expansive mission: "the attainment by all peoples of the highest possible level of health" through fighting disease and encouraging conditions that ensure good health.

A permanent staff works at world headquarters in Geneva. An annual World Health Assembly meets each year with representation from all UN members. In recent years, about one-half the WHO budget has been financed by nongovernment organizations, private foundations, and the pharmaceutical industry, who have collectively taken on much of the responsibility for global health.[50]

By the 1960s, with UN membership nearly universal, the WHO was often thought of as the world's public health authority. However, it suffered from inadequate enforcement power, and was occasionally hampered by politics and bureaucracy. Its decentralization into six autonomous regional offices (Africa, the Americas, Eastern Mediterranean, Europe, South East Asia, and Western Pacific) probably spared it the worst consequences of global power politics. The regional directors supervise the WHO representative offices in the member countries, which often serve as important advisers on health matters to local governments.

In its 60-year history the WHO has gone through several changes in emphasis. It began by pursuing the traditional approach it inherited from the predecessor organizations, relying on international sanitary regulations to limit the spread of certain epidemics across international borders. The world health community eventually recognized that this approach had failed, due in part to reporting failures (even countries that overreacted to reports of disease in neighboring countries were reluctant to report epidemics in their own territory) and to the explosion of travel and trade. The rise of new epidemics in the 1980s (AIDS), the 1990s (hemorrhagic fevers in Africa), and the new millennium (SARS in China), as well as reemergence of old plagues, such as cholera in Peru in 1991, plague in India in 1994, and diphtheria in the former Soviet Union in 1995,[51] were new crises that did not fit into the old model, yet cried out for a global response.

In 1995 the agency began a long process of drafting new international health regulations; they were finally adopted by its assembly in 2005, and implemented in June 2007. The new rules would give a greater role to preventive measures within countries, and require reporting for a wider range of diseases and syndromes.

Starting in the 1950s, the WHO developed a more ambitious agenda, designed to combat major epidemic diseases one at a time through vaccination campaigns, pest elimination, systematic reporting, and, where appropriate, isolation. A global Malaria Eradication Program, begun with great fanfare in the 1950s, made much progress but eventually petered out into smaller local campaigns in the face of funding problems, pesticide controversies, and poor health infrastructure in many tropical countries.[52]

On the positive side of the ledger, the organization scored a spectacular success when it sponsored the global effort to eradicate smallpox. Begun in 1967, the intense campaign centered on "ring vaccination" of all those living near each new reported case. Large-scale positive publicity managed to win wide cooperation all over the world, even in the face of wars and cultural or political opposition. The last natural case was reported in 1977. Not a single naturally occurring case has emerged since then, and none is expected, since no animal reservoir exists for this disease, which has killed untold millions throughout history. In 1978 a worker died of smallpox in Birmingham, England, due to inadequate safety procedures at a lab. In 1980 the WHO officially proclaimed that smallpox was eradicated.

THE NEW MODEL—THE CURRENT GLOBAL RESPONSE

WHO continues to play an active role in fighting epidemics, but only as one player in a complex network of government agencies, NGOs (nongovernmental organizations), and private foundations. The UN itself created a new agency to deal with AIDS apart from the WHO—UNAIDS (Joint United Nations Programme on HIV/AIDS, founded in 1995).[53] It coordinates the work of 10 other UN agencies (each of which has health-related programs of its own). Observers sometimes complain that the proliferation of agencies is inefficient and can even distort priorities. For example, UNAIDS has been criticized for overestimating the incidence of AIDS in East and West Africa.[54]

In practical terms, the world's first line defense against new or revived epidemic disease resides in an interlocking network of national, international, and nongovernmental bodies. Among the major data-collection and reporting bodies are the U.S. Centers for Disease Control and Prevention (CDC),[55] the new European Centre for Disease Prevention and Control (ECDC),[56] and the Public Health Agency of Canada, whose Global Public Health Intelligence Network (GPHIN) monitors the Internet continuously.

GPHIN is the source of 20 to 40 percent of the WHO's disease outbreak information.[57]

The WHO helps coordinate all this information via online collections such as WHONET, which monitors evidence of resistance to antibiotics and other medicines, and the Global Influenza Surveillance Network, which helps decide what flu strains should be included in each year's flu vaccine. "ProMed-mail" [Program to Monitor Emerging Diseases], run from Harvard University by the International Society for Infectious Diseases, is an open database where health professionals around the world can post daily updates about emerging diseases and toxins.

In recent years, the developed world seems to be paying more attention to the epidemics and endemic diseases that routinely devastate many tropical countries. Since the 1990s, efforts have proliferated both to slow the spread of disease and to treat those already infected. The foreign assistance budget of the United States has increased substantially in the new century, with an emphasis on health care programs such as the Bush administration's Emergency Plan for AIDS Relief. In the European Union, traditionally more generous, the national government programs are now being supplemented by new programs run by the supranational European Commission.

More and more players have jumped into the game, such as the Global Fund to Fight AIDS, Tuberculosis, and Malaria, founded in 2002, which collects and redistributes several billion dollars a year; the Bill and Melinda Gates Foundation, which has pledged billions of dollars to fight epidemics, such as by developing a vaccine against HIV/AIDS; and thousands of smaller groups, working in particular countries or against particular diseases. Doctors Without Borders, founded in France, has helped redefine the old humanitarian and emergency tradition of religious missions (which live on in their own right). It has placed thousands of health professionals in scores of countries on the frontlines of the struggle for better health, particularly in areas of conflict. It has also inspired activists in wealthier countries to demand more cooperation and support from government and the private sector for this struggle. Pharmaceutical and other corporations around the world have responded to public pressure by making some drugs and other resources available at a lower price in countries unable to afford even a fraction of the market price, and by allowing drug companies in poorer countries to manufacture their drugs without paying royalties.

A new model has emerged of decentralized, entrepreneurial work at the local level, linked by complex international funding and information networks. This model encourages creativity and healthy competition, and it widens the support base of volunteers and contributors around the world. It also can suffer from duplication of efforts and inefficiency, occasional amateurism, and the lack of clout when small, independent groups try to fight entrenched interests. Time will tell if the benefits outweigh the costs.

Proud Successes

Most of the "easy" work has already been done. Smallpox, one of the major historical killers, has been eliminated. Polio is also on the way to oblivion and measles has been practically eradicated (at least in most of the world). These jobs have been relatively "easy" because effective vaccines exist for all three of these viral diseases, and because there are no animal reservoirs where the viruses can hide to return in the future.

Smallpox was eliminated in a 10-year program initiated by the WHO in 1967, at a time when the disease was killing 2 million people a year and disfiguring or blinding millions of others. Earlier campaigns had failed, but new freeze-dried vaccines and better injection systems made the goal seem reachable. It also had full support from the two superpowers: the Soviet Union, which had originally pressed for the program, and the United States.

The initial strategy of 100 percent mass inoculation was soon modified under the difficult conditions prevailing in Africa and especially southern Asia. In one region of western Nigeria, for example, where 90 percent of the population had gotten the vaccine, an outbreak still occurred in 1966. An ad hoc strategy of surveillance and containment succeeded in eliminating the disease from the region, and this became the model for the national programs in India and elsewhere. At the first report of an outbreak, containment teams would visit the affected area, inoculate everyone in the immediate vicinity, and undertake careful searches, often house-to-house, in a wider radius.[58]

The program was characterized by a great deal of local initiative and experimentation, often implemented by lower-level staff. In the end, only a portion of the population was ever inoculated, but within 10 years the disease had been eliminated. After the last victim recovered in Somalia in 1977, no more cases were reported, although tragically another case occurred the following year when an accidental viral escape from a lab in Birmingham, England, killed a laboratory worker.

The apparent elimination of smallpox in nature, the first infectious disease to be completely conquered, raises important questions. Does the virus still exist in a carrier or an isolated population, or will it ever be used by terrorists or rogue states? To prepare for such possibilities, should medical researchers continue to maintain stocks of the virus? How much vaccine should be produced, refined, and kept ready for possible outbreaks?[59]

A similar success against polio seemed at hand by 2003, with only isolated hot spots reported in several countries, among them Nigeria. The 15-year $3 billion Global Polio Eradication Initiative (run jointly by WHO, the United Nations Children's Fund [UNICEF], Rotary International, and the U.S. CDC) had reduced the number of cases each year from 350,000 in 125 countries in 1988 to just 784 individuals in 2003.[60] The disease primarily affects children under the age of five, often resulting in paralysis and sometimes death.

Unfortunately, in October of that year the governors of three northern Nigerian states suspended the vaccination campaign. Popular Muslim preachers had spread rumors that the vaccines had been tainted by Christian conspirators in the West with chemicals that would render women infertile, or that the vaccines would infect people with HIV/AIDS. By the following year, the Nigerian strain had reinfected several neighboring countries that had been polio-free. It also apparently spread during the pilgrimage to Mecca, as hundreds of cases turned up in Yemen and Indonesia, the first in a decade. An intense information campaign by the Nigerian government convinced opponents to relent after several months, and the campaign resumed the following year.[61] However, lingering suspicions continue to hamper the campaign, as did an unfortunate incident in 2007 when 70 Nigerians contracted polio from a mutant virus in their vaccine.[62] In 2006 Nigeria reported 1128 cases, nearly 60 percent of the world's remaining polio burden, with a few clusters remaining in India, Pakistan, and Afghanistan.[63] The new target for global eradication was set for 2008.

In 2001 a worldwide Measles Initiative was set up by the American Red Cross, the United Nations Foundation, the U.S. CDC, WHO, and UNICEF. By 2005, it had achieved its aim of cutting measles deaths in half; from a 1999 world total of 871,000 deaths the numbers declined to 345,000 by the target year. Vaccination efforts were concentrated in the 47 countries that accounted for 98 percent of the 1999 toll. Some 500 million children were vaccinated by 2004, many with supplementary doses ("booster shots"). The program included treatment of victims with nutritional supplements, and surveillance efforts.[64] The disease was eliminated from the Western Hemisphere in 2002, and deaths declined by a stunning 91 percent in Africa between 2000 and 2006. India, where supplementary vaccinations are not universal, still suffered about 100,000 deaths in 2005.[65]

In February 2007 a group of wealthy nations led by Italy launched the Advanced Market Initiative, a 1.5 billion Euro program to develop inexpensive vaccines for children in developing countries. The goal is to prevent 5.4 million deaths by 2030. The first vaccine to be developed will fight pneumococcal disease. The donor countries have promised participating drug companies that they will purchase as much of the vaccines as are needed in the developing countries.

---

[1] Stacey L. Knobler, Alison Mack, Adel Mahmoud, and Stanley M Lemon, eds. *Threat of Pandemic Influenza: Are We Ready? Workshop Summary*, Washington, D.C.: National Academies Press, 2005. p. 72.

[2] John Barry. *The Great Influenza: The Epic Story of the Deadliest Plague in History*. New York: Viking, 2004, p. 392; some experts believed that "few victims had escaped without some pathological changes."

[3] Charles C. Mann. *1491: New Revelations of the Americas before Columbus*, New York: Alfred A. Knopf, 2005, p. 93.

[4] For example, see D. L. DeVincenzi, H. P. Klein, and J. R. Bagby. *Planetary Protection Issues and Future Mars Missions* [microform]. Springfield, Va.: National Technical Information Service, 1991.

[5] Frank Ryan. *Virus X. Understanding the Real Threat of Pandemic Plagues*. London: HarperCollins, 1996, p. 285.

[6] P. Martens and A. J. McMichael, eds. *Environmental Change, Climate and Health: Issues and Research Methods*. Cambridge: Cambridge University Press, 2002.

[7] Mark Williams. "The Knowledge." *MIT Technology Review* (March/April 2006).

[8] Norman F. Cantor. *In the Wake of the Plague: The Black Death and the World It Made*. New York: Free Press, 2001, p. 227.

[9] I. Edward Alcamo. *AIDS: The Biological Basis*. Boston: Jones & Bartlett Publishers, 2003, pp. 16–18.

[10] Beth Ann Hill. *Multiple Sclerosis Q & A: Researching Answers to Frequently Asked Questions*. New York: Penguin, 2003, p. 20.

[11] Helen Pearson. "Island-Hopping Virus' Ferocity Exposed." Available online. URL: http://www.nature.com/news/2006/060522/full/060522-4.html. Accessed May 23, 2006.

[12] Ian Glynn and Jenifer Glynn. *The Life and Death of Smallpox*. New York: Cambridge University Press, 2004, pp.225–226.

[13] Dixie Farley. "Treating Tropical Diseases." Available online. URL: http://www.fda.gov/fdac/features/1997/197_trop.html. Accessed July 7, 2006.

[14] World Health Organization Fact Sheets. "Yellow Fever Fact Sheet." Available online. URL: http://www.who.int/mediacentre/factsheets/fs100/en/. Accessed May 19, 2006.

[15] Stephen Jay Gould. "Planet of the Bacteria." Available online. URL: http://www.stephenjaygould.org/library/gould_bacteria.html. Accessed May 19, 2006.

[16] National Information Program on Antibiotics. "Bacteria." Available online. URL: http://www.antibiotics-info.org/bact01.asp. Accessed May 18, 2006.

[17] Neil A. Campbell et al. *Biology*, 7th ed. Menlo Park, Calif.: Addison Wesley Longman, 2005.

[18] Celia W. Dugger. "WHO Backs Wider Use of DDT vs. Malaria." *New York Times*, September 16, 2006.

[19] Jacqueline Ruttimann. "Drug Companies Slow to Adopt Malaria Treatment Plan." Available online. URL: http://www.nature.com/news/2006/060515/full/news060515-5.html. Accessed May 16, 2006.

[20] Jorge M. de Freitas et al. "Ancestral Genomes, Sex, and the Population Structure of *Trypanosoma cruzi.*" *PLOS Pathogens* 2, no. 3 (March 2006).

[21] Global Alliance to Eliminate Lymphatic Filariasis. Home page. Available online. URL: http://www.filariasis.org/index.pl Accessed May 19, 2006.

[22] World Health Organization Fact Sheets "Schistosomiasis." Available online. URL: http://www.who.int/mediacentre/factsheets/fs115/en/index.html. Accessed May 19, 2006.

[23] Steven S. Morse. "Factors in the Emergence of Infectious Diseases." In Andrew T. Price-Smith, *Plagues and Politics: Infectious Disease and International Policy.* New York: Palgrave, 2001.

[24] World Health Organization. "Onchocerciasis Control Programme." Available online. URL: http://www.who.int/blindness/partnerships/onchocerciasis_OCP/en/. Accessed May 22, 2006.

[25] Donald G. McNeil, Jr. "Dose of Tenacity Wears Down a Horrific Disease." *New York Times*, March 26, 2006.

[26] World Bank Group. "Saving Children." Available online. URL: http://devdata.worldbank.org/wdi2005/Section1_1_4.htm. Accessed May 23, 2006,

[27] Donald G. McNeil, Jr. "WHO Approves Rotavirus Vaccine." *New York Times*, February 13, 2007.

[28] Christopher Wills. *Yellow Fever Black Goddess: The Coevolution of People and Plagues.* Boston: Addison Wesley, 1996, p. 23.

[29] For example, see SciFLO Brazil. "Prehistoric Tuberculosis in America: Adding Comments to a Literature Review." Available online. URL: http://www.scielo.br/scielo.php?script=sci_arttext&pid=S0074-02762003000900023. Accessed June 6, 2006.

[30] For example, see Charles Greenblatt and Mark Spigelman, eds. *Emerging Pathogens: The Archaeology, Ecology, and Evolution of Infectious Disease.* New York: Oxford University Press, 2003, p. 6; University of Chicago at Illinois Department of Oral Sciences. "Paleopathology/Disease in the Past." Available online. URL: http://www.uic.edu/classes/osci/osci590/6_1Paleopathology%20Disease%20in%20the%20Past.htm. Accessed June 6, 2006.

[31] Arno Karlen. *Man and Microbes: Disease and Plagues in History and Modern Times.* New York: Simon & Schuster, 1996, p. 61.

[32] Thucydides. *The History of the Peloponnesian War.* Trans. David Grene. Chicago: University of Chicago Press, 1989, pp. 115–118.

[33] R. S. Bray. *Armies of Pestilence: The Impact of Disease on History.* Cambridge: James Clarke & Co., 2004.

[34] Wendy Orent. *Plague: The Mysterious Past and Terrifying Future of the World's Most Dangerous Disease.* New York: Free Press, 2004, pp. 74ff; Edward Marriott. *Plague: A Story of Science, Rivalry, and the Scourge That Won't Go Away.* New York: Metropolitan, 2002, pp. 111–114.

[35] Norman F. Cantor. *In the Wake of the Plague: The Black Death and The World It Made.* New York: Free Press, 2001.

[36] Mann. *1491: New Revelations*, pp. 55, 92–93.

[37] Mary Lucas Powell and Della Collins, eds. *The Myth of Syphilis: The Natural History of Treponematosis in North America*. Gainesville: University Press of Florida, 2005.

[38] J. N. Hays. *The Burdens of Disease: Epidemics and Human Response in Western History*. Piscataway, N.J.: Rutgers University Press, 1998, pp. 62ff.

[39] Sharon LaFraniere. "Circumcision Studied in Africa as AIDS Preventive." *New York Times*, April 28, 2006.

[40] Stephen H. Gehlbach. *American Plagues: Lessons from Our Battles with Disease*. Amherst: University of Massachusetts Press, 2005.

[41] Gehlbach. *American Plagues*, pp. 28, 29; National Library of Medicine. "Smallpox: A Great and Terrible Scourge." Available online. URL: http://www.nlm.nih.gov/exhibition/smallpox/sp_variolation.html. Accessed Oct. 18, 2002.

[42] Wills. *Yellow Fever*, pp. 109–116.

[43] Meyer Friedman and Gerald W. Friedland. *Medicine's 10 Greatest Discoveries*. New Haven, Conn.: Yale University Press, 1998, pp. 55–64.

[44] Edward Marriott. *Plague: A Story of Science, Rivalry, and the Scourge That Won't Go Away*. New York: Metropolitan, 2002, pp. 111–114.

[45] Gehlbach. *American Plagues*, p. 64.

[46] Judith Walzer Leavitt. *Typhoid Mary*. Boston: Beacon Press, 1996.

[47] Laurie Garrett. *Betrayal of Trust: The Collapse of Global Pubic Health*. New York: Hyperion, 2000.

[48] Marriott. *Plague*.

[49] J. Gordon Melton. "Medical Missions." *Encyclopedia of Protestantism*. New York: Facts On File, 2005.

[50] For full information on WHO's mission, structure, and function, see its Web site: URL: http://www.who.int/en/.

[51] Simon Carvalho and Mark Zacher. "The International Health Regulations in Historical Perspective." Andrew T. Price-Smith, ed. *Plagues and Politics: Infectious Disease and International Policy*. New York: Palgrave, 2001.

[52] Javed Siddiqi. *World Health and World Politics: The World Health Organization and the UN System*. Columbia: University of South Carolina Press, 1995, pp. 161–178.

[53] See UNAIDS. "Uniting the World against AIDS." Available online. URL: http://www.unaids.org/en. Accessed April 20, 2006.

[54] Craig Timberg. "How AIDS in Africa Was Overstated." *Washington Post*, April 6, 2006.

[55] Centers for Disease Control. Home Page. Available online. URL: http://www.cdc.gov. Accessed April 8, 2006.

[56] European Centre for Disease Prevention and Control. Home Page. Available online. URL: http://europa.eu/agencies/community_agencies/ecdc/index_en.htm. Accessed May 4, 2006.

[57] Carvalho and Zacher. "International Health Regulations," p. 254.

[58] Chun Wei Choo. "The World Health Organization Smallpox Eradication Programme." Available online. URL: http://choo.fis.utoronto.ca/fis/courses/lis2102/KO.WHO.case.html, Accessed July 19, 2006.

[59] See Cynthia Needham and Richard Canning. *Global Disease Eradication: The Race for the Last Child.* Herndon, Va.: ASM Press, 2003.

[60] World Health Organization. "South Asia Slashes Polio Cases by Nearly Half." Available online. URL: http://www.who.int/mediacentre/news/releases/2005/pr08/en/index.html. Accessed July 19, 2006.

[61] IRIN News. "Muslim Suspicion of Polio Vaccine Lingers On." Available online. URL: http://www.irinnews.org/report.asp?ReportID=39593&SelectRegion=West_Africa. Updated Feb. 19, 2004.

[62] Donald E. McNeil, Jr. "Polio in Nigeria Traced to Mutating Vaccine." *New York Times,* October 11, 2007.

[63] UNICEF. "Facts on Children." April 2007. Available online. URL: http://ww.unicef.org/media/media_36235.html. Accessed June 17, 2008.

[64] World Health Organization. "Global Measles Deaths Plunge by 48% over Past Six Years." Available online. URL: http://www.who.int/mediacentre/news/releases/2006/pr11/en/index.html. Accessed March 10, 2006; Celia W. Dugger. "Global Battle against Measles Is Said to Save 2.3 Million Lives." *New York Times,* January 19, 2007.

[65] Celia W. Dugger. "Mothers of Nepal Vanquish a Killer of Children." *New York Times,* April 30, 2006.

2

Focus on the United States

The United States is perhaps the most ethnically diverse country in the world. Native Americans, colonists and refugees, enslaved people in bondage, and armies of immigrants from every corner of every continent contributed to the mix. As a microcosm of the human race, the American people are as vulnerable to infectious diseases as any other population. In fact they have undergone many deadly epidemics, from smallpox and yellow fever in the colonial era, through the mass deaths of the 1918 influenza pandemic (which probably emerged first in the United States before it swept through the world), through the crippling polio epidemics of the mid-20th century, up until the contemporary AIDS pandemic, which originated in Africa but first became widely known in the United States.

Like the fortunate citizens of the other developed countries, however, today's generation of Americans has been shielded from most of the crippling and deadly epidemics that still plague the developing countries. Most deadly bacteria and viruses are kept at bay through routine measures such as government-funded vaccination of children and other at-risk groups, careful treatment of drinking water, comprehensive laws protecting the food supply, an abundance of antibiotics and antiviral drugs, and hospitals equipped with vast quantities of throwaway masks, gowns, hypodermic needles, and other equipment. In addition, the temperate climate of the United States leads to a "winterkill" of disease-bearing insects. Even HIV/AIDS, which has killed over half a million Americans since 1981, has been contained to a degree—though not defeated.

However, all these measures might not be enough to protect against new disease agents—or old microbes that have learned to get around our defenses. Toward that end, the federal government maintains a system of laboratories under the Centers for Disease Control and Prevention (CDC), an agency of the Department of Health and Human Resources. The CDC keeps in constant touch with public health officials and health care workers all across the country and the world. It tries to keep up with any signs of new or revived epidemics—such as the SARS pandemic, which it helped to contain and defeat. Hopefully, this system will spare the country some of the horrors it experienced in the past.

EPIDEMICS IN U.S. HISTORY

Smallpox

In the spring of 1721 the colonial town of Boston, with its 11,000 citizens, was struck with a smallpox epidemic, brought to the city on a British ship. By the fall, over 100 people were dying every day. Commerce died off, and about 1,000 people fled to the countryside. In all, 5,980 people came down with smallpox and 844 died.[1]

The epidemic can be seen as an important milestone in the development of medicine and medical research, thanks largely to Reverend Cotton Mather. A prominent citizen of Boston, Mather, notorious for his support of the Salem witch trials, played a far more positive role in this episode. The famous minister had lost three children to previous epidemics of the disease. When the 1721 epidemic struck, he had already become familiar with the practice of inoculation—in which pus from a smallpox sore is introduced into a scratch on a healthy person's skin, to allow the healthy person to develop immunity. Mather first learned of the practice from his servant Onesimus, who said it was widespread in his native Africa, and he later read about similar attempts in Europe. Mather now publicly threw his support behind the practice, despite fierce opposition from nearly all of Boston's doctors and most of the public, who considered the idea foolish and primitive.

Mather (backed by the town's other ministers) enlisted Doctor Zabdiel Boylston to try the technique. Boylston inoculated his own son and a few other volunteers. When all of them survived, public opinion began to turn. Boylston eventually inoculated 248 people, only 2 percent of whom died (compared with 9 percent of people who had not been inoculated). In the face of this scientific evidence, Americans came to accept inoculation. A century later it was replaced by vaccination, in which pus from a much less dangerous cowpox sore is used.

Yellow Fever

Yellow fever, a painful and often fatal disease, is today thought of as a tropical or subtropical disease. Yet it routinely felled many Americans in cold as well as warm states. In 1793, a yellow fever epidemic struck Philadelphia, killing 4,000 citizens—and also stimulating a public controversy about the cause of the disease.[2] Many believed the old "miasma" theory, that foul odors from decaying garbage, sewage, and animal carcasses caused the disease while others counted themselves among "contagionists." They pointed to a sudden influx of refugees, many of them sickly, who had fled from a Caribbean rebellion and arrived in town just before the epidemic began. The state legislature, unsure of the truth but unwilling to take chances, imposed a quarantine on arriving ships—but too late to be of much help.

The famous physician Benjamin Rush, a miasmist, met the epidemic head-on with a bold treatment plan. He bled his patients (opening veins and draining significant quantities of blood) and "purged" them (feeding them calomel, a white powder containing mercury, to stimulate violent diarrhea). The idea was based on a "rational" rather than an experimental approach, based on a theory that fevers were caused by spasms of the arteries. Most Philadelphia doctors followed Rush's lead. The maverick publisher William Cobbett then distributed pamphlets with statistics showing that the death rate shot up after this treatment was introduced. Rush sued for libel, bankrupting Cobbett and driving him from the country. In the long run, however, Cobbett's statistical approach became an important principle in epidemiology, and Rush's ideas became discredited.

Cholera

Cholera is caused by a bacteria found in contaminated water. The bacteria release toxins into the digestive system that keep the body from absorbing liquid. The patient suffers from severe diarrhea; about half of untreated patients die of dehydration. Countries that enjoy safe, treated drinking water rarely see much cholera, and if they do, patients can almost always be saved by giving them plenty of clean water mixed with sugar and salts.

Cholera was introduced to the United States in 1832 by immigrants, just after the second world cholera pandemic swept through Europe. It killed more than 3,000 people in New York City that year, 3,000 in Montreal and Quebec, and more than 4,000 in New Orleans. These unclean, overcrowded cities provided the ideal host for the disease. New pandemics hit the country in 1849, 1866, and 1873, once more apparently entering through the major port cities and quickly spreading, mostly along waterways. In 1849, for example, 8,000 people died in Cincinnati and 900 in Buffalo. By this time, many of the victims were being poisoned with mercury, an ingredient used in calomel, the most prescribed (and useless) anti-cholera drug of the time.

From the start, observers suspected that good sanitation would help curb the disease. This guess was confirmed by the 1850s, and public pressure for improved water and sewer systems soon prevailed in most of the country.[3] By the turn of the 20th century, cholera had become a disease of the past in the United States.

Tuberculosis

Tuberculosis (TB), a bacterial disease which usually attacks the lungs, kills some 1.7 million people a year in poor countries.[4] The bacteria is said to be present, at least in dormant form, in one-third of all human beings alive today. The disease has become quite rare in the United States, although those with weak immune systems, such as AIDS patients, do occasionally get sick. In the 19th century, however, it was the most widespread and deadly infectious disease in the country, responsible for nearly one in four deaths every year.[5] The bacteria was endemic; it was a constant danger for the urban poor in particular, who lived in crowded, unventilated slums where the disease could quickly spread via coughing.

Before the 1820s doctors did not always understand that tuberculosis was a separate disease. They believed the victims were suffering from pneumonia, influenza, or other diseases. When it was recognized as a specific disease, it came to be called "consumption," as the body became gradually consumed. The bacteria that causes the disease was isolated in the early 1880s by the celebrated German scientist Robert Koch, who won the 1905 Nobel Prize for the discovery.

Bad living conditions (for example, exposure to coal fumes) and a poor diet could weaken the patient. Although no class was immune, and some famous people died of the disease (from the 19th-century composer Franz Schubert to the 20th-century writer Franz Kafka), many people came to think of TB as a poor man's disease. Sometimes the poor were even blamed for getting sick, as if the disease were caused by their supposed bad habits and immorality. Housing laws gradually reduced crowding and improved air quality for the poor, and public education about contagion helped reduce the spread of TB, for example, laws against spitting in public were widely publicized and enforced.

For the many people who still came down with the disease, a new treatment emerged in the late 19th century—the sanitarium. The idea, first developed in Europe, was that patients would improve if they could spend time (or live permanently) in rest homes in the country, with clean air, rest, moderate exercise, and a decent diet. Some doctors advocated mountain air, others sea air, still others a dry, desert climate. Most patients did in fact improve, at least temporarily. Clean air, rest, and good food strengthened the patients. Charitable people raised funds to build such homes for the poor while wealthier people retired to private health resorts. At their peak, TB sanitariums in the

United States contained over 130,000 beds[6]—even though no careful research had demonstrated any lasting effect. By the mid-20th century, effective vaccines and antibiotics had all but eliminated the disease in developed countries, and TB sanitariums became a quaint relic of the past.

A mini-epidemic of TB came back in the 1980s in the United States among people whose immunity had been damaged by AIDS, but it was quickly suppressed. In the 21st century, strains of the TB bacteria emerged that were resistant to antibiotics, although few cases have yet reached North America. In one widely reported exception, a Georgia patient Andrew Speaker who was diagnosed with nonsymptomatic multiple drug-resistant TB caused a minor panic in mid-2007 because of his unsupervised travels to Europe and Canada.

Polio

The mid-20th-century campaign against polio was the first coordinated national effort in the United States against an epidemic disease. The campaign mobilized the public as well as the medical community and eventually defeated the often fatal or paralyzing disease.

Polio made its first epidemic appearance in the 1880s, in Europe. An epidemic struck rural Vermont in 1894, larger than any reported until that time, bringing the malady to wider attention. It killed one out of seven of those taken ill and paralyzed most who survived, either temporarily or, in many cases, permanently.[7] Most of the victims were children.

Larger and larger epidemics began occurring with increasing frequency in the United States and around the world in the following decades. According to one theory, improved sanitation made matters worse. In the past, infants would be exposed to the virus through unclean water, but they would fight off the disease due to their natural immunity, inherited from their mothers. Now, children would not be exposed until they left the sheltered nursery environment, by which time their maternally transferred immunity had disappeared.

By careful epidemiological research, scientists eventually learned that the disease was caused by a virus, that it was spread by drinking water contaminated with feces (often found in lakes or swimming pools). Most people who become infected did not show any serious symptoms; they became "carriers" who spread the disease unknowingly.

In a stroke of "good luck," one polio victim, Franklin D. Roosevelt, was elected president of the United States in 1932 and reelected to three more terms. Roosevelt lent his name to the effort to raise public consciousness about the disease. For several decades, millions of citizens participated in a yearly "March of Dimes" to raise money for polio research.

Early attempts to develop vaccines proved fatal—several volunteers were paralyzed and several others died. However, continued research eventually yielded an injected "killed virus" vaccine, developed by Dr. Jonas Salk. It was first tested in 1953, just as the disease emerged on a massive scale—there had been 22,000 cases of paralysis the previous summer. To ensure that the vaccine did in fact prevent polio, the largest medical test ever devised began: 1.8 million children in schools across the country were given a series of injections containing either the new vaccine or a placebo. It was a widely celebrated, unifying national project.

The vaccine (and other, even more effective vaccines released in following years) completely eliminated naturally occurring polio in the United States by 1980, and in the rest of the Western Hemisphere by 1991. A global program by the WHO seems likely to eliminate the disease from the entire world in the near future.

Two Scares: Legionnaires Disease and Swine Flu

Perhaps lulled into a false sense of security thanks to the success of the anti-polio campaign and of the many new antibiotics, the American public in the late 20th century sometimes reacted with unnecessary panic when suddenly confronted with new, mysterious threats of infectious disease.

In July 1976 the American Legion held a convention in Philadelphia to celebrate the nation's bicentennial. To the horror of the delegates, within two days hundreds of them had taken ill with acute pneumonia, and 34 of them soon died. A "swine flu" epidemic was just starting to emerge in Asia, and the media around the world speculated that the Philadelphia outbreak marked its arrival in the United States, more deadly even than had been feared.

President Gerald Ford and Congress approved a national immunization program against the flu, about which little was yet known. In the meantime, researchers led by the U.S. Centers for Disease Control scoured the convention facilities and examined the survivors and the dead. Not until January of the following year did they find evidence for a new type of bacteria in the convention hotel's air-conditioning system; it was named *Legionnella*. Once the microbe was isolated, doctors realized that it was fairly common, and was the cause of several thousand cases of pneumonia per year—about a quarter of them fatal. The bacteria grows best in standing water in plumbing and air-conditioning systems.[8]

In the meantime, the swine flu inoculation campaign went into full gear. Despite delays and controversies, about a quarter of the U.S. population received the vaccine. The epidemic never in fact showed up, but about 25 people died from complications of vaccination (as is inevitable in such a large program). The episode educated the medical profession and the public toward a greater degree of caution in responding to new threats.

STILL FIGHTING: THE CURRENT SITUATION

The history of American epidemics can be written as a series of medical victories combined with luck—when epidemics petered out naturally on their own. The fight waged through history, however, has not ended. The country, along with the rest of the world, still must contend with a variety of present and potential infectious disease threats.

HIV/AIDS

A strange new chapter in the age-old story of deadly epidemics opened in the United States in 1981. HIV, the virus that causes AIDS, does not as a rule kill directly. Rather, if untreated by antiviral medicines, it slowly and almost inevitably destroys its human host's immune system, leaving patients susceptible to a wide variety of both common and rare ailments.

Because HIV is spread silently and often unknowingly by carriers who appear healthy, its pandemic career has been unique. Bubonic plague, smallpox, or influenza followed predictable life cycles. They would quickly sweep across continents, killing large numbers of people in a year or two. They would then retreat to a dormant stage, only to reemerge at some later date, often in a slightly different form, when conditions were ripe. HIV/AIDS, by contrast, took decades to spread quietly around the world, unknown to medicine, until it emerged in a single, horrifying pandemic cycle, spreading to more and more millions of people every year. HIV-positive people (who have the virus in their blood) remain asymptomatic for several years—they do not know they are HIV-positive, appear healthy, and they typically infect other people unknowingly.

Despite its rapid spread, HIV/AIDS is actually difficult to catch. Even those in close daily contact with patients, such as health care workers, can avoid infection if they take simple precautions. As a result, the risk of HIV infection is concentrated largely among certain high-risk groups, such as intravenous drug users or those who practice unsafe sex. Those not in such groups tend to be unafraid—and, if they choose to be, callously unconcerned. Although the death toll may soon exceed that of any pandemic in history, both in the United States and around the world, HIV/AIDS poses a unique moral challenge. So far, Americans have been willing to support generous efforts to control the disease both domestically and abroad. It is hoped that they will continue to help even if they themselves no longer feel threatened.

HIV (human immunodeficiency virus) probably emerged first in Africa sometime in the first half of the 20th century.[9] However, the first diagnosed cases of AIDS (acquired immunodeficiency syndrome, the disease caused by HIV) were identified in New York City in 1981. Nearly all the diagnosed American patients in the first few years were men who participated in a culture of casual male-to-male sex, which had taken hold in urban gay communities in the previous decade. In Belgium and in France in 1982 a few male and female African patients were diagnosed as having the disease.

The fact that the world first learned of HIV/AIDS as a "gay epidemic" had very important consequences. In a positive sense, a natural constituency emerged to agitate for treatment and research to combat the disease—the new gay organizations and media that had sprung up in the 1970s, especially in New York and California, the most prominent communications centers in the world. In a negative sense, the disease acquired a stigma, since homosexuality was regarded by many people with disdain and disapproval. No one is ashamed to visit a doctor to check if he or she has the flu, but people around the world resisted being tested for HIV. Many have died as a result, or infected others who died in their turn.

Another negative impact was that the gay community, fearful of government repression, fought against the time-tested public health tactics of tracing sexual contacts, testing all hospital admissions for the new disease, and closing down venues where casual sex was practiced.[10] Nevertheless, fear and education programs soon brought changes toward safer sexual behavior. Widespread use of condoms and more discriminate sexual behaviors eventually led to a reduction in the rapid spread of HIV in this community. In 2006, the CDC finally recommended that HIV tests be given routinely to all Americans—a policy that could, it said, save thousands of lives.

In the early years of the epidemic, some people acquired the disease through blood transfusions, and a few were infected by accidental sticking with hypodermic needles at health facilities. But blood supplies are now checked, and discarded if HIV is found, and health workers have become more careful with "sharps." Today, most people are infected via sex—not always casual sex; they are sometimes faithfully married or cohabiting partners whose spouses were unknowingly infected before marriage. Many others are infected through sharing needles while using illegal intravenous drugs. Tragically, several million children around the world have been infected in the womb, during the birth process, or through breast-feeding. This has become rare in the United States, due to widespread testing and antiviral drug treatment before delivery. Malawi doctors reported in 2008 that infant infections can be further reduced if mothers continue to take drugs during breast-feeding.

Focus on the United States

The HIV/AIDS epidemic has stimulated new models of treatment and education in the United States. Much of the care has been delivered through community-based organizations such as Gay Men's Health Crisis in New York, in part because the public's fear of contagion at the start of the epidemic led to cases of discrimination against AIDS patients, even within the health care system. These groups, financed by public as well as private funds and staffed in part by volunteers, also funnel social and housing assistance to people disabled by AIDS, a group that has thankfully shrunk due to more effective medicines.

Despite the stigmas associated with AIDS, and the reluctance of the Reagan administration to publicly discuss it, the disease soon attracted an unprecedented amount of federal funding, at first for research (largely coordinated through the National Institutes of Health), and later for treatment. In 1990, the Ryan White Act was passed by Congress. It was named in honor of an Indiana schoolboy who had been infected with HIV during a blood transfusion, and subsequently expelled from his school; White died in 1990. The act made available federal financial support to state, local, and private programs helping people with AIDS. It included funding for ADAP, the state-administered AIDS Drug Assistance Program, which ensures that anyone without adequate health insurance will receive the best available treatment, including expensive antiviral drugs.[11] Ryan White has recently been funded at around $2.5 billion per year.

In the United States, HIV/AIDS has increasingly become a disease of poverty. In the early years, public opposition to needle-exchange programs (which provide drug abusers with free, clean needles) helped the virus spread among poor male and female drug users, who were most likely to share needles. In 2005 African Americans comprised about half of all new diagnoses of HIV/AIDS, although the group constitutes only 13 percent of the overall U.S. population. Of those under the age of 25 diagnosed that year, 61 percent were African American.[12] However, for several years the total number of new cases has been declining in this population group as well. The introduction of rapid HIV tests in recent years, which show results in under 30 minutes, has helped make testing more widespread, and get more people on antiviral treatment; this has probably helped to reduce the number of infections passed along by people who did not know they were HIV-positive.[13]

As of mid-2006, a quarter century into the epidemic, 550,000 Americans had died of AIDS, slightly more than half of all those who contracted the disease. In recent years, the annual death toll has fallen to around 15,000. The CDC estimates that over 1 million Americans are HIV-positive, and that about one quarter of these do not know they are positive.

Today, an HIV-positive status, and even a diagnosis of AIDS, is not usually a death sentence. If properly treated and carefully monitored, the majority of individuals can lead productive lives for years. However, there is no reason to be complacent. The improvement has been caused largely by a handful of drugs, which are not effective for all patients. Besides, the HIV virus easily mutates, and it has begun to acquire resistance to some of these medicines. Unless an effective vaccine is found, or until medicines can be found that clear HIV out of the many hiding places it finds within the body, HIV/AIDS is likely to constitute the greatest infectious disease danger the country faces—unless or until pandemic influenza strikes.

Hepatitis A, B, and C

Hepatitis is a general term for an infectious disease of the liver. Most cases are caused by one of three common viruses, called Hepatitis A, B, and C. Hepatitis A, the most common, can cause widespread local epidemics; it is generally spread through intimate contact including sexual relations, but it can also be spread in food and water. There is no treatment available, but most cases last a few months at most, and give the patient lifelong immunity. Vaccines are available for Hepatitis A and B, and Hepatitis C vaccines are in the process of clinical testing as of 2007.

The B and C viruses are spread through exposure to the blood of an infected person, either during unprotected sex, the sharing of needles, or medical accidents. Either type can be treated with antiviral drugs, which eliminate the virus in about half of all cases. If untreated, they both can cause severe, long-term illness including cirrhosis, cancer, and liver failure. Together they kill about 15,000 people a year in the United States. Vaccines are available for types A and B; they are routinely given to newborn babies and children, to people who may be at risk due to unsafe sex or intravenous drug abuse, to health workers, and to travelers. The vaccine is safe for use by anyone.[14]

Influenza (Flu)

According to the CDC, every year between 5 and 20 percent of the American population comes down with the flu. It is caused by one of a number of related viruses, which are easily transmitted through coughing, sneezing, or touching. It causes severe, sudden inflammation of the nose, throat, or lungs, and it is usually accompanied by fever and body aches. Most people recover after a week or two, but 200,000 people must be hospitalized each year in the United States and about 36,000 die—mostly infants, elderly people, and people weakened by chronic diseases.

Each year a different set of virus strains prevails, and each year a different vaccine is made available based on the prevailing strain. In the United States, the Food and Drug Administration decides which strains to use, in consultation with the World Health Organization and other bodies. The FDA currently authorizes three drug companies to produce some 80 to 120 million doses yearly.[15]

From time to time, flu viruses emerge that are particularly dangerous. In 1918, the "Spanish flu" killed more than half a million Americans, and as many as 100 million people worldwide. Scientists fear that certain contemporary strains of "avian flu," which originated among wild birds and poultry, have the potential to become very dangerous as well.[16]

Health Care–related Infections

Today's hospitals are far safer than they used to be before Florence Nightingale began her famous campaigns to reform hospital sanitary procedures in mid-19th-century England.[17] Nevertheless, "health care–associated infections" still kill thousands of vulnerable patients and health care workers every year. The CDC estimates that some 1.7 million people pick up preventable infections during hospital stays each year, and 99,000 die.[18] Many infections are transmitted to patients while using respirators, catheters, and dialysis equipment. The CDC has established programs to try to reduce these numbers, but some of the microbes most common in health care facilities have developed antibiotic resistance, such as strains of *Staphylococcus* and *Streptococcus* bacteria.

Rare but Deadly Diseases

A number of rare but deadly diseases are endemic in various parts of the United States. They are transmitted only from animals to people, either directly or through an insect vector. Though they cause few deaths, they all require significant government expenditures for surveillance and control.

RABIES

Rabies is a viral disease that attacks the brain. If the patient is not rapidly given preventive treatment with rabies immune globulin, rabies causes severe symptoms of mental instability and kills the patient, usually within 10 days of the first appearance of symptoms. The virus was once fairly common among house pets, but today it is confined mostly to wild animals such as raccoons and bats, largely thanks to vaccination of cats and dogs. It is endemic at a low level in the United States. At most one or two people die of rabies each year in the United States.[19] Anyone who has been bitten by a wild animal or had contact with its bodily fluids should seek immediate treatment, which is now painless and effective.

HANTAVIRUS

First recognized in 1993, hantavirus pulmonary syndrome is a rare disease transmitted to humans from rodents—those found in the wild and those that infest homes, throughout North and Central America. Nearly half of the more than 200 cases reported in the United States in the 1990s proved fatal; no bite is necessary to transmit the disease—it is sufficient to breathe in aerosol particles emitted by a diseased rodent. There are a large variety of hantavirus species around the world. They are all carried by rodents, and many of them can cause various types of fatal illness.[20]

ROCKY MOUNTAIN SPOTTED FEVER

First seen in the 1890s when it was called "black measles" due to its characteristic rash, this bacterial disease is spread by a tick that is endemic throughout the western United States, Canada, and Central America. It responds well to antibiotics, but it is often fatal if untreated.[21]

LEPROSY

This bacterial disease, potentially disfiguring or fatal, was once endemic in Hawaii. It now infects some 25 American-born individuals across the country each year, in addition to over 100 immigrants from countries where the disease is more common.[22] The disease is successfully treated with antibiotics. The first such drug was developed by U.S. Public Health Service doctors working at the Carville, Louisiana, isolation facility.[23]

PLAGUE

The bacteria that killed millions of people in the Middle Ages is still endemic in the wild, and it has been found among rodents at many sites in the western United States. About 10 to 15 people are infected in the United States each year via flea bites. Antibiotics are effective against this threat, which can cause severe illness and death if untreated.

WEST NILE VIRUS

A deadly microbe usually transmitted through mosquito bites, the West Nile virus thrives in birds, which constitute the main disease reservoir. Most humans infected suffer mild or no symptoms, but in about 1 percent of cases, the virus can affect the central nervous system, especially among elderly patients or those who have had organ transplants.

The virus, fairly common in parts of East Africa, has been found on nearly all continents. It first hit the United States in 1999, infecting patients in the New York City area. The sudden appearance of dead birds in towns around the country caused a media sensation in 2001/2002. The CDC reported 174 deaths from the disease in 2006, among 4,261 infected individuals.

LYME DISEASE

Lyme disease has become endemic in large parts of the United States in recent decades. Originally diagnosed near Lyme, Connecticut, in 1975, the infection has now been detected in every region of the country. It is caused by a bacterium whose complicated life cycle passes through deer, ticks, and people.

When diagnosed right after infection—usually via a characteristic red, circular rash—the disease can be treated effectively with antibiotics. Because the flulike symptoms resemble those of other diseases, Lyme disease has generated controversy among doctors and patients. The number of yearly cases is disputed; estimates range from 25,000 (based on cases reported to the CDC) to roughly 10 times that number. Those who believe the higher number to be correct usually favor longer term antibiotic treatment (of up to four years), even after the bacteria can no longer be found using presently available tests. Most established medical authorities are fairly skeptical about these claims. Both camps agree that the bacteria, if untreated, can cause serious heart, neurological, and other illnesses.

WHO PROTECTS US?

The health care system in the United States is complex, diverse, and expensive. The country as a whole spends about 16 percent of its national product on health expenditures, the highest of any major country, amounting to $1.9 trillion in 2004.[24]

The government plays a huge role. In one way or another, it pays perhaps 60 percent of all health care expenditures each year.[25] The bulk of this figure represents direct federal or state payments for health care for the poor (Medicaid), the elderly (Medicare), veterans, new mothers, children, and other special groups. The government also subsidizes private insurance and medical costs through generous tax deductions. In addition, the U.S. government supports a vast complex of agencies in medical research, health education and control, and surveillance—many of them crucial to the fight against infectious disease and epidemics in the country and around the world.

Agencies in Medical Research, Health Education and Control, and Surveillance

CDC: CENTERS FOR DISEASE CONTROL

The country's first defense against pandemics is the Centers for Disease Control and Prevention (CDC). An agency of the Department of Health and Human Services, the CDC defines its goals as "Health promotion and prevention of disease, injury, and illness," and "preparedness" against potential threats to health.[26] Its programs to prevent, monitor, and fight infectious disease are conducted by three related agencies: the National Center for Infectious Diseases (NCID), the National Center for Immunization and Respiratory Disease, and the National Center for HIV, STD (sexually transmitted diseases), and TB Prevention. The agency was called the Communicable Disease Center from 1946, when it was founded with a mission to combat malaria, until 1970.

Most of the CDC's 9,000 employees are based at headquarters in Atlanta, but many others are stationed within state and local health agencies in the United States and counterpart agencies around the world. The agency provides informative Web sites for the public, and it publishes both the science journal *Emerging Infectious Diseases* and the celebrated *MMWR*, the *Mortality and Morbidity Weekly Report*, which keeps tabs on infectious disease development around the world.

The CDC's "Bio-Safety Level 4" laboratories monitor and research extremely dangerous microbes, including possible bioterror agents, and they contain the only U.S. stores of smallpox virus. In 2003 a CDC lab was one of the first two labs in the world to identify the cause of the SARS (Severe Acute Respiratory Syndrome) epidemic.

The NCID maintains dozens of surveillance systems for various categories of disease, working together with state and local public health departments, hospitals, doctors, and laboratories to provide updated information and training on new or existing diseases. It has become a key player in the global fight against epidemics, in cooperation with the WHO and national agencies around the world. The CDC's National Center for Health Statistics is another valuable resource for professionals, scholars, and the general public.

NIH: NATIONAL INSTITUTES OF HEALTH

The National Institutes of Health in Washington, D.C., is the major supporter of medical research in the country. It maintains its own elaborate network of laboratories and supplies billions of dollars in annual grant money to universities and other laboratories across the country. Prominent among its two dozen institutes and centers is the National Institute of Allergy and Infectious Diseases, which also focuses on the body's immune system.

Over the decades, the NIH has played an important direct role in understanding and combating AIDS, flu, and other major epidemics. It also helps set priorities for such research nationwide, both through allocating grants to research projects and through a variety of initiatives and cooperative programs.

FDA: FOOD AND DRUG ADMINISTRATION

The Food and Drug Administration has two key roles: It monitors the country's food supply, a key item on any health agenda, and it regulates the use of legal drugs. The latter role is extremely important due to the global consequences of its actions. All new drugs and medical devices must pass its muster for safety and effectiveness before they can be marketed. Its decisions on approving or rejecting drugs place it in the center of many controversies, in which it can be accused of being too cautious—or too hasty in granting approvals. For example, in recent years some critics have accused it of delaying the "morning after" contraception pill on political grounds, while others say it fails to monitor drugs adequately after their approval, allowing drugs like the arthritis medicine Vioxx to be prescribed even when serious side effects began to emerge. In general, however, the agency is widely admired for fairly weighing the often diverging interests of various drug companies, patients, doctors, and politicians.

HHS: HEALTH AND HUMAN SERVICES

While the NIH researches infectious disease, and the CDC keeps tabs on existing and potential pandemic threats, responsibility for responding to epidemic breakouts as well as bioterror attacks resides in their parent agency, the Department of Health and Human Services (HHS). For example, in December 2005 Congress allocated $3.3 billion to the department to prepare plans for responding to the threat of avian flu. The money is being used for "monitoring disease spread to support rapid response, developing vaccines and vaccine production capacity, stockpiling antivirals and other countermeasures, coordinating federal, state and local preparation, and enhancing outreach and communications planning."

PHS: U.S. PUBLIC HEALTH SERVICE

The federal government role in fighting infectious disease goes back to 1798, when a system of marine hospitals was set up to take care of seamen.

It later developed into the uniformed, 6,000-member U.S. Public Health Service. Led by the surgeon general, the doctors, nurses, and other health professionals of the service played an important role throughout the 19th and early 20th centuries in keeping epidemic diseases at bay through quarantine, examination of immigrants, and medical care during natural disasters. Today, PHS clinics and personnel work in underserved communities such as Indian reservations. Many of them are stationed at various offices of the CDC, the Food and Drug Administration, and other health agencies, wherever clinical physicians are needed.

The Rest of the Picture: Local Agencies and Nonprofits

Under the federal system, state and local governments maintain their own health agencies. They often work in tandem with each other and with federal agencies, sometimes duplicating work, at other times initiating research and practical programs. These local agencies deserve most of the credit for the improvements in sanitation and housing conditions that helped defeat such 19th-century scourges as TB and cholera.

Local agencies continue to play a major role in combating sexually transmitted diseases through education and clinics. They also focus on diseases or environmental issues specific to their locales. For example, the Maryland Department of the Environment monitors shellfish for bacterial levels;[27] and Washington State's Animal Disease Diagnostic Laboratory conducts testing of cattle for mad cow disease, in cooperation with the U.S. Department of Agriculture.[28]

The nonprofit sector plays an important auxiliary role, largely in the field of public education. U.S. religious and secular charitable foundations are playing a major role in financing the worldwide efforts against AIDS and other pandemic diseases.

---

[1] Stanley M. Aronson and Lucile F. Newman. "Boston's 'Grievous Calamity of the Small Pox.'" *New York Times*, December 17, 2002.

[2] Stephen H. Gehlbach. *American Plagues: Lessons from Our Battles with Disease*. New York: McGraw Hill, 2005, pp. 1–20.

[3] Charles E. Rosenberg. *The Cholera Years: The United States in 1832, 1849, and 1866*. Chicago: University of Chicago Press, 1987.

[4] World Health Organization. "Tuberculosis Fact Sheet." Available online. URL: http://www.who.int/mediacentre/factsheets/fs104/en/#global. Updated March 2007.

[5] Gehlbach. *American Plagues*, p. 152.

[6] S. A. Rothman. *Living in the Shadow of Death: Tuberculosis and the Social Experience of Illness in American History*. Baltimore: Johns Hopkins University Press, 1994, p. 198. Cited in Gehlbach. *American Plagues*, p. 153.

[7] Gehlbach. *American Plagues*, pp. 157–181.

[8] Laurie Garrett. *The Coming Plague: Newly Emerging Diseases in a World Out of Balance.* New York: Farrar, Straus & Giroux, 1994, pp. 153ff.

[9] See section "AIDS and Africa" in chapter 3.

[10] Randy Shilts. *And the Band Played On.* New York: St. Martin's Press, 1987.

[11] Johns Hopkins AIDS Service. "Ryan White Care Act." Available online. URL: http://www.hopkins-aids.edu/manage/ryan_white.html. Accessed May 17, 2007.

[12] Centers for Disease Control and Prevention. "Fact Sheet: HIV/AIDS among African-Americans." Available online. URL: http://www.cdc.gov/hiv/topics/aa/resources/factsheets/aa.htm. Accessed May 17, 2007.

[13] D. A. MacKellar et al. "Rapid HIV Test Distribution." *Morbidity and Mortality Weekly Report.* June 23, 2006.

[14] Immunization Action Coalition. "Hepatitis A, B, and C." Available online. URL: http://www.immunize.org/catg.d/p4075abc.pdf. Accessed January 2007.

[15] Food and Drug Administration. "Meeting the Challenge of Annual Flu Preparedness." Available online. URL: http://www.fda.gov/cber/summaries/nfid051806jg.htm. Accessed May 18, 2006.

[16] See section "Avian and Other Flus" in chapter 3.

[17] Hugh Small. *Florence Nightingale: Avenging Angel.* New York: Palgrave Macmillan, 1999.

[18] Centers for Disease Control and Prevention. "Estimates of Healthcare-Associated Infections." Available online. URL: http://www.cdc.gov/ncidod/dhqp/hai.html. Accessed October 31, 2007.

[19] Centers for Disease Control and Prevention. "Rabies Information." Available online. URL: http://www.cdc.gov/ncidod/dvrd/rabies/introduction/intro.htm. Accessed December 1, 2003.

[20] Centers for Disease Control and Prevention. "All About Hantaviruses." Available online. URL: http://www.cdc.gov/NCIDOD/diseases/hanta/hps/noframes/millstestimony.htm. Accessed June 23, 1999.

[21] Centers for Disease Control and Prevention. "Rocky Mountain Spotted Fever Overview." Available online. URL: http://www.cdc.gov/ncidod/dvrd/rmsf/overview.htm. Accessed May 20, 2005.

[22] Centers for Disease Control and Prevention. "Leprosy in America: New Cause for Concern." Available online. URL: http://jscms.jrn.columbia.edu/cns/2005-03-15/whitford-americanleprosy. Accessed March 15, 2005.

[23] National Institute for Allergy and Infectious Diseases, Division of Microbiology and Infectious Diseases. "Leprosy—Hansen's Disease." Available online. URL: http://www.niaid.nih.gov/dmid/leprosy/. Accessed August 22, 2006.

[24] National Coalition on Health Care. "Health Insurance Cost." Available online. URL: http://www.nchc.org/facts/cost.shtml. Accessed May 17, 2007.

[25] Asaf Bitton and James G. Kahn. "Government Share of Health Care Expenditures." *Journal of the American Medical Association* (March 5, 2003).

[26] Centers for Disease Control and Prevention. "The Futures Initiative." Available online. URL http://www.cdc.gov/futures. Accessed August 26, 2006.

[27] Maryland Marine Notes Online. "Seafood Safety in Maryland: So Far, So Good." Vol. 15, no. 6 (November/December 1997). Available online. URL: http://www.mdsg.umd.edu/MarineNotes/Nov-Dec97/index.html. Accessed October 21, 2007.

[28] Washington State Department of Agriculture. "Expanded BSE Testing." Available online. URL: http://agr.wa.gov/FoodAnimal/AnimalFeed/BSE.htm. Accessed July 5, 2005.

3

Global Perspectives

Chapter 2 dealt with pandemics and public health from the perspective of the United States. This chapter will explore the wider world. The first three sections will deal with individual regions or countries and the ways they have dealt with particular epidemic diseases. The final section deals with influenza and the ever-present danger of a flu pandemic.

SARS, CHINA, AND THE WHO

Introduction

In recent decades China has begun to reclaim its historic place as a major economic and technological power. Economic growth through unrestrained private enterprise has brought greater prosperity for the majority of citizens, better health, a longer life expectancy, and impressive advances in medical and scientific research. This should be good news on the pandemic front—a country that has been the source of some historic pandemics now has the resources to fight them at the source.

Unfortunately, the public health infrastructure has not kept pace with rapid social change. Hundreds of millions of people have migrated from rural areas to overcrowded cities, where they face dangerous industrial pollution, poor sanitation, and a barely regulated food industry—all factors that encourage infectious disease and limit health gains among this population. At the same time, the government has come to expect that doctors, hospitals, and even government health agencies support themselves through fees, a policy that can lead to the neglect of preventive care and public health.

The political system concentrates power and information in the hands of a secretive and insecure Communist Party leadership, which has often chosen to suppress information about health dangers rather than deal with them. For example, AIDS was neglected for years.[1] When finally moved to action, however, this centralized system still displays an ability to mobilize the entire population to a degree that few other countries can match.

The brief, terrifying epidemic of SARS (Severe Acute Respiratory Syndrome) in 2002–03 showed both the strength and the weakness of the Chinese political and health care delivery systems. A few months of inaction and disinformation allowed a new and deadly disease to spread within and beyond the country. Fortunately, when cases began appearing outside the country, the international public health community, led by the UN's World Health Organization (WHO), sprang into action to encourage and assist China and other countries to identify the virus, isolate all those infected, and cut off the threat of a more widespread epidemic. In the face of internal panic and international pressure, the Chinese government responded with a massive campaign that quickly suppressed the SARS virus at its source.

The lesson of SARS is that the free, frank, and rapid exchange of information is a vitally important requirement in the fight against pandemics in today's interconnected world. The epidemic served as a dry run for new methods of international cooperation.

The Ecological Background

In the early decades of Communist rule, China dispatched barefoot doctors to rural areas all over the country. These public health workers, who had some six months of clinical training, eliminated or sharply curtailed traditional plagues such as smallpox and sexually transmitted diseases. The program eventually fell apart, due to mass migration, a loss of revolutionary zeal, and the shift toward privatization of medical care. In recent decades multiple-drug-resistant tuberculosis and hepatitis B have surged—the latter infecting an estimated 130 million people, and schistosomiasis is spreading once again.[2]

The teeming Pearl River delta region of South China's Guangdong Province, where SARS first appeared, has seen outbreaks of measles, dengue, malaria, and encephalitis. Contact tracing, a key tool in fighting epidemics, becomes extremely difficult when much of the population consists of migrants who do not have fixed addresses. In October 2003 a Chinese official government report to the WHO admitted that "the public health system is defective, the public health emergency response system is unsound and the crisis management capacity is weak."[3]

A complicating factor in Guangdong is the local taste for "wild flavor"—food made from wild rather than domestic animals and said to confer good luck, prosperity, or virility. Once the preserve of the wealthy few, wild flavor restaurants appeared by the thousands all across the region to cater to the vast new middle class. As prices rose, millions of wild animals were brought each year from across the country and abroad. Kept alive in crowded cages under unsanitary conditions, in close proximity to one another and to traders and restaurant workers, these animals posed at least a theoretical threat of interspecies transmission of new and mutated viruses. In the past, many human plagues originated among animals living in close contact with people. Microbes that make the transition to a new species are often particularly devastating to their hosts. That seems to have been the case with the SARS virus: Virus particles isolated from palm civets in January 2004 were an almost perfect match with similar particles isolated from patients that same month.[4]

The Epidemic Emerges

No one can know exactly where and when the virus first jumped to infect a human being, but the first cases of a puzzling new type of pneumonia appeared in hospitals in several Guangdong cities in November 2002. On November 16, for example, a 46-year-old government official was admitted to a hospital in Foshan, a city about one hour's trip from Guangzhou, the provincial capital, suffering from a severe, unusual pneumonia. He had also infected five other family members.

In December a 36-year-old butcher who worked at a wild flavor restaurant in Shenzhen on the Hong Kong border was admitted to a hospital in his native Heyuan, 60 miles north of Shenzhen, and then transferred to Guangzhou, where he recovered after being on a respirator for three weeks. In his work, he would routinely slaughter and cut up some 50 animals a night in an unventilated kitchen, constantly exposed to blood, feces, and urine.[5]

These early cases were diagnosed at the admitting hospitals as "atypical pneumonia," a catchall term for lung inflammations caused by several rare microbes such as Legionnaire's bacteria. However, the disease did not respond to antibiotics, as atypical pneumonia usually does, and the symptoms were more severe, including high fever, cloudy chest X-rays, complete exhaustion, and slackened face muscles due to lack of oxygen. Furthermore, the patients did not fit the profile of pneumonia patients, who were usually infants, the elderly, or other immune-compromised individuals. Instead, the majority had been strong, healthy adults. Doctors used anti-inflammatory drugs and oxygen with some success, but in many cases they had to put patients on respirators; even then, a disturbing number of them died.

From the start, one of the most terrifying aspects of the new disease was that the microbe seemed to be targeting health care workers. Many of the early victims were the doctors and nurses who treated the patients; they represented about 20 percent of the total caseload throughout the epidemic. The first fatality among health care workers was that of an ambulance driver who brought an early patient to the Third Affiliated Hospital of Zhongsan University in Guangzhou. That patient, a seafood trader, infected 28 staff members in the 18 hours he spent at that hospital; he was transferred to two other hospitals, where he infected another 60 people.[6]

The devastating effect on the health care system certainly complicated the early attempts at diagnosis and treatment. However, it also ensured that the city and provincial health authorities took notice more quickly than they might have had the disease been restricted to a small number of puzzling cases in random hospitals. A similar pattern emerged when the disease spread beyond China. As one observer noted, "It was the stunning specter of large numbers of hospital workers falling gravely ill" that got attention.[7]

Even before the authorities could react, rumors about a new epidemic began to spread in Guangdong and elsewhere in China. In November, WHO representatives attending a regular influenza meeting in Beijing, China's capital, were told by Guangdong doctors that a respiratory outbreak was raging in rural hospitals; they were assured, however, that the cause was a routine A-type flu virus, similar to the flu viruses that infect millions of people all over the world each winter, without causing much mortality. The WHO was on the alert for the possible appearance of avian influenza (bird flu), which had jumped to humans in Hong Kong in 1997, killing a third of the 18 people infected. Nevertheless, as WHO Beijing mission chief Henk Bekedam later said, "This is China. Do you know how many rumors we hear?"[8]

The first mention of the epidemic in the Chinese media took the form of a denial. On January 5, 2003, the *Heyuan Daily* ran a front-page notice: "Regarding the rumor of an ongoing epidemic in the city, Health Department officials announced at 1:30 A.M. this morning, 'there is no epidemic in Heyuan.'"[9] Given the widespread press censorship in China, such a denial is often considered by readers to be coded confirmation that a rumor is true. More than a month passed until the next public announcement.

Most of the province's newspapers are privately owned and compete for readers, often by running investigative stories, but epidemics and other disasters are among the many topics usually considered off limits. Nevertheless, reporters raced around the province collecting information and passing it along to editors. On February 8, two major papers in Guangzhou reported that a mysterious illness was affecting local hospitals. That day the Communist Party regional propaganda department sent notices to all media organizations asking them to avoid any mention of the disease to prevent "public fear and instability." Two days later another memo barred reporters from interviewing staff or patients at the hospitals, and on February 10 the papers were even banned from reporting on panic buying of staples and medicine.[10]

China's media policy tries to limit "negative news" that might undermine the government, social stability, or the political standing of local or national leaders. Reporters and editors can be disciplined for violating the policy. Thanks to the national political changes that eventually occurred during the SARS epidemic, some official light has been shed on these practices. The authoritative *People's Daily* in Beijing wrote on June 9, "The belated, incomplete reporting resulted in the government's failure to fully carry out its duties in the initial, but crucial period of the SARS outbreak. Unfortunately a long-held but outdated conviction among many top public servants dictated that information could also cause possible social panic and disorder. Hence, information was controlled, which was just what happened at the onset of the SARS outbreak."[11]

By that time, panic had taken hold in various cities in Guangdong Province, as rumors spread, mostly via telephone text messages. Stores ran out of vinegar (whose fumes are considered antiseptic in China), antibiotics (which can be purchased over the counter), traditional Chinese herbs used for respiratory ailments, and even food staples. Higher prices brought shipments from neighboring provinces, causing shortages there as well. Reports about these shortages reached Hong Kong in January, alerting news agencies that something unusual was going on. Masked policemen began appearing at train stations in Guangzhou, moving people along to prevent crowds from assembling.

China Responds

Provincial authorities had in fact taken notice and had begun to take necessary measures to contain the epidemic—all under the cloak of secrecy. The measures eventually contained the epidemic in Guangdong, but the secrecy allowed it to spread to other parts of the country and abroad.

On January 3 the Guangdong Department of Health sent a team of respiratory specialists and epidemiologists to Heyuan to investigate the new outbreak. They collected specimens for antibody tests against known disease agents, and wrote what became the first official SARS report, essentially a summary of symptoms. As the epidemic had not spread beyond the hospital, no alarms were sounded.[12]

According to government protocols in effect at the time, all medical personnel were required to report certain infectious diseases such as plague, cholera, dengue fever, and polio up the chain of command. However, the provision did not apply to any new outbreak that did not fit into the required categories. In any case, Chinese officials later told investigators from the U.S. Congress that their national disease surveillance system, established in 1998, had proved ineffective. Reporting followed a one-way route, from lower to higher rungs in the hierarchy, and it took at least seven days for information to work its way up.[13] Besides, local health authorities reported first of all to the provincial Communist Party secretary before notifying their health agency superiors in Beijing. In Guangdong that secretary was the powerful Zhang Dejiang, a member of the national Politburo. Even the national minister of health could not bypass his authority. Zhang later claimed that he had informed the State Council in Beijing on February 7, but that was more than a month after the epidemic was discerned in Guangdong.[14]

On January 20, following new reports from Shenzhen and other cities, and a new round of hoarding, the Health Department team was reconvened, with a delegation from the national Center for Disease Control and Prevention (CDC) in Beijing. The Chinese CDC,[15] whose national offices are modeled on the U.S. agency of the same name, incorporated the old network of local epidemic prevention stations, which were mostly involved with pest control. Most of its 3,000 offices need major upgrades to be genuinely effective. By early February the Guangdong CDC was feverishly trying to isolate the disease agent, without success. Following the SARS epidemic, the government instituted a program to upgrade CDC labs in the 300 largest cities.[16]

The provincial health system now went into action, under the leadership of Zhong Nanshan, the charismatic head of the Guangdong Institute of Respiratory Diseases. By February hospitals were given strict guidelines for isolation, infection control, and contact tracing, and doctors shared their hard-learned knowledge of the best treatment protocols (including respirators and steroids when necessary); heroic volunteer doctors and nurses were recruited across the province. Facilities that were not adequately equipped were ordered to transfer patients to those that were; rural hospitals had to report new cases within 12 hours—urban hospitals within six hours.[17] Unfortunately, the guidelines, reported up to the national minister of health on January 23, were still marked "top secret" in accord with government rules, and they were delivered only to key officials within the province—some of whom were away on extended Chinese New Year holidays. Hong Kong's 7 million people, by then officially citizens of China and intimately connected with Guangdong (400,000 people crossed the border every day), were still being kept in the dark, as was Taiwan, which also has close ties to Guangdong, and the WHO.[18]

On Febuary 10 the official Xinhua News Agency briefly announced in Beijing that an outbreak of atypical pneumonia had been brought under control. On February 11, the Guangdong provincial government staged a press conference about the epidemic, in response to growing demands from local and international reporters. Public health officials presented an accurate account of the epidemic's early course, but they claimed falsely that it was over.

In fact, local hospitals were diagnosing over 40 new cases a day in Guangdong at the time. Nevertheless, the government decided to reopen schools and universities after New Year's Day, and officials allowed the millions of migrant workers who had gone home for the holidays to return to the province. This dangerous policy was based on fear of unrest combined with the relentless need to maintain economic growth. Zhang Dejiang told Chinese TV in June, "If we made a contrary decision, it would have been impossible to achieve a GDP growth rate of 12.2 percent."[19] After all, a localized plague epidemic in India in 1987 that had been widely reported in the media cost that country $2 billion in output.[20]

In late February a senior microbiologist at the Chinese CDC's Institute of Virology in Beijing isolated chlamydia in patient samples. This bacteria is best known as a common cause of sexually transmitted disease, but it is also known to cause pneumonia. Over the objections of Guangdong doctors, the epidemic mystery was officially declared solved, and all other labs in China were now denied samples. It was left to labs outside the control of Beijing, in Hong Kong and the United States, to discover the true cause, a previously unknown coronavirus.

Breakout to the World

Had SARS been kept within the confines of Guangdong Province, the world might never have known about this deadly new virus. Perhaps that was the hope of the secretive local and central authorities, but ironically their secrecy insured its spread. Beginning in late February a handful of carriers unknowingly spread the virus to 10 widely dispersed provinces and regions of China, and to some 25 countries in Asia, the Americas, and Europe.

On February 21 a Guangzhou respiratory specialist named Liu Jianlun, who had treated SARS patients, checked into the Metropole Hotel in Hong Kong to attend a wedding. He took violently ill, coughing and vomiting in a hotel corridor in the presence of several other guests, including an American businessman about to depart for Singapore and several visitors from Toronto. The businessman took ill aboard his plane and was taken to a hospital in Hanoi, Vietnam, where he infected several doctors and nurses. Hanoi physicians reported the undiagnosed infection to the WHO representative in Hanoi and to the WHO Western Pacific regional office in Manila, the Philippines—the first official notification outside China. Dr. Carlo Urbani, a famed veteran of many battles against epidemics in poor countries, decided to visit Hanoi to investigate personally. He himself soon picked up the virus, and he carried it with him to Bangkok, Thailand, where he died. China no longer enjoyed the option of secrecy.

A total of 16 guests at the Metropole fell ill after returning to Singapore and Toronto, where they in turn infected hundreds of other people. Worst affected was Hong Kong itself; Liu was the first known case, but others soon began cropping up. As in Guangdong, the first cases spread the virus rapidly through the city's hospitals. Panic intensified when over 100 residents of one housing project, Amoy Gardens, became ill, suggesting that the microbe could be transmitted through the air. Eventually investigators concluded that contaminated moisture droplets from improperly sealed wastewater pipes were the likely agent of transmission in Amoy Gardens.

Guangdong doctors visited Hong Kong when Liu's case was reported to collect samples, but they maintained their silence about their own province. By now, late February, sensationalist media coverage around the world, fed by several weeks of vague but alarming rumors out of China, left no doubt that a dangerous epidemic had broken out. Authorities in all the epidemic locales outside China acted quickly to contain the damage. Special hospitals were set up in Singapore and Taiwan, and home quarantines of varying severity were put in place for people who had been exposed. Schools were closed for extended periods in both Singapore and Hong Kong. In Toronto, a total of 7,000 potentially exposed individuals were eventually subjected to quarantine.

The epidemic spread within China by much the same pathway—a small number of "superspreaders" infected others, especially health care workers. The virus apparently reached Beijing via a businesswoman from Shanxi in northwest China. She had become infected during a visit to Guangdong in February, and, after infecting several family members and doctors in Shanxi, she traveled to Beijing in early March, hoping to get better treatment. Admitted to an army hospital, she helped spark a local epidemic of well over a thousand cases in Beijing, with those victims spreading the disease to Tianjin city on the coast and to Inner Mongolia. In Beijing, world-class doctors and hospitals had to work in the dark at first, without benefit of the accumulated Guangdong experience.

The World and the WHO Respond

Anyone looking for reasons to be optimistic about the future health of the human race should note the rapid and inspiring response of the world community to the SARS epidemic. Scientists and health care workers in many countries jumped into the fray. Once the news had escaped the control of the Chinese government, the Internet, e-mail, and teleconferencing ensured that every bit of relevant knowledge was shared. The UN's World Health Organization deserves special mention for quickly grasping the serious nature of the crisis and coordinating the world's response.

The WHO had been criticized in the past for its relatively slow response to the AIDS crisis. To be fair, it had its hands full dealing with age-old scourges such as tuberculosis, malaria, cholera, and influenza. According to some, its quick action on SARS can be credited to a renewed emphasis on activism and greater initiative brought about by former AIDS program chief Jonathan Mann. Mann was a visionary who had quit the agency and prodded it from the outside until his death in 1998.[21]

WHO staff had heard rumors of a major respiratory outbreak in southern China as early as November 2002, perhaps several weeks after the first cases cropped up in Guangdong. By early 2003 these rumors were spreading around Hong Kong, where scientists had heard from colleagues across the border about a large number of sick medical staff, and about the serious symptoms the pneumonia patients presented. On February 5 the WHO received an e-mail from a former employee in Guangdong about possible avian flu. ProMed, a respected disease surveillance Web site based at Harvard University, quoted a report from a China Web site claiming that hundreds had already died.

The WHO was repeatedly assured by contacts in Beijing that the situation was under control; its requests to send specialists to Guangdong were repeatedly deferred. Fears of an avian flu outbreak were spurred by reports of wild duck and geese die-offs in the waters in and around Hong Kong, which appeared starting in December 2002. But when local virologists from the Pandemic Preparedness in Asia project in that city were unable to isolate avian flu viruses from any of the remains, the concerns died down.[22]

On February 10, five days after receiving the e-mail from the former employee, the WHO regional office in Manila asked Beijing to comment on a text message that had leaked out of Guangdong about a mutant influenza epidemic; it was the first official request for information about the epidemic from outside China.[23] According to procedure, as long as the victims were confined to one country, the WHO had no powers to take action without the approval of the national government. The stunning spread of SARS from the single case at the Metropole Hotel, however, created a media frenzy that could not be ignored. Within a few days nearly the entire Hong Kong population donned surgical masks, and airline and airport personnel in Asia and elsewhere began imposing screening methods (forehead temperature scanning in Hong Kong and Singapore) and detaining passengers deemed to be ill—all in response to an epidemic whose parameters were still completely unknown to the wider world.

On March 11, Carlo Urbani, before himself taking ill, managed to persuade top Vietnamese health officials to take action. They called in an international team of experts and imposed a strict quarantine on the two designated SARS hospitals. The epidemic in that country was completely suppressed within two months. Urbani's collapse in Bangkok later that day rang all the alarm bells at the WHO. The agency immediately notified its Global Outbreak and Response Network (GOARN), an international coalition of 110 national governments and scientific institutions that was set up in 2000 to respond to just such a crisis. Members were asked to scour every possible source of information and to gather samples from exposed or symptomatic individuals.

On March 15, two days after the first patients in Hanoi and Toronto died, the WHO held an emergency teleconference with national health agencies around the world. Immediately following this meeting U.S. CDC director Julie Gerberding convened experts at a secure communications center set up in Atlanta following the anthrax bioterror attacks of 2001, which she now dedicated to the SARS fight. The center united a host of federal, state, and local health, emergency, and intelligence agencies.

Still on the 15th, top WHO figures met in Geneva to issue a "worldwide health threat," their first ever. The bulletin gave a name to the epidemic—Severe Acute Respiratory Syndrome or SARS. It warned against the disease's relatively long incubation period and its ability to transmit via very casual contact, and it called for isolation of patients and "barrier nursing." In this practice, patients are isolated in individual rooms or behind screens, and all those who come in contact wear gowns, masks, and rubber gloves. The agency also distributed tissue samples from victims to 12 leading labs around the world to help isolate the microbe that had so far eluded detection at several labs, even a Hong Kong lab that was using mucus smuggled out of Guangzhou.

Two labs almost immediately isolated a paramyxovirus similar to measles; the family is known to cause pneumonia on occasion, but this finding turned out to be irrelevant, as no other labs confirmed that finding. On March 24 both the U.S. CDC and the Hong Kong Preparedness Project announced they had found a previously unknown coronavirus in tissue samples; further tests proved this to be the real culprit, and other tests in China and Japan found similar viruses among domestic animals, strengthening fears of an animal-to-human jump. In 2004 Chinese military researchers told U.S. Congress investigators that they had isolated coronavirus from SARS cases a few weeks earlier, but they had been told to suppress their findings in deference to the earlier official Chinese line that the culprit was chlamydia.[24] Doctors were frightened: other cornaviruses are among the most common cause of colds, and they are known to live on surfaces for hours.

On March 24, GOARN confirmed 456 cases and 17 deaths in 14 countries. Under global pressure, China now admitted to 792 cases and 31 deaths, but it still refused WHO access to Guangdong. A March 26 global WHO teleconference gave doctors comprehensive information about the course of the disease and the best appropriate therapy. Urbani died on the 29th after an 18-day struggle; his foresight and heroism probably saved thousands, if not millions, of lives.

The U.S. CDC and WHO quickly developed an intimate daily partnership, using satellite broadcasts and Webcasts to share X-rays and other clinical information with doctors and public health officers around the world. Never before had an outbreak been so thoroughly and accurately monitored. The CDC sent 12 investigators to SARS hot points, distributed hundreds of thousands of alerts to Americans who had traveled there, and helped enforce stringent hospital controls.

On March 27, the WHO urged that all airline passengers be screened for symptoms, not just those traveling to or from the affected countries. On April 2, for the first time in its 50-year history, the WHO issued a travel advisory, telling nonessential travelers to avoid Guangdong and Hong Kong. The advisory was later extended to Singapore and Toronto.

A WHO team was finally allowed to visit Guangdong from April 3 to 10, after it threatened to pull out of the country. The representatives were impressed by the province's efforts to suppress the epidemic. Meanwhile, the scientific knowledge base rapidly expanded. By April 7 three diagnostic tests had been developed to positively identify SARS cases, labs had learned to reproduce the virus, and a U.S. Army facility began testing antivirals. On April 12 the British Columbia Cancer Agency announced it had decoded the SARS virus genome, a feat duplicated by the CDC, which made its announcement the next day. On the 16th, the WHO announced that primates infected by the virus in Rotterdam had taken ill with the appropriate symptoms, thus proving beyond a doubt that the virus was the disease agent.

China Turns a Corner

In late April China's approach to SARS took a sudden, dramatic turn. Foreign journalists speculated that a top-level power struggle in Beijing helped explain the change. While the struggle raged earlier in the year neither faction was willing to abandon the old policy of secrecy and face charges of endangering national security. However, once President and Communist Party Secretary Hu Jintao and Premier Wen Jiabao emerged triumphant, they used the epidemic as a club to attack former party chief Jiang Zemin and his ally, Health Minister Zhang Wenkang. Zhang and Beijing mayor Meng Xuenong were dismissed on April 20. That day the government held an extraordinary press conference admitting the earlier missteps and deceptions and dramatically raising estimates of the scope of the epidemic nationally and within the capital city.[25]

Only 10 days before, the authorities had been trying to stonewall reporters. After the courageous Beijing chief of surgery Jiang Yanyong and a few other whistleblowers broke silence in early April to report on the growing crisis in the city, the government allowed interested foreigners to visit Beijing hospitals, but only after first removing patients and staff infected with SARS and sending them on dangerous ambulance trips around the city.[26]

In a complete about-face, on April 18 Hu and premier Wen began a highly publicized fact-finding "tour of the South." All television stations were preempted for 24-hour SARS coverage. Zhong Nanshan and other doctors active in the fight were turned into national heroes. Citizens committees were formed, theaters and public buildings closed, and "snooping grandmas" (used in the past to control dissidents) were mobilized to enforce home quarantines (some 30,000 exposed individuals were quarantined in Beijing alone). Beijing took on the look of a ghost town, as at least a million residents fled and others stayed home.

A national "strike SARS hard" campaign went into effect, especially in the affected provinces. Roadblocks were placed all over to prevent travel by sick people, and unknown individuals were barred from most villages. The campaign's strict surveillance, rapid reporting, and contact tracing quickly brought the epidemic under control; no cases were reported between July 2003 and January 2004, when the final three cases emerged. National reporting regulations were strengthened; it became illegal for government officials to withhold epidemic information from higher authorities—although the public still does not enjoy the legal right to know.

In early May 2003 Zhong Nanshan won approval for Hong Kong researcher Guan Yi, who had helped isolate the virus, to take samples from traders and livestock in the Guangzhou "wild flavor" markets. Guan Yi quickly isolated the virus in several animals, most of them palm civets. Eleven of the traders were antibody-positive carriers, meaning they had acquired the virus but had not fallen ill. The lesson was clear: The disease had jumped from animals to humans. On the recommendation of the WHO, the government closed down the wild flavor markets nationally for a few months, and thousands of animals were slaughtered.

In August, after the epidemic seemed to be over, and under pressure from the industry, the general ban was lifted, even though infected animals continued to be discovered. However, in January civet cats were once more ordered killed on all farms and markets, after a handful of new human cases were reported. The species jump has not recurred in the three years that have passed since then.

Following the epidemic, Guangdong Province, Hong Kong, and Macau signed an agreement for monthly sharing of information on a list of 30 infectious diseases. In 2004, WHO officials praised the Chinese government for a greater degree of transparency and willingness to work with international experts.[27] Other observers, however, charged that China was still being less than frank in its statements concerning a minor avian flu outbreak that year.[28] In addition, citizens' groups involved in HIV/AIDS education and assistance continued to complain of government opposition as late as 2007.[29]

Conclusion

By the middle of 2003, when the epidemic was essentially contained, nearly 8,500 people had been diagnosed with SARS, and over 900 had died. The real toll may be somewhat higher, as some cases were excluded from the total for lack of evidence, especially among the early victims in China. The disease caused economic losses of some $30 billion, and subjected local populations to the ancient terrors of plague.

It could have been much worse. It is to be hoped that the world's governments have learned the lesson that transparency and cooperation are essential to protect their populations from infectious disease. The tools and procedures developed or refined in those frightening months should come in handy in the face of any new emerging disease.

AIDS AND AFRICA

Introduction

HIV, the human immunodeficiency virus that causes the disease AIDS (acquired immunodeficiency syndrome), probably did not exist until about 60 or 70 years ago. However, it has already killed more than 25 million people. Additionally, more than 33 million are infected with the virus, and many of them are likely to develop AIDS and die before treatments can reach them. Thus, the current AIDS pandemic has already become one of the most deadly in history, and it is far from over. In 2007, some 2.5 million additional people became infected with the virus; several million other people who were already infected with the virus came down with AIDS that year, and about 2.1 million people with AIDS died. These numbers reflect the latest United Nations estimate, issued in November 2007 in the UNAIDS report, "07 AIDS Epidemic Update." In that report, the agency somewhat reduced the numbers it had earlier released. The new figures reflect more accurate nationwide surveys in Africa and India. In India, the numbers were cut nearly in half, as it became apparent that the epidemic was confined largely to high-risk groups and was not spreading to the general population.[30]

No country has emerged unscathed, but the greatest losses have been in sub-Saharan Africa, where the virus first emerged. Unfortunately, the region includes some of the poorest countries in the world, with some of the least developed health care delivery systems. The combination of large caseloads and inadequate medical care has produced a tragedy of historic proportions, which has set back economic development and political stability and demoralized much of the continent.

North Americans are rightly concerned about potential dangers such as avian influenza or bio-terrorism. However, there is nothing potential or hypothetical about AIDS—it is causing untold suffering to a sizable part of the world's population. The good news is that the wider world is finally taking note, and beginning to help. The tragedy is that so much more needs to be done, and there is no guarantee that it will be done.

Researchers are following several promising paths toward an effective vaccine to protect people against the HIV virus, but years of work remain. Unfortunately, the most promising vaccine trial ended early in September 2007 following poor results.[31] A cure for AIDS is probably even further away. Fortunately, a large variety of effective medicines and treatment protocols have become available to keep people with AIDS alive and relatively healthy. Most people with AIDS in the wealthier countries, and a lucky minority in all countries, are surviving for years and leading productive lives. The challenge is to get these treatments to *all* the sufferers in Africa and Asia as well, as quickly as possible. It will require tens of billions of dollars, and a massive government and private effort to develop the educational and health programs and facilities. But *it is doable.* Peter Piot, executive director of UNAIDS, has written, "there is overwhelming evidence that the AIDS epidemic can be controlled—but only when governments make fighting AIDS a priority."[32]

History

AIDS first came into view in 1981, in the United States. A number of sexually active gay men in New York City and San Francisco suddenly showed up at doctors offices and hospitals with rare and severe ailments that are associated with a weakened immune system. By the end of the year hundreds of other cases were reported, and the U.S. CDC recognized that a new disease had emerged. Most of the original patients died after a year or two of painful illness. Within two years, the HIV virus was isolated from the blood of AIDS patients, convincing scientists that the disease was contagious. HIV was soon shown to be the cause of the disease, in the opinion of nearly all scientists and doctors. A tiny minority of scientists and a larger group of conspiracy theory buffs still maintain that HIV does not cause AIDS; almost none of the patients have embraced that point of view.

Scientists eventually found that HIV is very similar to a virus still found among chimpanzees in Cameroon in West-Central Africa.[33] Based on slight variations among the different strains of HIV, scientists speculate that the virus crossed over to humans on a few different occasions sometime in the period from the 1920s to the 1940s, probably when hunters entered isolated forests to kill, butcher, and eat infected chimps. The earliest confirmed case of HIV infection was that of a man in Kinshasa (in today's Democratic Republic of the Congo [DRC], a 500-mile boat trip from Cameroon), who gave a blood sample in 1959, which was stored and reexamined in the 1980s. Other early cases have been found in blood samples in the United States (1969) and Norway (1976).

Thus, it took about 50 years for the first few cases to spread to epidemic proportions—probably because the virus is difficult to catch. Unlike most infectious diseases, casual contact is not enough. By far the most common mode of transmission is sexual relations. Whenever there is sexual penetration of any kind and the couple does not use condoms, if one partner is already infected with HIV, there is a chance that it will be transmitted to the other partner, whether the couple is heterosexual or homosexual. A minority of cases are transmitted through blood, via transfusions, medical accidents, or injection. The highest risk occurs when needles are shared by drug users, administered by poorly trained "injectionists" or by informal or "folk sector" healers, or reused by medical staff who lack new or sterile syringes. The many children infected by HIV generally acquired the virus during the birth process or via breast-feeding; this is still a significant transmission path in sub-Saharan Africa.

How did the early cases escape detection for so long? If cases were confined to remote rural areas, few modern doctors would have seen them. Local people often attributed their disease to witchcraft or other nonscientific causes. Besides, AIDS does its damage by weakening the immune system and allowing many different diseases to flourish. Different patients show different infections, depending on age, location, gender, and chance. Finally, it can take up to 10 years or more for a person infected with HIV to develop the symptoms of AIDS. Doctors had little reason to connect one puzzling case with another that had occurred a year or two before.

The virus spread quietly through travel, migration, war, long-distance trade, prostitution, and blood transfusions. The process of transmission soon became very complex. For example, even though the virus began its journey in Africa, non-African tourists, business people, diplomats, or others who visited the continent may well have picked up HIV in one country and brought it to another, or even spread it between people in one country. It is believed that infection became widespread sometime in the 1970s. In 1981, after the initial appearance in the United States, doctors began to notice cases in the Americas, Africa, Europe, and Australia.

By 1982 several African countries reported clusters of cases. In Uganda the syndrome was commonly called "slim" or "wasting disease," due to rapid weight loss among those infected. Zambia, Rwanda, and Congo reported many cases in 1983, while others were showing up among African nationals living in Europe. Doctors in Zaire (now the DRC) realized that early cases had actually occurred in Kinshasa in the late 1970s, showing up either as "slim" or as meningitis.[34] In Africa, unlike in developed countries, most patients seemed to be heterosexual men and women, and most cases seemed to have been transmitted through heterosexual sex. This pattern has continued to the present. Scientists believe that when common sexually transmitted diseases such as gonorrhea go untreated, as is common in Africa, HIV is far more likely to spread during intercourse.[35] In the 1980s, fewer than 100,000 cases of AIDS were officially reported in Africa, but observers believed the true number was far higher; they estimated over 650,000 cases of AIDS by the end of 1991, among more than 5 million people infected with HIV.[36]

By 1990 several drugs had become available that could slow down the course of the disease, and doctors had learned how to treat some of the "opportunistic infections" that afflicted people with AIDS. However, the drugs were expensive and the treatments required advanced medical facilities. Only a tiny minority of black African people with AIDS benefited from these advances before the start of the 21st century. In 1995 the South African Ministry of Health reported that 8 percent of pregnant women in that country were HIV-positive, but very few of them were being given AZT, a drug that had recently been shown to be effective in preventing the transfer of the virus to a baby during birth. The ministry estimated that 850,000 people, over 2 percent of adults, were HIV-positive.[37]

Also in 1995, the first of a new class of very effective AIDS drugs, called protease inhibitors, was approved. For people in the developed world, a diagnosis of AIDS ceased to be an automatic death sentence. Meanwhile, in 1998, an estimated 70 percent of all the world's new HIV infections were occurring in sub-Saharan Africa, amounting to several million people, according to UNAIDS, and almost none of them were being treated.[38]

In 2000 the 13th International AIDS Conference was held in Durban, South Africa, the first time it had been held in a developing country. In response to public skepticism by the country's president, Thabo Mbeki, about the role of

HIV as the exclusive cause of AIDS, 5,000 doctors from around the world signed a statement (called the Durban Declaration) affirming that HIV was indeed the culprit.[39] They feared that debates over questions that had already been settled would only get in the way of meeting the ever-growing crisis.

As the new century unfolded, some progress was reported. Several African governments such as Uganda, which had long pursued prevention and treatment programs, were witnessing a slowdown of the epidemic. New sources of funding appeared, including a massive increase in aid from the U.S. government and from private charities, also largely American. Pharmaceutical companies in the West and in India were browbeaten into dramatically cutting the price of their drugs for Africans, who could never buy them at market price in any case. The virus continued to spread in Africa, but at a slower pace; the prevalence of HIV (the percentage of the total population that is infected) probably peaked in the late 1990s.[40] In addition, new, more accurate statistics based on cross section population surveys showed that HIV was less prevalent in West Africa, in rural areas, among older age groups, and among men than had been feared.[41] Even with the revised estimates, southern Africa continued to face the biggest crisis.

In 2006 the number of African AIDS patients being treated with the new antiviral medications surpassed 1 million for the first time;[42] by 2007 the number had reached 1.3 million.[43] Cynical observers could well say, "too little, too late," but given the technical and social challenges of delivering these drugs in the African setting, the accomplishment is impressive. If the political will in Africa and the West continues to be focused on AIDS, it may be possible to build on this base of progress and bring relief and hope to the peoples of Africa.

By late 2006 another important tool against HIV emerged—male circumcision. Apart from Muslims, most of whom live in the northern parts of the continent, the majority of African males are not circumcised. In 2005 and 2006 several large-scale trials conducted in South Africa, Uganda, and Kenya confirmed earlier hopes that the practice can reduce transmission of HIV during sex by at least 50 percent. Most areas of Africa lack sanitary facilities and trained personnel for this type of outpatient surgery; but the effort to build networks for this purpose might earn a very good return for the money, until an AIDS vaccine can be found, which may be far in the future.

Impact

By 2006, over 20 million people had died of AIDS in sub-Saharan Africa, where it was the leading cause of death. Two million died in 2005 alone. About 24.5 million were infected with HIV at the end of 2005, 2 million of them children under 15 years old.[44]

The pandemic has put tremendous strains on the region's hospitals. A shortage of beds means that only very sick people are admitted, at a stage where medicines do not always work. Many health care workers are themselves ill with AIDS, or have experienced "burnout." The pressures have contributed to emigration of health care workers, who are much in demand in the West.[45] In response, churches and other nongovernmental organizations have helped patients develop community and home-based care programs, which has eased the burden somewhat on hospitals.[46]

AIDS has increased the percentage of African families living in poverty, due largely to the loss of income by patients and those caring for them. In the 15–24 age bracket, AIDS claims three women for every man in the region. So many young women have died that some 12 million African children have become orphaned. Many are adopted by relatives, but many others have to fend for themselves.

The education system has been negatively affected in several ways. In Zambia in 2004 some 20 percent of teachers were found to be infected with HIV.[47] The loss of teachers through death and illness leaves many classes untaught. In addition, children with AIDS or orphaned by AIDS are far less likely to attend school. Ironically, the deterioration of schools undermines AIDS prevention programs, which hope to reach teenagers, who are so much at risk for the disease.

Economic activity has been depressed by AIDS, since most victims are young adults, in their most productive years. AIDS has reduced the rate of economic growth in sub-Saharan Africa as a whole by 2 to 4 percent, according to various estimates. By 2010, South Africa, by far the most important economy in the region, is expected to have 17 percent lower economic output than it would have had without AIDS.[48] In Africa, people with AIDS are more likely to be urban residents and to be better educated. As these people took ill and died in large numbers, economic life and government services visibly suffered. Large and small businesses report major cost increases due to absenteeism, the expense of training replacement workers, and health care, funeral, and related costs. In response, many larger businesses, especially those with skilled work forces, have begun workplace AIDS programs, covering education, prevention, and treatment.

Many African countries have seen sharp declines in the "Human Development Index" published by the United Nations Development Program and based on life expectancy, domestic economic production, and literacy.[49] Life expectancy in sub-Saharan Africa had fallen to 47 in 2002 (the average newborn child could expect to live that long); without AIDS, the figure might have been 62 years if pre-AIDS improvements had continued. In South

Africa, according to one estimate the figure is expected to drop from 68.4 before the epidemic to 36.5 in 2010.[50]

International Response

Faced with the sudden appearance of AIDS, even the resource-rich nations of Europe and North America needed several years to develop the technology and expertise to begin to contain the epidemic. Africa, with far fewer resources and with a much larger HIV burden, desperately needed help from outside the continent. No other region was more dependent on the good will and competence of foreign governments, international bodies, NGOs, and private charities. No other region has so large a stake in the international anti-AIDS campaign.

The WHO began its Global Surveillance of AIDS in 1983, two years after the epidemic emerged, at a time when the biology of the disease and its international scope were as yet unclear. The first International Conference on AIDS was held in April 1985 in Atlanta, the home of the U.S. CDC. The 2000 attendees focused primary on scientific research, and the World Health Organization decided to organize a conference to discuss coordinated action against the epidemic; by 1986 it had set up a separate program to deal with the disease, the Global Program on AIDS, under the leadership of the dynamic CDC alumnus Jonathan Mann. Mann won large budgetary increases, and he fought for both increased spending by governments and attention to the needs and rights of HIV-positive individuals, who often faced fear and discrimination. In 1996 the UN combined several subagencies on AIDS into a superagency called UNAIDS, based in Geneva.

The decision to build a separate agency for AIDS has attracted some criticism over the years, as annual deaths from AIDS in the developing world remain less than half of the deaths from preexisting preventable scourges such as malaria, tuberculosis, childhood diarrhea, and complications of pregnancy and childbirth.[51] On the other hand, none of the other diseases has increased so dramatically as AIDS, or has the potential to kill such a large part of the human population.

In part, to meet these objections, the Global Fund to Fight AIDS, Tuberculosis, and Malaria was formed in 2001, with the help of the World Bank, the UN, governments, and NGOs. It serves as a conduit for the growing amount of funding made available from the UN, the European Union, the U.S. Congress, businesses, and private sources. By 2007 the Global Fund had disbursed more than $3 billion and committed $8.4 billion to grants in 136 countries. It aims to help fund proven, practical programs in target countries.[52] However, even these large sums are only enough to fund about one-third of the valid proposals the Global Fund receives.

The total funding available for HIV/AIDS activities increased dramatically in 2003 when the U.S. Congress approved President George W. Bush's proposal for a President's Emergency Program for AIDS Relief (PEPFAR), a five-year, $15 billion international relief program, most of it "new" money, added to existing programs; the bill covers spending for malaria and tuberculosis as well. Although many critics are skeptical of the unpopular Bush administration and oppose the program's bilateral orientation (separate programs for each of the 15 recipient countries, 12 of them in Africa), as well as its emphasis on abstention as one of the main prevention strategies, the money has begun to make a significant difference in several countries.[53] In 2007 President Bush requested an additional $30 billion from Congress to cover the years 2009–13.

The struggle against AIDS has attracted a host of celebrities, including such figures as England's Princess Diana, whose visit to an AIDS clinic in 1987 drew massive worldwide news coverage. In the early years, many were responding to the heavy toll the disease took in the entertainment industry in the developed world. In time, however, they helped create an international culture of awareness and concern about health crises and other problems in the developing world. Many politicians and business people were now committed to helping—or eager to avoid the appearance of standing in the way.

This climate eventually helped convince the pharmaceutical industry to relax its patent rights on AIDS drugs and to sell its products at steep discounts to AIDS programs in poorer countries. In South Africa in 2001, for example, international drug companies dropped their lawsuits against a program to produce inexpensive generic AIDS drugs in the country. Two of the generics produced in South Africa won approval from the U.S. Food and Drug Administration in 2006, along with an American-made generic drug, making them all eligible for PEPFAR funds.

Since 2003, the William J. Clinton Foundation, run by former U.S. president Bill Clinton, also played an important role in negotiating several major deals with private-sector companies to provide discounts on AIDS drugs, HIV tests, and chemicals used in making generic drugs. On March 29, Clinton publicly supported mandatory HIV testing in the most affected countries—in part because these countries could now afford the reduced cost of HIV tests and of the antivirals that could counter HIV and AIDS.

Country Surveys

Each country in Africa, as elsewhere, has responded in its own characteristic way to the HIV/AIDS epidemic. The cases of Uganda and South Africa, both controversial in different ways, shed light on the various political and ideological factors that can complicate the struggle.

UGANDA

Of all the countries in sub-Saharan Africa, Uganda is often cited as the most successful in meeting the challenge of HIV/AIDS. Clear-sighted leadership, mobilization of public opinion, and prompt action probably reduced the scale of the epidemic significantly, although the virus has continued to spread.

Some recent observers question the degree of progress in Uganda. A few suggest that the epidemic was never quite as widespread as originally believed, so that the decline in HIV prevalence is partly a "statistical artifact." In other words, the high prevalence rates in the early years may have been based on limited studies within high-risk communities, while the current lower rates are based on more comprehensive national data.[54] In addition, controversy has raged in the anti-AIDS community about the contributions that sexual abstinence and monogamy campaigns have made to the country's successes.[55] However, few observers deny the main achievement: Uganda has leveraged its limited resources in effective ways that have helped preserve social stability and kept a lid on both the disease toll and its impact on the country.

The AIDS patient load in Uganda was small through the early 1980s, but tests found high levels of HIV infection. The Ugandan Red Cross found that 12 percent of blood donors in Kampala, the capital, tested positive for HIV.[56] In 1986 President Yoweri Museveni, who had taken office in a coup in January, personally launched an anti-AIDS program in visits around the country. He said that it was a "patriotic duty" for citizens to remain free of HIV.

Ugandan doctors were at the forefront in developing affordable approaches to care and treatment for opportunistic infections. But nothing could be done at the time to control the underlying disease. Museveni stressed prevention above all. His approach became known as ABC—abstain from sex before marriage (especially if you are young), be faithful to your partner, and use condoms. While many African leaders (and even those in the West) avoided the topic as an embarrassment, Uganda's health minister spoke about AIDS at the WHO annual assembly that year. The Ministry of Health set up a program to ensure a safe blood supply.[57]

In the next few years Ugandan AIDS activists formed the AIDS Support Organization, or TASO, a community-based AIDS program,[58] and an official AIDS information center was established with British assistance to provide testing and counseling.[59] In 1987 the military began efforts to prevent the spread of HIV within its ranks. Nevertheless, a national survey in 1988 found that 9 percent of the population tested positive for HIV.

In other important moves, the government set up AIDS control projects in various ministries (Justice, Agriculture, etc.) to address different sectors; took out a World Bank loan in 1994 to finance a "Sexually Transmitted Infections" project, which encouraged those suffering from endemic sexually transmitted diseases (STDs) to seek treatment;[60] and ran an important large-scale test in 1997 to demonstrate that antiviral drugs successfully prevent mother-child transmission of HIV during delivery. The following year a Drug Access Initiative was started to press for lower prices for antiviral drugs and to build infrastructure to distribute those drugs to patients when they became available. In 1999 the Ministry of Health set up a voluntary door-to-door HIV screening program, with mobile screening centers offering rapid tests to 100 people a day.[61] These programs brought a long-term decline in the prevalence of HIV. Fewer healthy people were being infected with HIV; as AIDS patients died, the HIV-positive population began to shrink.

Uganda's relative success in containing the epidemic has not protected it from the political and ideological controversies that embroil the AIDS community. By giving equal prevention roles to abstinence, monogamy, and condom use, Uganda attracted great interest among Christian medical aid groups. After all, they noted, the breakdown of traditional Christian and tribal sexual mores, both among newly urbanized Africans and among gay men in the West, had greatly facilitated the rapid spread of the epidemic.

American Christian groups, who staff and support a large number of clinics throughout Africa, were the key constituency pushing the Bush administration to launch its multibillion-dollar PEPFAR program. As a consequence, PEPFAR includes a provision mandating that one-third of the funds going to AIDS prevention programs must be devoted to abstinence and faithfulness education. This provision has been a red flag for many AIDS activists. At the Sixteenth International AIDS Conference in Toronto in August 2006, Stephen Lewis, United Nations special envoy on AIDS to Africa, called the PEPFAR provision "incipient neocolonialism,"[62] since it can be seen as dictating policy to the recipient country. Bush administration spokespersons (and many other AIDS activists) replied that by law only 7 percent of PEPFAR money goes to abstinence and faithfulness education, that Uganda had in fact pioneered the concept of abstinence and faithfulness ("zero grazing") on its own years ago with apparent success (including a rise in the age of first sex[63]), and that no AIDS program anywhere ignores abstinence.

Thanks to the controversy, the always uncertain country statistics for HIV prevalence have now become a political football—supporters of PEPFAR stress the positive figures that have been reported in Uganda for years;

while opponents now point to those statistics that contradict claims of a "Ugandan miracle." In the end, the controversy may not have any great impact in the field. As long as PEPFAR continues to offer billions of dollars to buy drugs, its programs will be welcomed; those who mistrust its programming or disparage abstinence education may prefer to work with the other funding programs that have become available in recent years. The two camps do not differ either on the ultimate goal or on the general requirements to meet that goal.

SOUTH AFRICA

South Africa has the most developed economy and health care sector in sub-Saharan Africa. In the 1990s, after a long struggle against racial oppression, the country emerged as a stable multiracial democracy with a dynamic capitalist economy. Under a majority black government, nonwhites for the first time could look to a future of social and economic progress.

When the first free elections were held in 1994, the AIDS epidemic had already been raging for some years, but the total impact was not yet clear—the entire country had been focused on the struggle against apartheid (racial segregation and oppression), while AIDS seemed to most people to be a minor irritant. The first cases diagnosed in the 1980s occurred largely among gay men, often whites. Since 1990, however, the gay caseload has been far outnumbered by heterosexually transmitted cases. The epidemic has also been far more severe among blacks than among whites, Asians, or those of "Coloured" background (a distinct ethnic group in Cape Province). According to the country's 2005 National HIV Survey, 13.3 percent of blacks over two years of age were HIV-positive, compared with 0.6 percent of whites, 1.6 percent of Indians, and 1.9 percent of Coloureds.[64]

In South Africa, women are far more likely than men to be HIV-positive, and the disparity seems to be growing worse. The 2005 survey, using new lab procedures that can tell when a person has been infected, found that a shockingly high 6.5 percent of all women aged 15–24 became infected that year, compared with 0.8 percent of all men. The government reported that year that 30.2 percent of all pregnant women who visited prenatal clinics that year were infected.

Yearly surveys show that the incidence (the number of new infections) has been decreasing as a whole, but the confirmed HIV burden is enormous. Government statistics for mid-2006 show that 5.2 million people are HIV-positive—they constitute about 11 percent of the entire population.[65] About 350,000 South African children under 10 are also infected with HIV. The death toll has been enormous and is growing as well, as the huge reservoir of HIV-positive South Africans, few of them benefiting from antiviral drugs, continues to develop AIDS. Although AIDS was cited in only 13,590 death certificates in 2004, local and international agencies agree that the toll is far higher. Noting that the overall death toll among children and young adults has shot up, and that AIDS-related illness such as tuberculosis have soared as well, these researchers, including UNAIDS and the Medical Research Council of South Africa, estimate that well over 300,000 people died of AIDS in 2005.[66]

Of all the countries most afflicted with AIDS, South Africa has seen perhaps the greatest amount of controversy. Many local and international critics of President Thabo Mbeki accuse both him and his administration of making a bad situation worse through denial, inaction, and wrongheaded policies.

Anti-apartheid leader and future president Nelson Mandela addressed South Africa's first National AIDS Convention in 1992. The issue was not a high priority of the new government, but many steps were taken by the government, private citizens, and NGOs. In 1998, then deputy president Mbeki launched a Partnership Against AIDS, stating that over half a million people were being infected every year. Two years later the government set up a National AIDS Council to oversee a five-year program to combat AIDS and other STDs. In 1999, Parliament passed a law legalizing the production of inexpensive antiviral drugs in South Africa, and won agreement from the departing Clinton administration, which had initially opposed the measure.[67]

But in 2000, Mbeki, now the president of South Africa, startled the International AIDS Conference in Durban by focusing on poverty as the cause of AIDS. He then publicly consulted with a handful of prominent dissident scientists who deny that HIV causes AIDS. In a letter to world leaders in April, he defended his meeting with the dissidents as a blow for freedom of inquiry, and wrote: "It is obvious that whatever lessons we have to and may draw from the West about the grave issue of HIV-AIDS, a simple superimposition of Western experience on African reality would be absurd and illogical."[68] Mbeki then appointed several people who deny that HIV causes AIDS to his presidential AIDS advisory panel. The government also resisted demands that HIV-positive pregnant women be given a dose of an antiviral drug, a universal practice by then, charging that the drug was toxic.

Without doubt, poverty, poor education, and inadequate medical care are the main reasons that HIV/AIDS has hit Africa so hard, while richer countries have managed to contain the epidemic. AIDS workers also agree that prevention measures must take local culture and behavior into account. However, no racial or cultural difference has been found in the way HIV/AIDS enters or harms individual bodies, and anti-AIDS drugs and medical procedures are effective everywhere. Ten years of experience around the world proves that a regimen of antiviral drugs can turn severely ill AIDS patients into functioning individuals in a matter of weeks, whether they live in Paris or in a village in Africa. Furthermore, people who follow the ABC principles of sexual restraint, and who do not share needles for any purpose, never develop AIDS, no matter how many other diseases they may previously have suffered, and no matter how ill-nourished they may be. Throughout 2006 and 2007, national and international criticism of Health Minister Manto Tshabalala-Msimang mounted, after she publicly called for the use of beetroot, lemon, and garlic as effective AIDS remedies. In September of that year, Mbeki appointed a new, less controversial council of cabinet ministers to coordinate AIDS programming.[69]

Despite Mbeki's views, and long delays in implementing treatment programs, South Africa has begun producing cheap antiviral drugs with the acceptance of the leading international pharmaceutical companies. In November 2003, the government began an Operational Plan for Comprehensive Care and Treatment for People Living with HIV and AIDS, although only a minority of those who need antivirals were enrolled by 2007, some 300,000 out of perhaps 750,000 who could benefit. Additional controversy has swirled over access to antiviral drugs for HIV-positive prisoners in the country's prisons.[70]

In South Africa, as elsewhere on the continent, AIDS activists have learned to cooperate with traditional healers, in order to win their cooperation with drug therapy. In 2004 Parliament passed a Traditional Health Practitioners Bill to give them legitimacy and bring them into a regulatory framework. It is hoped that respected practitioners can help provide support and comfort, as well as instruct patients in preventive measures.

Conclusion

Scientists warn that an effective vaccine against HIV will not be available for at least several years. They have even less hope for an actual cure for AIDS. Thus, the simple lessons of prevention are as important as ever, especially safe sex. But unless human nature changes very quickly, the total number of HIV-positive people may well continue to rise, posing an enormous threat: If strains of HIV emerge that are resistant to antiviral drugs, AIDS may yet earn the dubious honor of becoming the worst plague in human history, and one of the worst catastrophes ever to hit Africa.

Still, the human race can congratulate itself on its progress so far—scientific progress in learning about the disease and its treatment, and social progress in mobilizing resources to contain the epidemic all around the world. So much more can be done, and must be done, with the tools already at hand. The evidence of the past decade gives grounds for hope that it will be done.

RIVER BLINDNESS AND WEST AFRICA

Introduction

In the fight against epidemic infectious disease, no victory comes easy. River blindness, the common name for onchocerciasis (on-ko-ser-ki-a-sis), provides a good example.

It took three decades of persistent hard work by a coalition of governments and international agencies, buttressed by continued medical and pharmaceutical research, to effectively eliminate the scourge as a major public health threat in the fertile river valleys of the West African savannah. Thanks to the Onchocerciasis Control Program (OCP), which formally ended in 2002, hundreds of thousands of people were saved from inevitable blindness, and 60 million acres of prime land were made safe for settlement and farming.

But this victory cannot be taken for granted, even where the disease has been practically eliminated. First, the black flies that transmit the disease between people range over vast parts of Africa, and they can travel for hundreds of miles in a single day. And second, the parasitic worm that causes the disease can survive for many years in its human hosts, even when the symptoms do not appear. Only continued efforts by the local population, supported by the world community, can keep river blindness at bay. In war-torn countries, such as Sudan and Sierra Leone, the task becomes much more difficult.

Furthermore, a somewhat milder form of the disease remains endemic in a broad swath of forest in Central Africa. Other foci include regions of Sudan, Ethiopia, and Yemen as well as isolated areas of Central and South America. International efforts aim to stop transmission of the parasitic *Onchocerca volvulus* worm in Latin America and thus eradicate the disease there, as it has been in parts of West Africa. Unfortunately, a similar goal seems unrealistic at this time for all of Africa, the home of the vast majority of victims.

Onchocerciasis—The Disease

Onchocerciasis is a chronic (long-lasting) illness caused by a parasitic worm, *Onchocerca volvulus*, that lives inside its human hosts. It is spread from one person to another by black flies belonging to the genus *Simulium*, which prey on humans for blood meals. The disease causes severe, disfiguring skin problems and secondary bacterial infections (when harmful bacteria invade the skin wounds). It commonly leads to inflammation of lymph nodes, which are part of the body's immune system and are needed to help fight disease. Its worst impact is on the eyes, where chronic infection and inflammation leads to damaged vision and eventual blindness.

While the disease is not by itself fatal, it shortens patients' lives by about 13 years on average.[71] It lowers resistance to other infectious diseases, which are fairly common in the subtropical and tropical conditions where the disease is endemic. Its victims find it more difficult to make a living, in part because of the social disgrace associated with the ugly skin eruptions and fear of contagion. A typical story is related on one Web site: "Her husband abandoned Marie when she was 30 years old. He left her with an empty house, no money, no food and three hungry children to raise on her own. He left her because her body was covered with horrible bumps, rashes, and discolorations that gave her skin the appearance of a mottled 'leopard's' hide. Her incessant scratching irked him."[72]

Impaired vision and blindness have obvious economic consequences. In certain areas heavily infested with black flies, whole families and villages have been stricken, leaving no social or economic safety net. Finally, blind individuals are more prone to accidents, especially in poor conditions.

HOW IT IS SPREAD

In the late 19th century Western doctors began to isolate nematodes (roundworms) from patients suffering from the disease, in Africa and later in Central America. Nematodes are one of the most common types of animal life. Biologists have identified some 20,000 species of nematode, most of them parasitic—since they have no respiratory or circulation systems they must get oxygen and food from host animals or plants. Related nematodes can cause elephantiasis (the enlargement and thickening of tissues) and other harmful conditions.

By the 1920s the black fly was identified as the disease vector or agent of transmission. Fortunately *O. volvulus* can live only in humans and black flies—there is no other animal "reservoir" of infection—which makes the battle against it a bit easier. At least 15 species of the fly can carry the parasite. The flies need fast-flowing rivers in which to breed, and thus their numbers may fluctuate with the seasons, depending on geography. They can fly hundreds of miles a day on the wind, and live about four weeks.

By now scientists have come to understand the entire life cycle of the parasite—although new surprises are always possible. For example, it was only in the past few years that microbiologists discovered the crucial role of

Wolbachia bacteria in the life cycle of the *Onchocerca* parasite. These bacteria are "endosymbionts" of *Onchocera*—they live inside ("endo") the parasite; they help it to reproduce while deriving food from it (in a "symbiotic" or mutually useful relationship). Scientists now believe that the bacteria may cause many of the damaging symptoms of the disease, in addition to the harm caused by the worm.

Following this discovery, medicine now has three avenues of attack against river blindness: (1) to eliminate the insect vector, the black fly, by spraying its breeding grounds with pesticides; (2) to inhibit or destroy the *Onchocerca* parasite within the human host by using antimicrobials; and (3) to attack the bacteria that help *Onchocerca* thrive and reproduce by using antibiotic drugs.

A patient is infected through the bite of an infected female black fly. The fly's saliva contains *O. volvulus* larvae (immature worms), which migrate under human skin and form hard protected nodules or knots in the head or pelvic regions. There they grow into threadlike adult worms after six to 12 months, the females reaching up to 20 inches in length, the males much shorter. After a pair mate, the female begins laying up to 3,000 eggs each day—for 15 years! These eggs become first-stage larvae called microfilariae, which are ingested by the next black fly that bites the victim. The larva begin the maturation process within the black fly, as they migrate to its salivary glands, ready to be passed along to the next human victim.

WHAT IT DOES

The microfilariae are the main cause of morbidity (the harmful effects on the body). The adults remain isolated in their nodules, but the microfilariae migrate to the skin, the lymph system, and the eyes. Early symptoms include extreme itching, swelling, and inflammation. The damage is probably caused not by the parasite itself, but by the intense reaction of the human immune system as the microfilariae die and release toxins into the body along with toxic products of *Wolbachia*. At various stages, the skin becomes brittle ("lizard-skin"), discolored ("leopard-skin"), and covered with raised bumps or plaques, especially on the legs.

In the eye, the inflammation causes temporary wounds, which at first clear up. If the infection persists (as it generally does), these wounds eventually harden, causing blindness. Even when drugs have cleared the microfilariae from the body the eyes may continue to deteriorate, as the overstimulated immune system continues to attack the eye's own tissues.

Although the disease is best known in the wider world as river blindness, only a minority of its victims lose their sight. But even for the lucky majority the parasite can have devastating effects, apart from the visible manifestations in the skin. *Onchocerca* can invade many different organs and can be found in blood and urine. It can cause bone and muscle pain and a reduction in the body mass index, which themselves can lower productivity at work. It is even suspected of causing epilepsy.

WHERE IT EXISTS

Onchocerciasis apparently originated in Africa, where it has been found in 30 countries. The African strains are the most damaging, and they affect by far the most people. A 2005 estimate, based largely on village surveys, found that some 37 million people were carrying the parasite, with 90 million more individuals living in endemic areas and thus at risk.[73] This was *after* the successful control program in West Africa.

The surveys used a tool called "rapid epidemiological mapping of onchocerciasis" or REMO. REMO begins by identifying geographical features like river basins where the disease is likely to be endemic. A sample of villages is visited in each of these regions; 50 residents are chosen at random in each village and examined for telltale nodes beneath the skin.[74]

In West Africa, before the OCP, at least 500,000 victims had severe visual impairment, and another 270,000 were blind. In some villages, over 90 percent of the population was infected, and more than a third of them were blind. Half the victims lived in Nigeria, additional large concentrations were in Burkina Faso and Mali. Men had higher infection rates for reasons that remain unclear.

The disease takes a different course in the forest regions of Central Africa, where the blindness rate is only one-seventh of that in the savannah. The reasons for this difference are not yet known. These areas may have different strains or varieties of *Onchoncerca* worms or black flies, or the victims may not be reinfected as often. Now that scientists recognize the important role of *Wolbachia* in the disease, some have speculated that *Onchocerca* in Central Africa carry a lower load of that bacteria.[75]

The disease long ago passed the narrow straits to take root in certain regions of Yemen at the southern end of the Arabian Peninsula, where the disease is called Sowda. Some 250,000 people live in the endemic regions, where past village surveys have found a high level of infection. A comprehensive control program began in 2001, aided by NGOs and donated medicine, using thousands of specially trained local volunteers. Program providers claim to have successfully treated over 75,000 infected individuals in its first two years.[76]

Onchocerciasis is also found sporadically in six Latin American countries. The parasite was apparently brought by Africans captured in the slave trade. Unfortunately, some of the local species of black fly proved to be able transmitters of the parasite, and the disease took root in various localized regions. Important focal points are found in Guatemala and Mexico, where the disease more often leads to blindness,[77] and in Colombia, Ecuador, Venezuela, and the state of Amazonas in Brazil.

An End to "Fatalism"—the OCP

In the field of infectious disease, one popular cliché is that the African response to endemic plagues like river blindness is "fatalistic." In the past little could be done in any case either to prevent infection or to help those infected, so people just "accepted their fate," or left their homes to seek safer ones. Vast fertile, well-watered river valleys in the French and British colonial lands in the interior of West Africa were nearly depopulated over the years largely for fear of the flies and the disease they brought.

However, this situation was intolerable to the new independent African governments that emerged in the early 1960s. Rapidly growing populations, combined with the ever-present threat of desert encroachment to the north, made it essential to regain use of the fertile valley lands. Not long after independence several West African countries attempted to drum up interest in a campaign to eradicate the flies. It was the era of "disease eradication," and a quick pesticide-spraying project seemed doable. A 1949 test in Kenya showed that spraying black fly breeding grounds with DDT could interrupt transmission of the parasite.

Tests in the 1960s in individual countries proved unsuccessful, as flies from neighboring areas would colonize areas freed from infestation by spraying. It became clear that the disease could be fought only by means of a regional-scale project. A meeting in 1968 at Tunis in North Africa between the World Health Organization (WHO), the U.S. Agency for International Development, and the Organisation de Coordination et de Coopération pour la Lutte Contre les Grandes Endémies, ended with a call for just such a large-scale program.

In response, the WHO launched the Onchocerciasis Control Program (OCP) in 1974 together with the World Bank, the United Nations Development Program, and the UN Food and Agriculture Organization. The ambitious goal was to eliminate transmission of the disease in an area of a half million square miles, in which 30 million people lived. The project began in seven countries and was later expanded to an additional four; nine of the 11 countries were former French colonies. Over the years dozens of other international sponsors were added, including governments, NGOs, and the private sector, all of them contributing funds, personnel, or expertise.

At first the program depended entirely on expensive weekly spraying of black fly breeding grounds with about a dozen different pesticides. Given the life expectancy of an adult worm, which churns out millions of microfilariae during its long life in its human host, it was considered necessary to continue spraying for at least 14 years, until the parasites would finally die out on their own in infected patients. Routine spraying continued until 2002 in the four extension countries.

NEW WEAPON IS ADDED—IVERMECTIN

A number of potent antiworm drugs were tested early in the program. Some of them did in fact kill the larval microfilariae, and one killed the adults as well. But they all had to be given in repeated doses and serious side effects emerged. When the two favored drugs were found to make the eye lesions (wounds) even worse, they were largely abandoned for this disease.

In 1982 the pharmaceutical company Merck introduced ivermectin, a safe antiworm medicine that was very effective against the *Onchocerca* microfilariae—reducing their count by 99.5 percent after three months. Not only did it kill the larvae, but it also inhibited reproduction by adult females. In 1987 the company began offering the medicine free of charge to developing countries, at that time an unprecedented step. For 20 years its "Mectizan Donation Program" has been distributing the drug to control programs and to national health ministries for use against onchocerciasis and also against lymphatic filariasis, which can cause elephantiasis.

Unfortunately, the drug does not kill the adult worms in the nodules, so follow-up doses are given at intervals of six to 18 months to suppress the new microfilariae before they can do harm. Often an anti-inflammatory drug is given alongside ivermectin, since the dead microfilariae and the associated *Wolbachia* release toxins and other products into the body that can cause severe allergic reactions.

In 2002 the OCP was declared officially complete, as the disease had been stopped in all 11 countries. Enough land had been freed up for settlement to feed an additional 17 million people each year, using local farming methods. As a result, the region has become a net exporter of food. About 18 million children have been born in the former endemic areas, all of them apparently free of parasites.[78] However, ongoing surveillance continues, as well as treatment in certain zones, mostly under the supervision of national governments.

Spreading the Benefits

Encouraged by the success of OCP, the African Program for Onchocerciasis Control (APOC)[79] was introduced in the mid-1990s to cover the remaining

African countries affected by the disease. The primary tactic was distribution of ivermectin. The drug is distributed by the communities themselves, with training and support from the international partners.[78] A large number of government, NGO, and private-sector players are involved, under the administrative umbrella of the WHO and the fiscal control of the World Bank. APOC is based in Burkina Faso, one of the original OCP countries.

The program was implemented beginning in 1996 in test districts. Over the past decade it has gradually been expanded to cover the entire region. By 2003, APOC had established 107 projects, which treated 34 million people in 16 countries. The original goal was to treat 90 million people each year in 19 countries—everyone in the affected regions. By the middle of the decade the program seemed on track. A phase-out period was to begin in 2008. It is hoped that by 2010 sustainable community-based drug-delivery programs will keep the continent free of any new transmissions. APOC, like OCP before it, was aided by elaborate computer modeling programs, which helped refine tactics in the fight.

A parallel program was introduced in Latin America in 1992.[80] Small-scale fly-control programs had proved only partially successful, as were campaigns to encourage nodulectomy (surgical removal of the worm nodules). The new Onchocerciasis Elimination Program in the Americas (OEPA) was set up in Guatemala with the participation of all six affected countries, the Pan American Health Organization, the U.S. Centers for Disease Control and Prevention, and various NGOs. The program aimed to provide twice-a-year doses of ivermectin to 85 percent of the 500,000 people living in the affected regions (180,000 of them infected). The ultimate goal was complete elimination by 2010; by mid-decade the goal seemed achievable, as six of the 13 regions apparently have no new cases.[81]

Sustainability—ComDT

One of the most exciting outcomes of the onchocerciasis control programs has been the successful development of community-directed treatment (ComDT). Under this program, village residents are responsible for collecting ivermectin from supply points, distributing them to all eligible recipients, and reporting any cases of adverse reactions. They also serve to counsel and encourage village residents and communicate relevant information.

Proven in test runs by 1995, ComDT might have been the only practical way of reaching the entire population, especially in rural areas where government health programs often do not reach. By 2007, ComDT was delivering periodic doses to some 65 million people across Africa.[82] Many are also receiving albendazole, donated by SmithKline Beecham, which is given alongside ivermectin to treat lymphatic filariasis, another nematode disease found in some of the same regions, which often leads to elephantiasis. Pilot projects are being designed to deliver other health interventions using the ComDT network, such as Vitamin A, a vital nutrient, praziquantel to fight schistosomiasis, and counseling and distribution of condoms against HIV/AIDS and for reproductive health.[83]

The average cost per person for ComDT for onchocerciasis has been calculated at 74 cents—less than a dollar to prevent blindness and a lifetime of disability.[84] Of course, no solution is without its own problems. Not all teams have won support from their villages, and there is not enough supervision from central authorities.

Conclusion

A generation ago, onchocerciasis was stubbornly endemic over vast areas of the African continent. In a remarkably short period of time it has been brought under control in much of its range, thanks in large part to the cooperation of untold thousands of local volunteers, and to the free distribution of ivermectin. At the OCP closure ceremony in December 2002, WHO director-general Gro Harlem Brundtland said, "The accomplishments of the [OCP] inspire all of us in public health to dream big dreams. It shows we can reach 'impossible' goals and lighten the burden of millions of the world's poorest people."[85]

Will it be possible to declare complete victory against river blindness in the near future? The better part of wisdom is to assume that the disease could make a comeback, if, for example, either the parasite or the black fly vector develops resistance against the drugs and pesticides used against them. (In certain areas, ivermectin has become less effective in suppressing reproduction by adult females after multiple treatments.) Even where transmission seems to have been stopped, constant surveillance and checkups are in order. In other countries, especially those containing war zones, one must assume that pockets of infection still exist. Studies still need to be done to determine when and how ivermectin treatment can be safely stopped.

The genomes of both *O. volvulus* and *Wolbachia* have been analyzed, opening up the possibilities of developing replacements drugs and even vaccines.[86] So far, the control programs have not decided to use the available generalized antibiotics against *Wolbachia* for fear of causing resistance to these vital drugs. Any further progress requires continued financial commitment from the world community. It would be tragic if the success of onchocerciasis control programs leads to a loss of interest by donors and researchers.

MALARIA AND INDIA

Introduction

The age-old war that civilization wages against epidemic disease has brought some heartening victories, such as against smallpox. Other battles are still in doubt, such as the worldwide struggle against HIV/AIDS, and the ever-present threat of deadly influenza. Between these extremes campaigns have been carried out where complete victory has seemed within tantalizing grasp, only to slip away. The viruses that cause polio and measles are in this category of moving targets.

The Indian experience with malaria falls into this third category. In the 1960s the disease seemed all but eliminated in the country, thanks to a determined campaign by the Indian national and local governments aided by the world community. Potent chemicals were sprayed to eliminate or keep away the mosquitoes that spread the disease from one person to another, and medicines were widely distributed to treat infected people and to keep uninfected people out of danger. These medicines proved very effective in stopping the parasitic protozoans (one-celled animals) from infecting or harming their victims. However, the deadly parasites soon reappeared, and the antimalaria campaign eventually lost steam.

While the outbreaks of recent years appear to be far smaller and less deadly than those of the first half of the 20th century (according to Indian government statistics), their very existence constitutes a threat that the bad old days could return. Many of the drugs and chemicals that led to the early successes are beginning to lose their effectiveness. Both the parasites and the mosquitoes are developing resistance. Furthermore, the very success of the early campaign means that few people in the country have a natural resistance to the parasite. How much time does humankind have left to deal a final blow to eradicate this scourge?

The Disease

Malaria has been one of the most destructive of all infectious diseases. During all of human history, and probably during prehistoric times as well, malaria was endemic in large parts of the world. In fact, strains of this common disease are found in birds, reptiles, and many mammals including chimpanzees, all caused by different species of the *Plasmodium* genus of protozoan.

Malaria was a leading cause of death for thousands of years in Asia, Africa, and the Mediterranean, and for hundreds of years in South and Central America. It even extended to North America and northern Europe, although the most deadly form, spread by *P. falciparum*, thrives only in certain warm or hot climates. It should be noted that even within the tropical malaria band many regions and districts are free of malaria, thanks to localized climate and topographic conditions. Rural areas are generally more likely to be affected than cities, due to the greater presence of untreated mosquito breeding grounds.

Historical estimates for malaria incidence are not too reliable, especially since the disease was sometimes hard to distinguish from other fevers. However, when medical statistics became dependable in the first half of the 20th century, it became clear that up to 10 percent of all deaths in the world could be attributed directly or indirectly to malaria. In parts of India, such as West Bengal and Uttar Pradesh, the disease was implicated in 50 percent of all deaths. In these areas, about 1.5 percent of the population died of malaria every single year.[87]

Epidemic outbreaks were common enough on all continents, but far more people died in periods between epidemics, in districts and regions where the disease was endemic. In such areas, everyone could expect to be bitten and infected sooner rather than later. Within six to 15 days of the first infection, the victim usually feels a sudden attack of chills leading to several hours of fever and sweating, accompanied by joint pain, vomiting, and the death of many red blood cells. With *P. falciparum*, *P. vivax*, and *P. ovale*, the cycle repeats itself every 48 hours; with *P. malariae*, every 72 hours. The two strains were known in ancient India and Greece as tertian and quartan fever (returning on the third and fourth days). Severe cases, usually caused by *P. falciparum*, involve intense headache, an enlarged spleen and liver, and a blockage of blood to the brain, often leading to coma. About one victim in five dies, even with intensive treatment.

While most adults survive an initial attack of either variety, many children succumb. Some children are born with a greater degree of resistance to malaria (for example, if one of their parents has the sickle-cell genetic mutation), but children in general have underdeveloped immune systems. Pregnant women are also vulnerable—and they are particularly attractive to mosquitoes. The disease can cause miscarriages, low birth weight, and infant and maternal mortality.

For those who survive, parasites can remain in the liver in dormant form, and victims often suffer relapses after a year or longer. The parasite can also cause damage to various body organs, including the kidney and the brain; children who survive the severe form of the disease are often developmentally impaired. Many chronic malaria patients suffer depression and irritability. Many people who die of other direct causes, such as malnutrition or respiratory disease, might have survived if their bodies were not weakened by repeated bouts of malaria.

Malaria can theoretically spread through blood transfusions, but it is never contagious between individuals. Without mosquitoes, the disease would die out within one generation. Adult females of any of 40 different species of *Anopheles* mosquitoes are the culprit. Every day at dusk, each of these mosquitoes begins to seek a meal of blood, most often from nonhuman animals. It will continue to search all night until it finds a victim; human victims are usually sleeping in their beds. If the human "donor's" blood contains *Plasmodium* gametocytes (reproductive cells), these cells travel to the mosquito's gut to reproduce. The "sporozoites," the next phase in the parasite's life, travel to the mosquito's salivary glands, and they are injected into the next victim.

These sporozoites enter the human victim's bloodstream and move to the liver. The protozoan then multiplies dramatically within the liver, and it bursts into the bloodstream, usually within several days (although a dormancy period of several months to three years occasionally occurs), where it begins to do much of its damage.

Different species of mosquitoes are more or less effective at spreading the parasites. *Anopheles gambiae*, widely present in sub-Saharan Africa, is a voracious biter and an efficient transmitter. It has a strong preference for humans, and it is very difficult to control. It can breed in even a hoofprint filled with water. People living in its habitat can be infected up to 1,000 times a year.[88]

Malaria tends to depress economic activity and development wherever it is endemic. A significant percentage of the population is sick or sickly at any one time, leading to repeated absence from work and school. In such circumstances, it is hard for people to be optimistic and take economic initiatives.

The Indian Case

The *Plasmodium* parasites that cause malaria have maintained their deadly human-mosquito-human life cycle in India for at least several thousand years. The most ancient Indian literature, the Vedas (3,500 to 2,800 years ago) frequently mention epidemics that seem akin to malaria. For example, the Atharva Veda offered incantations to propitiate the fever demon who returns every second day, and the one who returns every third day. The Atharva Veda also noted that fevers were particularly widespread after heavy rains or when grass grew very thick—conditions that encourage mosquitoes and that are still associated with malaria.[89] A malady called autumnal fever was considered the "king of diseases"; this is presumed to be malaria, which flares up during autumn conditions in much of India. As early as c. 800 B.C.E. an Indian medical work explicitly blamed mosquitoes for disease; their bites, it noted, can be followed by "fever, . . . pains, vomiting, diarrhea, thirst, heat, giddiness, yawning, shivering, hiccups, burning sensation, [and] intense cold."[90]

The disease (under various names) remained endemic in much of the Indian subcontinent throughout its long history. It struck down the mighty as well as the poor, including figures such as Muhammed bin Tughluk, the warlike sultan of Delhi, who died of malaria while fighting in Sind in 1351. Chronic malaria depressed the quality and length of life for untold numbers of Indians, and the infection sapped the country's economic productivity.

Malaria also took a dramatic toll among the European traders, soldiers, officials, and priests who began to set up colonies along the Indian coasts in the 16th century (as it had in Africa in the previous century). Many of the early Portuguese, French, Dutch, and English colonists lacked any immunity to one or another of the malaria parasites. As a result, epidemics were frequent and often devastating.[91]

By the early 1600s Europeans knew that the bark of the cinchona tree, a Peruvian Indian remedy, was an effective medicine for malaria, but the drug was relatively scarce and expensive. The active element was isolated by French researchers around 1820 and named quinine. Cinchona trees were exploited nearly to extinction in their original Andes habitat, but Dutch colonists managed to seed major plantations on Java. Exported to India, quinine dramatically reduced fatalities among the European population. By the mid 19th century the drug became common enough to be distributed as a preventative against malaria, often taken by British colonials in the form of gin and tonic (quinine water).

Quinine was apparently not common or inexpensive enough to distribute to the Indian masses, even for treatment during epidemics, and local remedies were not nearly as effective. Unfortunately, the number and intensity of malaria epidemics may have increased, and certainly did not decrease, as the British consolidated their rule in India.

The British Role

Epidemic malaria was becoming a worldwide problem in that era, perhaps triggered by population increases and greater mobility both within and between countries. In most of the tropical world, colonial empires created vast areas that were relatively safe for travel and trade. This may have allowed endemic parasitic infections to spread over wider areas. In addition, the spread of commerce, industry, and cash crops was often accompanied by disturbances to local land use that could facilitate the spread of dangerous mosquitoes.[92]

However, many Indians have long attributed the dramatic increase in reported malaria cases and fatalities over the 19th and early 20th centuries to specific policies and practices of the British colonial government, first in Bengal, where Britain ruled for 200 years, and then in the rest of the subcontinent in the 19th century. The huge malaria death tolls, which peaked in the first half of the 20th century, became an important issue for the Indian independence movement.

This was particularly noted in Bengal, where British Indian rule had its roots, and where malaria was particularly devastating. Much of Bengal, East and West, consists of a vast delta plain where the Ganges and Bramaputra River systems drain into the Bay of Bengal; it is also blessed (or cursed) with ample rainwater. Farmers have been cultivating this well-watered garden for millennia, aided since early historic times by large-scale hydraulic engineering projects, using the principle of "overflow irrigation." At certain seasons, government workers would make shallow cuts in the banks or levees of the major rivers, allowing silty water to overflow into a system of long parallel canals that eventually branched out into every field in the region. These canals also served to channel seasonal flooding and drain away excess monsoon rainwater.[93]

Bengal was the center of British rule from the 18th century until 1911 when the capital was moved to Delhi. It was also the center of Indian cultural and political life. From the middle of the 19th century many elite Indians in the province became convinced that British sins of omission and commission had undermined this huge hydraulic system, effectively blocking off drainage in many districts. Mosquito larvae thrive in standing or stagnant water, not in fast-moving rivers or seasonal floodwaters. The stagnant pools that were now becoming a feature of the landscape were ideal breeding grounds for mosquitoes. They also served as collect ponds for animal and human sewage and organic garbage, which had been previously flushed away by the overflow. The entire system began to silt up.[94]

According to Indian accounts, the traders of the British East India Company, who ruled Bengal for a century, considered flood prevention to be the main priority. They misunderstood the elaborate hydraulic system, which had been in disrepair in the troubled era when they first arrived and extended their control. The British also wanted permanent roads to reinforce their control, especially after the Indian Rebellion of 1857. In the topography of Bengal this meant raised and banked roadways. From midcentury a vast network of railroads were built in Bengal and much of the rest of the country. Culvert pipes were laid under the tracks, but they were inadequate to drain away the pools that formed all along the tracks, especially in the borrowpits dug to build up the embankments. Furthermore, jute production soared; its manufacture required a period of rotting in still water. In addition, dams built for fish farming and local crop irrigation added to the problem of still water. Finally, the large migrant labor forces that built the railroads, or were brought in to work cash crops, spread infection into previously clear areas.

Some British officials claimed that districts far from the railroads and other modern developments showed similar increased malaria rates, but other government studies found that new irrigation projects in the Delhi region seemed to encourage malaria. In 1870 the British sanitary commissioner of Hooghly (Calcutta region) conducted an inquiry into the recent epidemic fever. He found that the major rivers had "deteriorated into miles of damp naked ground" and polluted pools. Staggering case loads were reported elsewhere in the country as well. The Punjab epidemic of 1892 killed 283,000.[95]

By the early 20th century, one expert estimated that malaria contributed to about half of all deaths in India, either directly or in conjunction with undernourishment and other debilitating diseases.[96] Regional epidemics killed hundreds of thousands, but even more died of endemic malaria, which existed in most of the country, acting in concert with other diseases and inadequate nutrition. In 1921 730,000 died of malaria in Bengal. Similar numbers died there in each of the two war years of 1943 and 1944, when food was scarce and malnutrition increased.

Counterattack

To give credit to the government of British India (staffed by Indian as well as British civil servants), there were many efforts to understand and combat the problem. India became an important test bed for both scientific research in malaria and public health techniques to control its spread. In 1845 Surgeon-Major C. C. Dempster of the Indian Medical Service (IMS) developed methods of accurately diagnosing malaria. In 1897 British physician and microbiologist Ronald Ross, who began working for the IMS in 1881, was the first to prove that mosquitoes were the vectors, or transmission agents, of malaria, as many scientists and lay people already suspected. He worked out the entire disease cycle of the parasites within both mosquitoes and the people they infected. In 1902 he was awarded the second Nobel Prize in medicine for this work. Ross helped found antimalaria organizations in India, which still honor his memory.

In 1901, two British doctors backed by hundreds of soldiers launched an ambitious pilot project to eliminate the disease at Miran Mir, a heavily irrigated and highly infected rural district near Lahore (in present-day Pakistan) and the site of a British military base. They filled in ditches and puddles to keep mosquitoes from breeding; evacuated infected people from the worst areas to prevent transmission to healthy people; and distributed quinine for treatment and as a preventative.

The program was overwhelmed by a massive epidemic throughout the Punjab in 1908 and 1909, but it proved a good model for later, more successful efforts. That year, the government established the Central Malaria Bureau in Kasauli, which eventually developed into the National Institute of Communicable Diseases in Delhi. Today the institute has programs in training and research, and helps provincial authorities track and combat disease outbreaks.[97] In 1927 the bureau was expanded and renamed the Malaria Survey of India. In 1935 the agency published a groundbreaking report, "What Malaria Costs India: Nationally, Socially, and Economically."[98]

In the face of massive outbreaks during World War I, the military and the railroads set up special malaria boards that sprayed kerosene and other larvicides (pesticides that kill insects in their larval or immature stage) near bases and railroad stations across the country. Similar programs continued after the war. In the 1920s the Rockefeller Foundation sponsored programs at tea plantations. Aerial spraying began in 1937, with the safe and relatively long-lasting insecticide Paris Green. The natural pesticide pyrethrum came into use in 1938. During World War II, when Indonesia's cinchona plantations were under Japanese occupation, nonimmune soldiers in the armies of the United States and Britain were exposed to devastating attacks of fever while slogging through the jungles of Southeast Asia and the Pacific. Desperate to combat the insects, the armed forces began using the synthetic pesticide DDT, whose effectiveness against mosquitoes had first been demonstrated in 1938. Industrial technology, which probably worsened the malaria problem, was belatedly offering a solution.

The DDT Controversy

DDT is generally nontoxic to people and animals when used in reasonable amounts for home spraying. As a cheap, very effective pesticide and insect repellent, it was the key weapon that finally eliminated malaria (and other mosquito-born diseases) in Europe and North America, saved millions of lives in India and other countries, and freed up substantial areas of the world for development.

In 1962, Rachel Carson wrote her best seller *Silent Spring*, which argued that wide use of DDT as an agricultural pesticide (to kill bugs that eat crops) had caused harm to several wildlife species, especially birds. She stressed that DDT persisted in the environment after spraying. If animals took it in with their food, it might be concentrated on its way up the "food chain," and eventually cause cancer in humans.[99]

Experience has not borne out her cancer fears, but the claims of wildlife damage have been verified. Public opinion came to see DDT as a highly dangerous poison, and over the next several years it was sharply restricted or banned in many countries—not only in agriculture but also in residential pest control. The Stockholm Convention of 2001 called for a worldwide ban against the chemical, except in controlled use in emergencies such as malaria.[100] Several respected environmental groups tried to impose a complete ban at that time.

The anti-DDT campaign had little impact on wealthy countries, which could afford more expensive measures to keep mosquito-borne diseases at bay. The impact on poor countries, especially where malaria still prevails, was greater. South Africa, Sri Lanka, and other countries saw a major resurgence of deadly malaria as soon as DDT spraying was stopped. Many critics have charged that environmental groups have been insensitive to the needs of these poor countries; they say that anti-DDT measures have imposed additional costs and bureaucratic requirements on very weak countries with few alternatives.

At a minimum, it is clear that the so far irreplaceable role of DDT against malaria was not fully appreciated by most environmentalists for many years.[101] In their defense, environmentalists have noted that residential DDT use was never banned in India and a few other countries where it had done the most good. Besides, many mosquito species have developed resistance to DDT, so that other pesticides or other approaches must be encouraged.

In September 2006 the World Health Organization formally called for increased use of DDT as an essential tool to revive the stalled effort against malaria in Africa. Dr. Arata Kochi, head of the WHO malaria program, called DDT the most effective insecticide against malaria, and he said that it posed no health risk when properly used.[102]

The Tide Turns

DDT was transferred to the civilian sector in India after World War II with revolutionary effect. In Bombay, where the marshy local terrain had fostered repeated epidemics, a single spraying in test homes rid them not only of mosquitoes but also of bedbugs, ticks, cockroaches, and lizards.

Local antimalaria pilot programs resumed in 1946 and were expanded under WHO auspices between 1948 and 1952. Mahatma Gandhi gave the program his blessing, despite the concerns of some Hindus about killing insects.[103] In the early test districts the reported incidence of malaria plummeted along with death rates, and the population of severely affected districts began to expand after years of stagnation.

In the early 1950s, an estimated 75 million Indians (in a population of 360 million) were still suffering from malaria attacks each year; 800,000 of them died. Encouraged by success in the test areas, the Indian national government launched a National Malaria Control Programme (NMCP) in 1953, in cooperation with the state governments. Units of between 130 and 275 people were created, and health care delivery teams fanned out to the most affected districts. They used all the now tried-and-true methods of draining, larvicide spraying, case-tracking, and medicine. However, the main focus now was a systematic campaign of "indoor residual spraying (IRS)" of the walls of every home in affected regions with DDT. If the mosquitoes could be stopped when they took their meals, the chain of infection could be broken.

Within five years some 165 teams were in place, and the results were astounding—the total malaria caseload for the entire country fell to below 50,000 by 1961; in 1965, not a single malaria death was reported in India.

In collaboration with the WHO, UNICEF, and the U.S. Agency for International Development, India pledged to eliminate malaria completely within seven to nine years. The government doubled the number of control teams to cover the entire country. Unfortunately, eradication proved to be too ambitious a goal in India as elsewhere. By 1965 the number of cases began to rise again; in 1971 it surpassed 1 million.

Many reasons have been given for the general failure to achieve eradication in India, a failure that was far more dramatic in Africa. It should be noted that some countries seem to have achieved nearly total eradication (Mexico, Egypt, and most of Brazil).[104] In early 2008, the WHO reported that mass distribution of insecticide-treated bed nets, and delivery of the new drug artemisinin to rural clinics, had reduced malaria deaths among children by more than 50 percent in four African countries where the disease was endemic.

After the intense first few years of the campaign in India it proved difficult to maintain morale among the control workers at the same fever pitch, especially once the Ministry of Health gave the teams responsibility for other diseases as well. Inefficient laboratories meant that cases of malaria were often diagnosed too late for treatment, allowing the cycle of mosquito bites to resume. Besides, the general population also became complacent about malaria, which was now less common than many other endemic diseases in the region. Middle-class and wealthy families, who could buy preventative drugs, began to refuse to admit sprayers. A "Modified Plan of

Operations" was implemented in 1977 that aimed at rekindling public support.[105]

The oil price shocks of the 1970s drove up the price of DDT, which is made from petroleum, and supplies of the pesticide became scarce. Resistance to DDT began to emerge in some mosquito species as early as 1959. At first driven back to isolated reservoirs, the mosquito population managed to regenerate, especially those carrying *P. falciparum*, the most deadly species of malaria parasite.[106]

Subsequent programs have followed one another with greater or lesser success. In 1971 a program was begun to cover cisterns and other water gathering spots in urban areas.[107] Malaria has not come back on a national level in India to match its tragic resurgence in Africa, where more than 1 million die every year. However, full eradication proved an elusive, frustrating goal despite the country's corps of talented doctors, researchers, and drug manufacturers, and despite its growing economy and improved literacy levels.

The government has reported about 1,000 deaths annually in recent years, but this does not include data from private and nonprofit facilities, or deaths in which chronic malaria may have been a contributing factor.[108] One alarmist report put out by antimalaria nonprofit groups states: "There could be more than 18 million malaria cases and about 130,000 malarial deaths each year" in India.[109] Another, more common estimate puts the numbers at 20,000 deaths.[110]

Future Prospects

As of 2005, India's National Malaria Control Programme maintains that the disease has been effectively contained in areas of the country covering 80 percent of the population. The program relies on "active detection"—about 100 million blood smears are taken each year in home fever cases; a diagnosis of malaria triggers drug treatment and case tracking. Selected areas are targeted for mosquito control, using indoor spraying with pesticides, larvicide spraying in stagnant water, and insecticide-treated bed nets (ITN's). Over 4 million bed nets were ordered in 2005, while indoor spraying declined by 50 percent over the recent past. In the most heavily affected states and regions the government claims to have provided over 98 percent of districts with fever treatment depots and drug distribution depots. Village health workers are charged with primary treatment and malaria education.

The country's National Health Policy of 2002 aims to cut back mortality (deaths) by 50 percent and achieve "efficient control of malaria morbidity (disease)" by 2010.[111] The antimalaria efforts are supported by research in all facets of the disease conducted by the National Institute of Malaria Research, located in Delhi.[112]

New weapons have been found in the struggle—or rather traditional weapons that have been revived and improved. Chinese researchers developed a new drug, artemisinin, derived from a shrub used in traditional Chinese medicine. It is very effective against *P. falciparum*, although it must be used in combination with other drugs to keep the parasite from developing resistance. In February 2007, a powerful new antimalaria combination drug designed for children was introduced; it will be sold at cost in poor countries.[113] In 2004 India's Malaria Control Institute reported the results of several successful experiments using guppies and other larva-eating fish to destroy mosquitoes before they hatch, a traditional local strategy of pest control. A World Bank project called for extending this practice to 100 districts.[114]

The Indian Ministry of Health announced in 2005 that it was planning a major test of two promising new malaria vaccines beginning in 2007.[115] Early tests of one vaccine in Africa in 2007 showed it to be effective in infants and small children.[116] No one should underestimate the enemy—either the *Plasmodium* parasite or the mosquito vector; but there are at least grounds for hope that the last battles in the war may be at hand.

AVIAN AND OTHER FLUS: THE NEXT PANDEMIC?

Introduction

Influenza or the flu is a common infectious disease of humans, other mammals, and birds. It is caused by a particular family of viruses known as Orthomyxoviruses. It usually brings a variety of unpleasant symptoms including fever, muscular aches and pains, headaches, sore throat, coughing, and a general feeling of exhaustion. It can often also lead to pneumonia (caused by the flu virus itself or by bacteria). It is especially dangerous for people whose immune system is not working well. Young children, older people, and those suffering from chronic diseases are all considered to be "high risk"; for them, the flu can even lead to death.

Most strains of flu are extremely contagious. The disease usually passes between people through coughs and sneezes, which shoot tiny aerosol particles containing live virus into the air. Anyone with the flu (or even a cold) should have tissues handy to cover their mouths when they cough or sneeze, out of consideration for others. A person may be contagious even before symptoms appear, and will continue to be contagious for five to 10 days thereafter. The virus can also be passed in saliva or other body fluids, and it can survive for as long as a week on many surfaces at room temperature, including bedsheets, doorknobs, utensils, and other common objects. Fortunately, it can be killed by ordinary detergents or disinfectants.

Vaccines have been developed against the flu, and doctors recommend that anyone in a high-risk category be vaccinated every year (via injection). These vaccines do not always prevent the flu, in part because it is hard to tell which strains of the flu virus will spread in a given year. However, those who are vaccinated will generally suffer milder symptoms even if they do get sick. Every year, scientists at the World Health Organization and the various national health agencies (such as the U.S. Food and Drug Administration) make judgment calls about which strains will spread the following year, and they use such predictions to create that year's vaccine. In recent years, a nasal spray vaccine has also been developed, made of weakened but live virus. It is recommended for people *not* in the risk groups, although one major study showed it effective for young children as well.[117] Some antiviral medicines (such as Tamiflu) appear to be effective in preventing flu or reducing symptoms, although they have side effects and should not be used unless prescribed by a doctor.

Commercial poultry such as chickens and turkeys are often vaccinated as well, since influenza is often fatal in birds. The strain of avian (bird) flu that showed up in 1996 in East Asia, and that has caused much international concern, seems to kill almost all domestic birds it infects.

A SURPRISE EVERY YEAR

People exposed to a flu virus, whether or not they become ill, usually acquire immunity—the same strain of virus will no longer make them sick. Unfortunately, flu viruses frequently mutate or change, and new strains and varieties emerge every year. In most years, the changes are relatively minor and are considered to be genetic *drift*; in such cases, people usually retain at least some of their immunity.

In some years a major change or *shift* occurs. This may happen when a flu strain jumps between species. Unlike most forms of life, the genetic material of flu viruses does not exist as one long strand of DNA. Instead, it consists of eight separate pieces of RNA. As a result, when two different flu viruses, such as a human and a bird flu virus, are both present in a cell, for example, that of a pig, their genes can recombine fairly easily to create a completely new virus. Scientists speculate that this may be the underlying mechanism for most major genetic shifts in flu viruses.

Whatever the cause, a virus that has undergone a genetic shift is usually quite virulent, since no one is immune. In the 20th century, each major shift caused a pandemic, in 1918, 1957, 1968, and 1977.[118] In each case, more people became sick than usual, and there were more deaths.

Every year, during the cold weather months (October to May in the Northern Hemisphere, May to September in the Southern Hemisphere), flu strains spread in epidemic form around the world, making millions of people sick. The virus seems to survive longer in the cool, dry air of winter. Under normal circumstances, only about one in a thousand flu patients die, but since so many are ill, this can amount to a worldwide toll of hundreds of thousands of people. In an average year in the United States, 5 to 20 percent of the population gets the flu, over 200,000 people are hospitalized, and about 36,000 die.[119]

For healthy people, the flu is usually nothing worse than an inconvenience that interferes with work, school, or family life. However, some strains of influenza can be deadly. The strain that caused the worldwide pandemic of 1918, for example, killed 5 to 10 percent of its victims, including millions of healthy young men and women. It may have left behind many cases of disability as well.[120] The avian flu that began to infect small numbers of people in East and Southeast Asia in 2003 appears to have killed more than half of all those who have taken ill so far—although other people may have had milder cases that escaped the attention of the medical community. Fortunately, the number of patients has remained quite small, as the virus so far has not learned how to spread effectively from one human host to another.

This odd history makes influenza the greatest puzzle and the most unpredictable threat in the entire field of infectious disease. What made the 1918 strain so deadly? Why has nothing comparable emerged since then? Will the recent deadly avian flu make a complete transition to human hosts? If so, will it remain as deadly or will it mutate into a more typical human influenza virus? Virologists, epidemiologists, and public health specialists disagree about all these questions. They all agree, however, that the world community must remain vigilant and must pursue the research that could help us meet the worst eventualities.

A Long History

BEFORE 1918

It is not easy for a doctor to diagnose the flu without a lab test. The typical symptoms can be caused by many other viral or bacterial diseases, which themselves are called by different names in different cultures. A mild case can look like a common cold; a severe case can look like tuberculosis or typhoid. A recent study found that most doctors fail to diagnose flu in children, even in severe cases that eventually lead to hospitalization.[121]

If that is true about a live patient before a doctor, the puzzle is even more confusing for medical historians, who cannot say for sure when influenza first appeared. Many suspect that the disease first crossed to humans with the domestication of animals some 8,000 years ago, since humanlike flu strains have been found in many farm animals such as poultry, pigs, and horses. The Greek physician Hippocrates recorded a serious epidemic in 412 B.C.E. that may have been caused by influenza. The Italian name "influenza" was not used for the illness until sometime in the late Middle Ages in Europe; it reflected the belief that infectious diseases were caused by the "influence" of planets and stars. Gradually it came to refer to a specific disease that seemed to occur in epidemics during the cold months.

In 1580 an epidemic spread to Europe from Asia Minor and North Africa that was probably influenza, judging by the symptoms and outcomes. At least three, and possibly five influenza pandemics took place in the 18th century. They were generally perceived as originating in China or Russia, spreading westward across Europe and then reaching the Americas, typically over a three-year period. The flu pandemic of 1781–82 was probably the most written about up to that time. It struck India, China, Europe, Africa, and the Americas—sickening tens of millions of people throughout the known world.[122] Even in the era before steamships and railroads, the flu could cover many miles in a single day. Few people died, and most of those were old or sickly individuals—or pregnant women. Another, similar pandemic was recorded in 1829–32. An epidemic that killed off many chickens in Italy in 1878 is now believed to have been a strain of avian influenza.

The influenza pandemic of 1889–90, known in Europe as "Russian flu," was the most widespread and the most deadly to be recorded up to that time, killing about 1 million people around the world.[123] It began in Central Asia and quickly spread throughout the world. The flu strains that appeared in the years between 1890 and 1918 were similar in causing higher death tolls than had earlier been the case.

THE GREAT INFLUENZA

But nothing prepared the human race for the influenza pandemic of 1918–20, generally called "the Spanish flu." The name took hold because the newspapers of Spain, a neutral country during World War I, were not under censorship and could freely report the ravages of the disease, whereas governments in the countries at war tried to limit bad news in order to keep morale high.

In fact, we will probably never know where and when the strain first arose, but the epidemic first surfaced at an army base in Kansas in the United States in March 1918. It spread quickly across the country and to Europe along with the rapidly deploying American troops. The "first wave" spread to several countries by June, but without causing many more deaths than usual for the flu. In late August, a far more deadly "second wave" appeared in Boston, in the French port of Brest, and in Freetown, Sierra Leone. It was this mutated virus that rapidly swept the world. The worldwide mobilization and movement of troops between the various outposts of European empires, and the concentration of thousands of troops in crowded ships and in narrow trenches, gave the pandemic much of its impetus.

The Spanish flu pandemic was one of the most widespread and most deadly in history—for any disease. None before had reached so far so quickly. The entire world had become closely knit by rapid, efficient transportation networks, and within months there were victims on every continent and in almost every country. Only a few island nations escaped unscathed—such as Iceland, American Samoa, and New Guinea and its nearby island groups, where effective quarantines had been strictly imposed. The disease was so contagious that even very slight human contact was enough to bring it to isolated Eskimo villages in Alaska and remote tribes in Africa.

Mortality varied widely. India lost 18.5 million people; 675,000 died in the United States. In northern Nigeria, 1.9 percent of the European population died together with 3.2 percent of Africans; in South Africa, the toll may have reached 4.4 percent. In one village in Alaska, 72 of 80 people died.[124] Deaths worldwide reached into the tens of millions. Epidemiologists still do not agree on the total number of deaths, and their estimates range from 20 to 100 million; the latter figures would be about one person in 20 alive in 1918.

Influenza had never before—or since—been remotely as devastating. About one of every three people in the world caught the flu. The virus was remarkably virulent, often killing victims within a day or two of the first symptom. Autopsies (dissection and analysis of corpses) sometimes revealed massive damage to organs all over the body and/or severe internal bleeding—all inflicted in a matter of hours. Remarkably, Spanish flu seemed to be most damaging to young adults—previously healthy men and women in their 20s and 30s. Perhaps, many scientists speculate, their healthy immune systems overreacted to the virus, producing too many inflammatory proteins known as cytokines (in a process known as a "cytokine storm"), damaging tissues and clogging the lungs. The disease respected no boundaries of race or even class. Most people fled to the relative safety of their homes, hoarding food, caring for their ill, and waiting out the storm.

The medical community was almost helpless. Since 1892, most doctors had mistakenly believed that influenza was caused by a bacteria, *Haemophilus influenzae,* which the noted German bacteriologist Richard Pfeiffer had isolated from the lungs of flu victims. That bacterium and others like it were probably responsible for many of the deaths; however, such microbes generally flourish only in bodies already ravaged by the flu virus, which was thus the real culprit. Quarantine was the only effective preventive measure. Schools, theaters, and businesses of all kinds were shut down in cities all over the world, and strict sanitary measures were imposed.

The pandemic played itself out by early 1919 in most locations, although it did not completely die out until early the following year. Within a few years, when subsequent flu seasons proved extremely mild, the event seemed to drop out of the public consciousness. If anything, it was associated with the other horrors of World War I rather than with the annual flu season.

DEMYSTIFYING THE VIRUS

Despite the public's amnesia, the terrifying pandemic stimulated rapid advances in virology. The human influenza virus was first isolated in 1933. The first flu vaccine became available in 1945, developed by epidemiologist Thomas Francis, Jr. at the University of Michigan at the request of the U.S. Army. It was composed of killed virus particles representing the three strains of influenza most common at the time.

Scientists learned that there are three major types of flu virus. Influenza A causes all the regular yearly epidemics and the major pandemics. The common animal flu viruses also belong to type A. Influenza B can cause isolated epidemics at sites such as nursing homes, but influenza C rarely causes illness. The flu vaccines offered to the public each year usually combine material from two types of A virus and one type of B.

Within type A, the viruses are further subclassified based on two proteins found in the outer membrane or covering of the virus particle. These are hemagglutinin (H) and neuraminidase (N). There are three common forms of hemagglutinin in human viruses, labeled H1, H2, and H3; more than a dozen types are found in viruses infecting other animals. There are two basic neuraminidases—N1 and N2. These are the facts behind the familiar virus names mentioned in news stories: H5N1 for the current avian flu variety, H1N1 for the 1918 pandemic, and so on.

The H and N proteins are both antigens, that is, they stimulate the human immune system. H tends to accumulate small mutations, causing "antigenic *drift*." "Antigenic *shift*" occurs when a completely new form of H appears and spreads. It is believed that the 10 flu pandemics of the past 250 years were all caused by such antigenic shifts.[125]

In 2004 and 2005 scientists were able to use new techniques to analyze the 1918 flu virus, using tissue samples from victims that had been preserved in U.S. Army labs and in a frozen burial plot in Alaska. They concluded that the 1918 strain was an avian subtype H1N1 that had mutated to a form that could easily infect humans. It bore some similarities to the deadly avian flu strain that has appeared in recent years, but it is definitely a different strain.[126]

TWENTIETH-CENTURY PANDEMICS: MARKING TIME?

Despite the accumulating knowledge, researchers have so far failed to discover any clear patterns that could explain the 1918 exception. Nor are they confident that they can predict future pandemics of a similar nature.

For many years experts expected genetic shifts and pandemics to happen on a regular basis, for example, every 20 or 30 years. However, the only known shifts in the 20th century came in 1918 ("Spanish flu"), 1957 ("Asian flu"), 1968 ("Hong Kong" flu), and 1976–77 ("Russian flu"); none has occurred in the subsequent 30 years. These dates do not yield any obvious pattern. In any case, none of the other shifts was nearly as deadly as that of 1918.

Of course, by 1957 antibiotics were widely used to treat the bacterial pneumonia often associated with the flu, and only about 2 million people died.[127] Perhaps, some researchers say, the death toll would have been much higher that year without these new "miracle drugs."[128] Others guess that many of those who died in 1918–20 were really felled by tuberculosis (TB); the TB bacteria was very common at that time, but is much less common today, at least in the developed world.[129] According to this theory, even the 1918 virus would not take such a large toll if it came back today, thanks to antibiotics and more accurate ways to diagnose pathogens.

The 1976 swine flu that turned up in the United States did not even cause an epidemic even though the virus showed a genetic shift. The federal government's program of mass vaccination turned out to be unnecessary. That experience undermined further attempts to predict the next lethal pandemic.[130]

Avian Flu—The Next Pandemic?

Since the 1950s researchers have isolated H5 type influenza virus among scattered bird populations around the world, but none of them spread beyond the initial discovery site, and none of them jumped to any human victim.[131] In 1996 a virulent H5N1 strain turned up in a goose on a farm in Guangdong Province, China. This time, the virus spread; its progress was apparently rather slow over the next few years, until it broke out in other parts of China and neighboring countries in 2003 and 2004. In 2005 it spread as far as the Middle East, Europe, and Africa, largely due to migration of infected wild birds.

Almost from the start, some people were infected as well as birds. Almost all the human victims took ill as a result of very close contact with infected birds, but a handful of individuals may have gotten the disease from close family members. Unfortunately, the H5N1 virus proved as deadly among humans as among birds. By late 2007, slightly over 200 people had died of the disease, out of 333 confirmed cases. Most of the victims lived in Southeast Asia, the original disease focus, but there were troubling localized human outbreaks in Egypt as well in 2006 and 2007.

FIRST HUMAN CASES

The world first took note during an outbreak in 1997 in Hong Kong (which adjoins Guangdong), where several thousand chickens died in March from H5N1 strains. In the course of the year 17 people took ill with similar strains of the virus, all of them after contact with live chickens. Six of them died, including a majority of the stricken adults. In reaction, authorities killed all 1.6 million chickens found in the city and banned any further shipments from surrounding areas. No more cases were reported.[132] In June 2008 Hong Kong once again ordered a kill of all chickens, after the flu was found in four different markets; no human cases were reported.

The virus spread quietly over the next six years. The deadly SARS epidemic that occurred in 2002–04 exposed a weakness in disease surveillance and reporting in China. These limitations make it very difficult to study H5N1's animal or human spread between 1997 and 2003. But in February 2003 three Hong Kong residents took ill after visiting nearby Fujian Province; the two who returned were diagnosed with H5N1, and one died. In November that year a Chinese resident from Beijing died of the virus as well; he was reported to be the 20th case uncovered in China. Early in 2004 China reported killing 9 million poultry infected with H5N1 in 16 provinces.

The Chinese government began a vaccination program that eventually reached billions of chickens, ducks, and other poultry.[133] Vaccination of birds is controversial. Some experts believe the complex process (requiring as many as three injections per bird) could make the virus tougher by encouraging resistance; this could be disastrous if the virus became truly contagious among humans.[134] In addition, vaccination might simply conceal the virus by reducing symptoms among infected birds.[135]

In December 2003 the disease was reported among domestic poultry in South Korea, not far from Beijing. All the infected chickens died or were killed, but new outbreaks continued in that country throughout 2004. That year proved a breakout period for the epidemic, as cases began to be reported all across East and Southeast Asia:

- Two lions and two tigers in a Thailand zoo died after eating freshly killed chickens in December 2003; H5N1 was isolated from their bodies. By early 2004 outbreaks were reported in Thailand among poultry in 32 provinces, and human infections were reported as well; through 2006 17 Thais died, out of 25 people infected.
- Early in January 2004 Vietnam reported the first cases of poultry and humans infected with H5N1. Despite massive kills and quarantines, small outbreaks continued over the next two years. Since the end of 2005, by which time 93 cases and 42 deaths had been reported, no more human cases have emerged.
- Minor outbreaks were reported around the same time in Malaysia, Laos, and Cambodia; all six reported human cases in the latter country were fatal.
- Japan reported several outbreaks in commercial poultry between January and March 2004.[136]
- In February 2004 Indonesia, which would become a major focus of the disease, reported poultry outbreaks in 11 provinces.

In a frightening report in August that year, the journal *Science* reported research that confirmed the rumors that domestic cats could acquire fatal infection of H5N1 and transmit it to other cats. This was the first proven case in which domestic cats took ill from any influenza A virus.[137]

GLOBAL SPREAD

The spread of H5N1 across East and Southeast Asia could be attributed to the widespread international trade in poultry. However, a frightening new vector (means of transmission) appeared in 2005—migrating flocks of wild birds. Presumably, the wild birds picked up the virus from domestic birds while visiting farms to take advantage of ready supplies of feed and water. China reported in April and May of 2005 that several thousand birds from a variety of species had died of the virus at Qinghai Lake in central China, a crossroads for several bird migration routes.[138] In June there were poultry outbreaks in Xinjiang Province at the western edge of China. Similar outbreaks in poultry or wild birds were soon reported in Russian Siberia, Kazakhstan, and Mongolia.

In October 2005 the geographic theater widened, as "highly pathogenic" H5N1 was discovered in poultry in Turkey and Romania and in wild birds in

Croatia. Other isolated cases cropped up in the next few months in other Middle Eastern and European countries, with a small number of human infections and deaths as well. Africa entered the picture in February 2006 with cases in Nigeria, Niger, and Egypt; outbreaks were reported later in the year in Burkina Faso, Sudan, Djibouti, and Cameroon. India reported its first cases in February 2006 as well.

The rapid spread of virulent H5N1 in wild bird populations to dozens of countries throughout Eurasia and Africa puzzled scientists. As a rule, flu strains in wild birds tend to be mild; fatal illness kills birds before they can move very far, long before they can complete intercontinental migration. In the current case, the flu may have spread in short hops; dying birds may have infected watering holes shared by varying species and flocks. Several of the outbreaks, however, occurred along road or railroad routes, a possible indication that the disease spread through the poultry trade.[139] In any case, no virus was detected in any of the migrating flocks that returned to Europe from Africa later in 2006; this may indicate that wild birds are not, after all, an efficient vector. The only findings reported in the Western Hemisphere were a mild strain of H5N1 in wild swans and ducks in Michigan, Pennsylvania, and Maryland in August and September 2006. This was apparently unrelated to the Old World epidemic.

GOVERNMENT REACTIONS

Most countries reacted to the findings with massive kills of wild birds and poultry in the areas where the virus was detected. In Germany, after several dozen wild birds were found to be infected in February 2006 on Rügen Island in the Baltic Sea, thousands of domestic poultry were culled, and a special army unit began disinfecting people and vehicles leaving the island for the mainland.[140] European Union countries are required to establish surveillance and buffer zones around any cases of H5N1; several of them responded to the threat by ordering that poultry flocks be moved indoors to prevent mingling with wild, possibly infected birds.

In the United States, the federal government issued a *National Strategy for Pandemic Influenza Implementation Plan* on November 1, 2005, as President George W. Bush asked Congress for $7.1 billion to fund the program. It included beefed up national and international surveillance, disaster recovery plans, money to develop and stockpile vaccines and antiviral medicines, and funds to expand research into new, rapid methods of vaccine development. The plan devolved much real-time crisis responsibility to state and local authorities. Congress followed up a few months later with a supplemental appropriation of $2.3 billion for influenza preparedness. Most state governments, as well as many businesses, institutions, and business and professional organizations in the United States have issued their own plans and guidelines to reduce the medical, social, and economic impact of any possible influenza epidemic.

Of course, not all countries have the resources or bureaucracy in place to enforce such measures. According to Dr. Joseph Domenech, chief veterinary officer at the United Nations Food and Agriculture Organization, "The close proximity between people and animals and insufficient surveillance and disease control capability in eastern African countries create an ideal breeding ground for the virus."[141]

Indonesia, which has had repeated local outbreaks and has reported over 100 human deaths by 2008, presents some particular problems. An archipelago of thousands of islands with a population of 220 million, the country has moved in recent years toward decentralization and greater democracy. The downside is that it is difficult for the central authorities to enforce health policies on the patchwork of local and regional agencies that govern the country. The Health Ministry director responsible for infectious disease control told a reporter in May 2006, "The local government has the money, thus the power to decide what to prioritize. If some district sees bird flu as not important, then we have a problem."[142] In addition, chickens are often kept as pets and for home consumption in backyards, making control all but impossible without mass participation. Some farmers have reportedly tried to conceal infected birds, charging that the government had failed to compensate farmers whose flocks had been killed.

In June 2006 the World Animal Health Organization charged that the Indonesian government was no longer reporting most animal outbreaks. Despite newspaper reports of thousands of poultry deaths in 29 of the country's 33 provinces, the government had only reported 800 chicken deaths in the previous year.[143] The government announced in September 2006 that it would vaccinate 300 million poultry against the disease.

STRENGTHENING THE MEDICAL ARSENAL

Influenza vaccines have been available since 1945, but in most years only a limited number of doses have been produced—enough to take care of the at-risk population in the developed countries. If a deadly pandemic flu were to emerge, authorities might well want to vaccinate the entire population, yet the facilities now available could not ramp up vaccine production fast enough. Ideally, authorities need to know about new strains as quickly as possible, yet the technology for rapid diagnosis of infected people is not available in many countries, and faster tests are needed. Finally, the arsenal of antiviral drugs that might be able to mitigate the symptoms of influenza is still quite limited.

During the "swine flu" scare of 1976, public health officials in the United States urged that every individual be vaccinated, and nearly one-quarter of the population received swine flu shots. However, the vaccine itself apparently caused several hundred cases of severe neurological disease and 25 deaths, more than were caused by the flu itself. After vaccine companies were hit with major lawsuits, Congress eventually provided for government compensation for most vaccine-related problems, but the combination of legal liability and generally low prices for vaccines led many companies to abandon production.[144]

By 2004 only two companies were still supplying flu vaccine to the United States; when the British government suspended the license of one of them for contamination issues, the U.S. supply was cut in half for that year.[145] In 2005 a vaccine industry spokesperson said that if an H5N1 pandemic should arise today, all the world's producers together would be able to produce only 225 million doses of vaccine in six months.[146]

In May 2006, the U.S. government awarded $1 billion in contracts to five U.S. and European pharmaceutical companies to develop vaccine production methods using cell cultures rather than fertilized eggs as is currently done. The companies pledged to build facilities in the United States that by 2011 would be capable of turning out 300 million doses within six months of an order.[147] The European Medicines Agency, in 2005 streamlined procedures and fees for vaccine approval as a preparedness measure against a possible flu pandemic. Mock-up vaccines are approved in advance; in the event of a pandemic, elements of the precise strain causing the illness can be added to the preapproved vaccine. In May 2008 the European Commission approved the distribution of a new human vaccine against the H5N1 strain.[148]

Recent advances in diagnostic technology may also help head off a pandemic, if they can be quickly deployed. For example, the U.S. National Institutes of Health and Centers for Disease Control and Prevention announced in August 2006 that a new microchip had been developed that can take a sample from a patient and diagnose any of 72 different influenza virus strains, including H5N1, within 12 hours—instead of a week or more as currently required. The tissue sample would not need to be refrigerated, and the equipment needed to read the results is available in most countries, at least in capital cities.[149]

Antiviral drugs can make a vital difference in treating avian flu. A study at Oxford University found that H5N1 reproduces very quickly in human patients, stimulating a cytokine storm of immune proteins that can quickly fill a victim's lungs with fluid—as happened during the 1918 pandemic.[150] Antivirals can reduce the "viral load," the number of virus particles, to a level that the body can handle, if taken within two days of the first symptoms. Several antiviral drugs are available, such as oseltamivir (Tamiflu), zanamir (Relenza), and amantadine, but stockpiles are not adequate to handle a serious pandemic, especially in poorer countries. Developed countries are now slowly building up stockpiles; the United States plans to keep enough antiviral doses for 25 percent of the population; other countries have targets of 20 to 50 percent.[151]

Treatment with antiviral drugs can also keep healthy people from being infected with the flu. However, the drugs must be taken for several days or weeks at substantial cost, and thus are not expected to replace vaccines as a preventive measure.

Conclusion: Are We Safe?

No book that deals with epidemics can avoid the big question: Can a deadly flu pandemic happen again? One answer that might satisfy the majority of experts is: "yes, but."

Yes: given the propensity of the flu virus to mutate, and given the constant growth in international travel, trade, and migration, sooner or later a deadly and contagious influenza virus may well emerge one year and begin to spread from one person to the next and from one region to another. But: the world community is becoming better equipped from year to year to meet such a threat. Better surveillance, international communication, diagnosis, genetic analysis, vaccine production, antiviral development, and antibiotics will probably prevent anything like the terrible toll of 1918. The longer such a threat can be postponed, the better prepared we are likely to be.

With regard to the threat of avian flu, in the 10 years since the pathogenic H5N1 virus emerged to infect its first human victims it has failed to develop permanent mutations that would allow it to spread more easily to people. However, this is not entirely a matter of good luck. Several mutations have emerged that are quite worrisome to scientists, but as far as we know, every single person infected with the mutated virus has been isolated and either recovered or died without passing the mutation on.

We must be grateful for the swift response of World Health Organization (WHO) teams who encouraged governments to impose quarantines and arrange for the treatment of everyone involved with antivirals. This quick response has denied the mutated viruses the opportunity to mix with human flu viruses to create a super-pathogenic strain, which probably happened sometime before 1918.[152] The world community must continue to be vigilant, however, and proactively help those countries that lack the resources to deal with the issue on their own.

There are pessimistic observers who believe that avian flu is indeed likely to cross over and cause pandemics. One study published in *PLoS Medicine* early in 2006 used epidemiological models to predict that multiple crossovers of different strains are likely, and can probably not be contained by current methods.[153] The WHO itself warned in 2005, "Since late 2003, the world has moved closer to a pandemic than at any time since 1968, when the last of the previous century's three pandemics occurred."[154] The organization's chief avian flu coordinator, Dr. David Nabarro, reported early in 2006 that he was "quite scared" due to the flu's rapid spread to Europe, Africa, and India and its severity among birds.[155] However, confirmed human cases declined from 115 in 2006 to 86 in 2007.[156]

On the other hand, there is some evidence that many rural Chinese people carry antibodies to H5N1, indicating that they had been infected recently without becoming seriously ill. In addition, most Americans carry some immunity to the N1 neuraminidase antigen; such immunity may be enough to provide some protection if Americans are infected with H5N1.[157]

Perhaps a good summary of mainstream opinion was made in February 2006. At that time, Anthony Fauci, director of the U.S. National Institute of Allergy and Infectious Disease, stated: "If a catastrophic pandemic occurred tomorrow, everyone in the world would be unprepared," yet "we're so much better off now than we were six months ago, a year ago." With sufficient vigilance, research, and public attention our ability to meet the threat of pandemic flu will probably continue to improve.

---

[1] Edmund Settle. "AIDS in China: An Annotated Chronology 1985–2003." Available online. URL:http://www.casy.org/chron/AIDSchron_111603.pdf. Accessed November 14, 2003.

[2] The Global Fund. "Fighting Tuberculosis in China." Available online. URL: http://www.theglobalfund.org/en/in_action/china/tbl/. Accessed March 16, 2006. Leslie Giorkatos. "Center Fights Hepatitis B in Asians." *The Stanford Daily*, March 2, 2006. Available online. http://daily.stanford.edu/article/2006/3/2/centerFightsHepatitisBInAsian. Accessed March 4, 2006. China Economic Net. "China to control spread of schistosomiasis in next decade." Available online. URL: http://en.ce.cn/National/Science/200501/10/t20050110_2800866.shtml. Accessed March 16, 2006.

[3] Karl Taro Greenfeld. *China Syndrome: The True Story of the 21st Century's First Great Epidemic*. New York: HarperCollins, 2006, pp. 36–38.

[4] Dennis Normile. "Viral DNA Match Spurs China's Civet Roundup." *Science*, January 16, 2004, vol. 303. no. 5656, p. 292.

[5] Greenfeld. *China Syndrome*, p. 39.

[6] Thomas Abraham. *Twenty-first Century Plague: The Story of SARS*. Baltimore: Johns Hopkins University Press, 2005, pp. 2, 19.

[7] Elinor Levy and Mark Fischetti. *The New Killer Diseases: How the Alarming Evolution of Mutant Germs Threatens Us All*. New York: Crown, 2003, pp. 2–3.

[8] Greenfeld. *China Syndrome*, p. 123.

[9] Greenfeld. *China Syndrome*, p. xix.

[10] Abraham. *Twenty-first Century Plague*, pp. 20–21.

[11] "SARS, a Valuable Lesson for Chinese Government to Learn." *People's Daily* (English edition), June 9, 2003. Available online. URL: http://english.peopledaily.com.cn/200306/08/eng20030608_117858.shtml. Accessed August 4,2006.

[12] Greenfeld. *China Syndrome*, p. 61.

[13] General Accounting Office. "Asian SARS Outbreak Challenged International and National Responses." Available online. URL:http://www.gao.gov/new.items/d04564.pdf. Accessed April 2004; p. 26.

[14] Abraham. *Twenty-first Century Plague*, p. 23.

[15] See their Web page. Available online. URL: www.chinacdc.net.cn/n272562/ Accessed August 20, 2006.

[16] U.S. Consulate General in Guangzhou. "China's Healthcare Construction Market." Available online. URL:http://www.buyusainfo.net/docs/x_8008917.pdf. Accessed August 18, 2006.

[17] Greenfeld. *China Syndrome*, p. 86. John Pomfret. "Signs of Improvement at Epicenter of SARS Outbreak." *Washington Post*, May 4, 2003.

[18] General Accounting Office. "Asian SARS Outbreak," p. 23.

[19] CCTV interview, June 9, 2003, cited in Abraham. *Twenty-first Century Plague*, p. 27.

[20] Abraham. *Twenty-first Century Plague*, p. 24.

[21] Elinor Levy and Mark Fischetti. *The New Killer Diseases: How the Alarming Evolution of F Mutant Germs Threatens Us All.* New York: Crown, 2003, pp. 8–9.

[22] Greenfeld. *China Syndrome*, p. 45 ff.

[23] Abraham. *Twenty-first Century Plague*, p. 22.

[24] General Accounting Office. "Asian SARS Outbreak," p. 23.

[25] Greenfeld, *China Syndrome*. pp. 342–344.

[26] Greenfeld, *China Syndrome*. pp. 324–337.

[27] General Accounting Office. "Asian SARS Outbreak," p. 31.

[28] Greenfeld, *China Syndrome*. p. 395.

[29] Howard W. French. "Citizens' Groups Take Root across China." *New York Times*, February 15, 2007.

[30] Statistics are from UNAIDS. "07 AIDS Epidemic Update." Available online. URL: http://data.unaids.org/pub/EPISlides/2007/2007_epiupdate_en.pdf. Accessed on December 10, 2007.

[31] Lawrence K. Altman and Andrew Pollack. "Failure of Vaccine Test Is Setback in AIDS Fight." *New York Times*, September 22, 2007.

[32] Peter Piot. "In Poor Nations, a New Will to Fight AIDS." *New York Times*, July 2, 2002.

[33] F. Gao, E. Bailes, D. L. Robertson, Y. Chen et al. "Origin of HIV-1 in the Chimpanzee Pan Troglodytes Troglodytes." *Nature* 397 (1999): 436–444, cited in Avert.org. "Origins." Available online. URL:http://avert.org/origins.htm. Accessed August 25, 2006.

[34] T. C. Quinn, J. M. Mann, J. W. Curran, and P. Piot. "AIDS in Africa: An Epidemiologic Paradigm." *Science* 234 (1986): 955–963, cited in Avert.org. "The History of Aids." Available online. URL: http://avert.org/his81_86.htm. Accessed August 25, 2006.

[35] Reuters. "Treating STDs and Reducing AIDS High Risk: Doctors in Study Find Higher HIV Exposure in Untreated Villagers." *Washington Post,* August 25, 1995, cited in Avert.org. "The History of AIDS." Available online. URL: http://avert.org/his93_97.htm. Accessed August 25, 2006.

[36] J. Chin. "Global estimates of AIDS cases and HIV Infections: 1990." *AIDS,* 1990, 4 Suppliment 1: S277–283.

[37] H. Pope. "AIDS Set to Engulf South Africa." *Independent,* March 8, 1995, cited in Avert.org, "History of AIDS." Available online. URL: http://avert.org/his93_97.htm. Accessed August 25, 2006.

[38] UNAIDS. "AIDS Epidemic Update." December 1998, cited in University of Pennsylvania. "Africa: HIV/AIDS Update." Available online. URL: http://www.africa.upenn.edu/Urgent_Action/apic_113098.html. Accessed July 15, 2006.

[39] See "Durban Declaration" in International Documents.

[40] UNAIDS. "Report on the Global AIDS Epidemic 2006," chap. 2, p. 15.

[41] Craig Timberg. "How AIDS in Africa Was Overstated." *Washington Post,* April 6, 2006; UNAIDS. chap. 2, p. 10.

[42] World Health Organization. "HIV Treatment Access Reaches Over 1 Million in Sub-Saharan Africa." Available online. URL: http://www.who.int/mediacentre/news/releases/2006/pr38/en/index.html. Accessed September 1, 2006.

[43] Craig Timberg. "Spread of AIDS in Africa Is Outpacing Treatment." *Washington Post,* June 20, 2007.

[44] UNAIDS. chap. 2, p. 15.

[45] Unsigned editorial. "Africa's Health Care Brain Drain." *New York Times,* August 13, 2004.

[46] Avert.org. "The Impact of HIV & AIDS on Africa." Available online. URL: http://avert.org/aidsimpact.htm. Accessed May 18, 2007.

[47] Allafrica.com. "AIDS Is Damaging Education System: Mocumpi." Available online. URL: http://allafrica.com/stories/200402090631.html. Accessed February 9, 2004.

[48] S. Rosen et al. "The Cost of HIV/AIDS to Businesses in Southern Africa." *AIDS,* 18, no. 2 (January 23, 2004): 317–324.

[49] UNAIDS. chap. 4, p. 82.

[50] Karen A. Stanecki. "The AIDS Pandemic in the 21st Century." "International Population Reports," U.S. Bureau of the Census. Washington: Government Printing Office, 2004. Available online. URL: www.census.gov/IPC/prod/wpo2/wpo2-2.pdf. Accessed July 30, 2007.

[51] WHO, *2002 World Health Report,* p. 186. Available online. URL: http://www.who.int/whr/2002/en/whr2002_annex2.pdf. Accessed April 15, 2006.

[52] See the Global Fund home page. Available online. URL: http://www.theglobalfund.org/en. Accessed October 31, 2007.

[53] John Donnelly. "And Now for the Good News." *Boston Globe*, August 20, 2006.

[54] Michael Marco and Edwin J. Bernard. "Is Uganda's HIV Prevention Success Story Unraveling?" Available online. URL: http://www.aidsmap.com/en/news/E7A3F648-945A-405D-BF00-89BA7E7FDCDF.asp. Accessed August 22, 2006.

[55] Craig Timberg. "How AIDS in Africa Was Overstated," *Washington Post*, April 6, 2006.

[56] Randy Shilts. "Fear of Epidemic in the Mud Huts." *San Francisco Chronicle*, October 5, 1987, reprinted June 4, 2006.

[57] Avert.org. "HIV and AIDS in Uganda." Available online. URL: http://avert.org/aidsuganda.htm. Accessed August 23, 2006.

[58] See TASO home page. Available online. URL: http://www.tasouganda.org. Accessed December 12, 2007.

[59] See AIDS Information Centre, Uganda. Available online. URL: http://www.aicug.org. Accessed May 18, 2007.

[60] World Bank. *Project Performance Assessment Report, Uganda Sexually Transmitted Infections Project.* Available online. URL: http://lnweb18.worldbank.org/oed/oeddoclib.nsf/24cc3bb1f94ae11c85256808006a0046/188e550a7572213f85257037004dd471/$FILE/ppar_32600.pdf. Accessed June 14, 2005.

[61] D. Gough. "Uganda Starts Door-to-Door HIV Testing." *Guardian*, April 10, 1999.

[62] Donnelly. "And Now for the Good News."

[63] Allan Guttmacher Institute. "A, B, and C in Uganda: The Roles of Abstinence, Monogamy and Condom Use in HIV Decline." Available online. URL: http://www.guttmacher.org/pubs/or_abc03.pdf. Accessed December 2003.

[64] Human Sciences Research Council of South Africa. *South African National HIV Prevalence, HIV Incidence, Behaviour and Communication Survey, 2005*. Available online. URL: http://www.hsrcpress.co.za/full_title_info.asp?id=2134. Accessed May 18, 2007.

[65] Statistics South Africa. "Mid-year Population Estimates, 2006." Available online. URL: http://www.statssa.gov.za/publications/P0302/P03022006.pdf. Accessed May 18, 2007.

[66] Avert.org. "South Africa HIV & AIDS Statistics." Available online. URL: http://www.avert.org/safricastats.htm. Accessed August 31, 2006.

[67] BBC News. "Africa AIDS Drug Trade Dispute Ends." Available online. URL: http://news.bbc.co.uk/2/hi/africa/450942.stm. Accessed September 18, 1999.

[68] BBC News. "Mbeki's Letter to World Leaders." Available online. URL: http://news.bbc.co.uk/2/hi/africa/720448.stm. Accessed April 20, 2000.

[69] Michael Wines. "AIDS Cited in the Climb of South Africa's Death Rate." *New York Times*, September 8, 2006.

[70] "Prison AIDS Death Angers TAC," IRIN news release. Available online. URL: http://allafrica.com/stories/200608170775.html. Accessed August 17, 2006.

[71] Sinha Smeeta. "Onchocerciasis." Available online. URL: http://emedicine.com/med/topic1667.htm. Accessed June 30, 2006.

[72] African Program for Onchocerciasis Control. "Some Stories." Available online. URL: http://www.apoc.bf/en/some_stories.htm. Accessed January 25, 2005.

[73] María-Gloria Basáñez et al. "River Blindness: A Success Story under Threat?" *PLoS Medicine* 3, no. 9 (September 2006).

[74] Research and Training in Tropical Diseases. "Rapid Mapping for Onchocerciasis." Available online. URL: http://www.who.int/tdr/about/products/mapping.htm. Accessed May 18, 2007.

[75] T. B. Higazi, A. Filiano, C. R. Katholi, Y. Dadzie, J. H. Remme et al. "Wolbachia Endosymbiont Levels in Severe and Mild Strains of Onchocerca Volvulus." *Molecular and Biochemical Parasitology* 141 (2005): 109–112.

[76] "Sowda Needs to Be Controlled." *Yemen Times*, June 19, 2003. Available online. URL: http://yementimes.com/article.shtml?i=643&p=health&a=1. Accessed August 16, 2007.

[77] Britannica Online. "Onchocerciasis." Available online. URL: http://www.britannica.com/ebc/article-9057110. Accessed August 16, 2007.

[78] World Bank. "Global Partnership to Eliminate Riverblindness." Available online. URL: http://www.worldbank.org/afr/gper/. Accessed September 5, 2006.

[79] See the group's Web site. Available online. URL: http://www.apoc.bf/en/. Accessed May 18, 2007. Also see World Health Organization. "African Program for Onchocerciasis Control." Available online. URL: http://www.who.int/blindness/partnerships/APOC/en. Accessed May 18, 2007.

[80] B. Thylefors. "Eliminating Onchocerciasis as a Public Health Problem." *Tropical Medicine and International Health* 9, no. 4 (April 2004): pp. a1–a3.

[81] Carter Center. "Onchocerciasis Elimination Program of the Americas." Available online. URL: http://www.cartercenter.org/health/river_blindness/oepa.html. Accessed March 22, 2007.

[82] World Bank Group. "Global Partnership to Eliminate Onchocerciasis." Available online. URL: http://www.worldbank.org/afr/gper/. Accessed March 22, 2007.

[83] World Bank Group. "The Opportunity of ComDT Add-on Interventions." Available online. URL: http://www.worldbank.org/afr/gper/addon.htm. Accessed March 22, 2007.

[84] African Programme for Onchocerciasis Control (2005). "Final Communiqué of the 11th Session of the Joint Action Forum (JAF) of APOC, Paris, France, December 6–9, 2005. Ouagadougou (Burkina Faso)." Cited in Basáñez et al., "River Blindness."

[85] Basáñez. "River Blindness."

[86] TDR—Research and Training in Tropical Diseases Web site. "Research Results—Onchocerciasis." Available online. URL: http://www.who.int/tdr/dw/oncho2003.htm. Accessed May 18, 2007.

[87] Richard Carter and Kamini N. Mendis. "Evolutionary and Historical Aspects of the Burden of Malaria." *Clinical Microbiology Reviews* 15, no. 4 (October 2002): 564–594.

[88] Cynthia A. Needham and Richard Canning. *Global Disease Eradication: The Race for the Last Child*. Herndon, Va.: ASM Press, 2002, p. 39.

[89] Richard Tren. "Malaria and Climate Change." In Working Papers Series; Julian Simon Centre for Policy Research, October 2002. Available online. URL: http://www.libertyindia.org/pdfs/malaria_climatechange2002.pdf. Accessed May 18, 2007.

[90] Malaria Site. "Malaria in Ancient India." Available online. URL: http://www.malariasite.com/malaria/history_literature.htm. Accessed April 14, 2006.

[91] Carter and Mendis. "Burden of Malaria."

[92] V. P. Sharma. "Malaria Control in India." Available online. URL: http://www.pitt.edu/~superl/lecture/lec17341/index.htm. Accessed January 4, 2004.

[93] Ahmed Kamal. "Living with Water: Bangladesh Since Ancient Times." In Terje Tvedt and Eva Jakobsson. *A History of Water: Water Control and River Biographies.* London: I. B. Taurus, 2006, pp. 194ff.

[94] G. C. Chatterjee. "The Battle of the Damoodar." Calcutta, India: Central Co-operative Anti-Malaria Society, 1930.

[95] Tren. "Malaria and Climate Change," p. 3.

[96] S. R. Christophers. "What Disease Costs India." *Indian Medical Gazette* 59 (1924): 196–200. In Carter and Mendis, "Burden of Malaria."

[97] Indian Society for Parasitology. "Parasitology Centers." Available online. URL: http://www.parasitologyindia.org/parasitology_centers.htm. Accessed December 13, 2006.

[98] R. S. Bray. *Armies of Pestilence: The Impacts of Disease on History.* London: James Clarke, 2004, p. 101.

[99] Rachel Carson. *Silent Spring.* Boston: Houghton Mifflin, 1962.

[100] Center for International Environmental Law. "The Stockholm Convention and DDT." Available online. URL: http://www.ciel.org/Chemicals/Stockholm_DDT.html. Accessed June 2, 2004.

[101] Richard Tren et al. *Malaria and the DDT Story.* London: Institute of Economic Affairs, 2001.

[102] World Health Organization. "WHO Gives Indoor Use of DDT a Clean Bill of Health for Controlling Malaria." Available online. URL: http://www.who.int/mediacentre/news/releases/2006/pr50/en/index.html. Accessed September 15, 2006.

[103] G. Harrison. *Mosquitoes, Malaria, and Man: A History of the Hostilities Since 1880.* London: John Murray, 1978, p. 241.

[104] Javed Siddiqi. *World Health and World Politics: The World Health Organization and the UN System.* Columbia: University of South Carolina Press, 1995, pp. 161–178.

[105] Michael W. Service. *Demography and Vector-borne Diseases.* New York: CRC Press, 1989, pp. 144–150.

[106] Tren. *Malaria and the DDT Story.*

[107] Service. *Demography,* p. 67.

[108] "India Country Profile." In *World Malaria Report 2005.* Available online. URL: http://www.rbm.who.int/wmr2005/html/exsummary_en.htm. Accessed October 17, 2006.

[109] Tren. *Malaria and the DDT Story,* p. 22.

[110] Sumana Bhattacharya. "Climate Change and Malaria in India," *Current Science* 90, no. 3 (February 10, 2006). A. K. Avasarala. "Mosquito Laughs at Man." Available online. URL:

http://www.publichealth.pitt.edu/supercourse/SupercoursePPT/25011-26001/25401.ppt. Accessed December 12, 2007.

[111] "India Country Profile." In *World Malaria Report 2005*. Available online. URL: http://www.rbm.who.int/wmr2005/html/exsummary_en.htm. Accessed October 17, 2006.

[112] India National Institute of Malaria Research. Available online. URL: http://www.mrcindia.org/. Accessed October 18. 2006.

[113] Associated Press. "Malaria Drugs Could Cut Deaths in Africa." *New York Times*, March 1, 2007.

[114] Richard Black. "Fish Eat Away at Malaria in India." Available online. URL: http://news.bbc.co.uk/1/hi/sci/tech/3369341.stm. Accessed January 5, 2004.

[115] Indo-Asian News Service. "India to Test Malaria Vaccine, Review Drug Policy." *Hindustan Times*, November 4, 2005. Available online. URL: http://www.hindustantimes.com/news/181_1537470,0050.htm. Accessed December 3, 2006.

[116] Donald G. McNeil, Jr. "New Malaria Vaccine Is Shown to Work in Infants Under 1 year Old, Study Finds." *New York Times*, October 18, 2007.

[117] Donald G. McNeil, Jr. "Flu Spray Most Effective for Children, Study Finds." *New York Times*, February 15, 2007.

[118] D. J. Alexander and I. H. Brown. "Recent Zoonoses Caused by Influenza A Viruses." *Revue scientifique et technique* 19, no. 1 (April 2000): 197–225.

[119] Centers for Disease Control and Prevention. "Key Facts about Influenza." Available online. URL: http://www.ded.gov/flu/keyfacts.htm. Accessed August 30, 2006.

[120] John M. Barry. *The Great Influenza: The Epic Story of the Deadliest Plague in History*. New York: Viking, 2004, p. 392. Barry reports that according to some experts, "few victims had escaped without some pathological changes."

[121] C. S. Conover, E. E. Whitaker, D. Ages et al. "The Underrecognized Burden of Influenza." *New England Journal of Medicine* 355, nos. 31–40 (July 6, 2006).

[122] Medical Ecology. "Influenza." Available online. URL: http://www.medicalecology.org/diseases/influenza/influenza.htm#sect2.3. Accessed December 18, 2006.

[123] Global Security Organization. "Pandemic Influenza." Available online. URL: http://www.globalsecurity.org/security/ops/hsc-scen-3_pandemic-influenza.htm. Accessed November 11, 2005.

[124] David Brown. "Killer Virus." *Washington Post*, June 4, 2004; H. Phillips. "'Black October': The Impact of the Spanish Influenza Epidemic of 1918 on South Africa." *International Journal of African Historical Studies* 24, no. 2 (1991).

[125] DIMACS Working Group on Genetics and Evolution of Pathogens. "Patterns of Hemagglutinin Evolution and the Epidemiology of Influenza." Available online. URL: http://dimacs.rutgers.edu/Workshops/Genetics/slides/dushoff.pdf. Accessed November 25, 2003.

[126] Nature. "Alarms Ring Over Bird Flu Mutations." Available online. URL: http://www.nature.com/news/2006/060116/full/439248a.html. Accessed January 19, 2006.

[127] GlobalSecurity Organization. "Pandemic Influenza."

[128] John W. Kimball. "The Flu." Available online. URL: http://users.rcn.com/jkimball.ma.ultranet/BiologyPages/I/Influenza.html. Accessed February 8, 2007.

[129] Global Security Organization. "Pandemic Influenza."

[130] W. R. Dowdle. "Influenza Pandemic Periodicity, Virus Recycling, and the Art of Risk Assessment." *Emerging Infectious Diseases* 12, no 1. (January 2006): 34–39.

[131] Sarah Webb. "Five Lessons from Avian Flu: Work, Watch, Wait, Worry, and Wonder." *Discover*, June 25, 2006.

[132] René Snacken, Alan P. Kendal, Lars R. Haaheim et al. "The Next Influenza Pandemic: Lessons from Hong Kong, 1997." *Emerging Infectious Diseases* 5, no. 2 (March–April 1999).

[133] World Health Organization. "H5N1 Avian Influenza: Timeline of Events." Available online. URL: http://www.who.int/csr/disease/avian_influenza/timeline2007_04_02.pdf. Accessed April 2, 2007. Daily News Central-Health News. "China Develops Live H5N1 Vaccine for Use with Farm Birds." Available online. URL: http://health.dailynewscentral.com/content/view/0002026/67. Accessed December 26, 2005.

[134] Deborah MacKenzie. "Bird Flu Vaccination Could Lead to New Strains." *New Scientist*, March 24, 2004.

[135] Tony Paterson and Stephen Castle. "Dead Swans Litter German Island as Bird Flu Spreads." *The Independent*, April 6, 2007.

[136] World Health Organization. "H5N1 Avian Influenza: Timeline of Events."

[137] Thijs Kuiken, Guus Rimmelzwaan, Debby van Riel et al. "Avian H5N1 Influenza in Cats." *Science*, September 2, 2004.

[138] World Health Organization. "H5N1 Avian Influenza: Timeline of Events."

[139] Wendy Orrent. "The Science of Avian Flu: Answers to Frequently Asked Questions." *Discover*, February 20, 2006.

[140] Elisabeth Rosenthal. "Whirlwind Spread of Avian Flu Surprises Scientists." *International Herald Tribune*, February 20, 2006.

[141] ———. "Africa May Face Risk for Bird Flu, Officials Fear." *International Herald Tribune*, October 19, 2005.

[142] Margie Mason. "Bird Flu Explodes in Indonesia." Available online. URL: http://breitbart.com/article.php?id=2006-05-31_D8HV5U3G0&show_article=1&cat=life. Accessed May 32, 2006.

[143] Donald G. McNeil, Jr. "Another Death in Indonesia Deepens Fears of Bird Flu's Spread." *New York Times*, June 16, 2006.

[144] Randolph W. Pate. "Vaccine Liability: Congress Should Give Vaccines a Shot in the Arm?" Available online. URL: http://www.heritage.org/Research/HealthCare/wm946.cfm. Accessed December 16, 2005.

[145] Anita Manning. "Three Strategies for Preventing Another Vaccine Shortage." *USA Today*, December 14, 2004.

[146] Deborah MacKenzie. "Tests Dash Hope of Rapid Production of Bird Flu Vaccine." *New Scientist*, December 16, 2005.

[147] David Brown. "$1 Billion Awarded for Flu Vaccine." *Washington Post*, May 5, 2006.

[148] Tony Scully. *Nature,* May 20, 2008.

[149] National Institutes of Health. "Quick Diagnosis of Flu Strains Possible with New Microchip Test." Available online. URL: http://www.nih.gov/news/pr/aug2006/niaid-28.htm. Accessed August 28, 2006.

[150] Donald G. McNeil, Jr. "Immediate Treatment Needed for Bird Flu Cases." *New York Times,* September 11, 2006.

[151] Elisabeth Rosenthal. "Better Planning Is Needed for Flu Drugs, Experts Say." *New York Times,* October 19, 2005.

[152] Donald G. McNeil, Jr. "Scientists Hope Vigilance Stymies Avian Flu Mutations." *New York Times,* March 27, 2007.

[153] C. E. Mills et al. "Pandemic Influenza: Risk of Multiple Introductions and the Need to Prepare for Them." *PloS Medicine,* February 20, 2006. Available online. URL: http://medicine.plosjournals.org/perlserv/?request=get-document&doi=10.1371/journal.pmed.0030135. Accessed June, 2006.

[154] World Health Organization. "Responding to the Asian Influenza Pandemic Threat." Available online. URL: http://www.who.int/csr/resources/publications/influenza/WHO_CDS_CSR_GIP_05_8-EN.pdf. Accessed May 18, 2007.

[155] Donald G. McNeil, Jr. "At the UN: This Virus Has an Expert 'Quite Scared.'" *New York Times,* March 28, 2006.

[156] Donald G. McNeil, Jr. "A Pandemic That Wasn't but Might Be." *New York Times,* January 22, 2008.

[157] Alan Zelicoff. "The Sky Is Falling and Millions of Us Are Going to Die." Available online. URL: http://www.bioterrorism.slu.edu/Newsletter/Fall05Newsletter/Fall05ZelicoffOp.htm. Accessed August 28, 2006.

PART II

Primary Sources

4

United States Documents

The primary sources reproduced in this chapter are divided into three sections: past, present, and future. The items are placed roughly in historical order. All selections have been excerpted from longer documents. Follow the references below each excerpt to check out an entire document or article.

HISTORICAL DOCUMENTS

Yellow Fever Attacks Philadelphia, 1793

Although we think of yellow fever and malaria as tropical diseases, they can attack wherever the right type of mosquitoes are found. Yellow fever killed 4,000 people in Philadelphia in 1793, one-tenth of the population at the time. It forced the new government under President Washington to flee the city, then the temporary capital of the United States. The following account is from the diary of a local merchant, Samuel Breck.

I had scarcely become settled in Philadelphia when in July, 1793, the yellow fever broke out, and, spreading rapidly in August, obliged all the citizens who could remove to seek safety in the country. My father took his family to Bristol on the Delaware, and in the last of August I followed him . . . I was compelled to return to the city on the 8th of September, and spend the 9th there. Everything looked gloomy, and forty-five deaths were reported for the 9th. And yet it was nothing then to what it became three or four weeks later, when from the first to the twelfth of October one thousand persons died. On the twelfth a smart frost came and checked its ravages.

The horrors of this memorable affliction were extensive and heart rending. Nor were they softened by professional skill. The disorder was in a great measure a stranger to our climate, and was awkwardly treated. Its rapid march, being from ten victims a day in August to one hundred a day in

October, terrified the physicians, and led them into contradictory modes of treatment. They, as well as the guardians of the city, were taken by surprise. No hospitals or hospital stores were in readiness to alleviate the sufferings of the poor. For a long time nothing could be done other than to furnish coffins for the dead and men to bury them. At length a large house in the neighborhood was appropriately fitted up for the reception of patients, and a few pre-eminent philanthropists volunteered to superintend it. At the head of them was Stephen Girard, who has since become the richest man in America.

In private families the parents, the children, the domestics lingered and died, frequently without assistance. The wealthy soon fled; the fearless or indifferent remained from choice, the poor from necessity. The inhabitants were reduced thus to one-half their number, yet the malignant action of the disease increased, so that those who were in health one day were buried the next. The burning fever occasioned paroxysms of rage which drove the patient naked from his bed to the street, and in some instances to the river, where he was drowned. Insanity was often the last stage of its horrors.

. . . Counting upon the comparative security of his remote residence from the heart of the town, (he) ventured to brave the disorder, and fortunately escaped its attack. He told me that in the height of the sickness, when death was sweeping away its hundreds a week, a man applied to him for leave to sleep one night on the stable floor. The gentleman, like everyone else, inspired with fear and caution, hesitated. The stranger pressed his request, assuring him that he had avoided the infected parts of the city, that his health was very good, and promised to go away at sunrise the next day. Under these circumstances he admitted him into his stable for that night. At peep of day the gentleman went to see if the man was gone. On opening the door he found him lying on the floor delirious and in a burning fever. Fearful of alarming his family, he kept it a secret from them, and went to the committee of health to ask to have the man removed.

That committee was in session day and night at the City Hall in Chestnut Street. The spectacle around was new, for he had not ventured for some weeks so low down in town. The attendants on the dead stood on the pavement in considerable numbers soliciting jobs, and until employed they were occupied in feeding their horses out of the coffins which they had provided in anticipation of the daily wants. These speculators were useful, and, albeit with little show of feeling, contributed greatly to lessen, by competition, the charges of interment.

The gentleman passed on through these callous spectators until he reached the room in which the committee was assembled, and from whom he obtained the services of a quack doctor, none other being in attendance. They went together to the stable, where the doctor examined the man, and then told the gentleman that at ten o'clock he would send the cart with a suitable coffin, into which he requested to have the dying stranger placed. The poor man was then alive and begging for a drink of water. His fit of delirium had subsided, his reason had returned, yet the experience of the soi-disant doctor enabled him to foretell that his death would take place in a few hours; it did so, and in time for his corpse to be conveyed away by the cart at the hour appointed. This sudden exit was of common occurrence. The whole number of deaths in 1793 by yellow fever was more than four thousand.

Source: Samuel Breck. In Albert Bushnell Hart, ed. "Yellow Fever Attacks Philadelphia, 1793," In Albert Bushnell Hart, ed. *American History Told by Contemporaries*. Vol. 3 (New York: Macmillan, 1929).

1849 Cholera Epidemic—Missouri, Ohio, New York

Cholera first came to American shores in 1832. A second wave hit in 1849, quickly spreading through all settled regions. The following three excerpts from local historical accounts may give some flavor of the disease's impact.

1849 Cholera Epidemic, St. Louis, Missouri

Although scientists discovered how cholera spread in the 1850s, public opinion already understood the health importance of sanitation by the time of the 1849 U.S. cholera epidemic. The terrible toll in St. Louis, then one of the nation's main cities, helped spark the construction of sewers there. The following excerpt is from the Metropolitan Sewer District of St. Louis Web site.

The 1849 St. Louis cholera epidemic claimed 4,557 lives out of a population of 63,000. This is a death rate equivalent to 72 out of every thousand people.

Cholera was rampant in many U.S. cities at the time, but the large cities of New York, Chicago, New Orleans and Cincinnati had smaller death rates of 11, 24, 30 and 39 respectively. Victims of the water-borne disease usually died within 24 hours of their diagnosis from severe diarrhea, vomiting and rapid dehydration.

In the mid-nineteenth century, before bacteria were known to be the cause, two principal theories of disease transmission were prevalent. The "contagion" theory said illness was acquired through close contacts whereas the "miasmic" theory stated gaseous airborne poisons, vapors and fumes from decomposing organic matter caused illness. Traditional protections were quarantined isolation and general cleanliness and sanitation.

The city of St. Louis, a long time advocate of a public sewer system, petitioned the 1849 Missouri General Assembly for authority to issue bonds for sewer construction. At that time, the only existing sewers were relatively small drains meant to accommodate traffic on the levee and waterfront (constructed from street and harbor funds). There were also a few privately constructed storm water drains.

Meanwhile, sinkholes in the city's interior were becoming clogged and "miasmic" (gaseous). Chouteau's Pond in the Mill Creek Valley was being polluted with organic and industrial wastes. The only "public" water supply was located in the city's center. Most domestic water came from private wells not protected from contamination of the inadequate waste disposal practices of the time.

Mention of the St. Louis cholera cases first appeared in The Missouri Republican in January 1849. Urging action by municipal government, the newspaper reported arriving steamboat passengers were bringing cholera to the city.

By March 12, 1849, the Missouri General Assembly—with extra pushing from St. Louis officials—passed "An act to provide a general system of sewerage (and its financing) in the city of St. Louis." Such a sewer system would alleviate both "contagion" and "miasmic" health concerns.

The Biddle Street Sewer was authorized in August 1849, but not under construction until March 1850. Also authorized in 1850 was the draining of Chouteau's Pond via the Mill Creek Sewer and other large public sewers. However, it was too late to stop the epidemic.

The week of June 24, 1849, cholera deaths rose to 601 and were occurring at a rate of 86 per day. A public meeting was held on June 25 at the Courthouse where a Committee of Public Health was formed and given almost absolute power to take action to abate the spread of the disease. The Mayor and Municipal Assembly essentially abdicated their responsibilities to the Committee. Committee members immediately ordered anti-contagion and sanitation measures that included quarantines, fumigations and general municipal cleaning.

Although still recorded through 1851, cholera deaths eventually dwindled to a manageable number. A later epidemic in 1866 was smaller in scope where the death rate was 17 per thousand. The water and sewer systems were more extensive and the prevention methods more efficient. Cholera bacterium was identified and isolated in 1884 and led to more effective prevention.

Source: Metropolitan Sewer District of St. Louis. "1849 St. Louis Cholera Epidemic Helps Initiate Sewer Construction." Available online. URL: http://www.msd.st-louis.mo.us/PublicComm/Pipeline/2-2000/S3.htm. Accessed September 2000.

1849 Cholera Epidemic, Gallia County, Ohio

The 1849 cholera epidemic reached Gallia County, Ohio, 150 miles upstream from Cincinnati on the Ohio River. The county seat of Gallipolis was largely spared, apparently due to timely improvements in sanitation. The following excerpt is from the Gallia County Genealogical Society Web site.

In July 1849, *The Journal,* Gallipolis' weekly newspaper, reported on outbreaks of cholera in Montreal, New York, New Orleans, St. Louis, Cincinnati and other American cities. In each case there were hundreds of people who had died. Around Gallipolis there had been only a few sporadic cases, and there had been four deaths in Coalport in Meigs County. The busier, more urban areas of Gallia County, however, were to be spared. It was in the backwater townships of Walnut and Harrison where cholera would wreak its havoc.

An account of this epidemic is recorded in the Hardesty History of Gallia County, published in 1882. The illness apparently entered the county when a Walnut Township resident, William Martt, assisted a family with a move in Lawrence County. He became ill immediately upon returning home. He was cared for by his family and neighbors. He died within a week. During that week other members of his family and friends came down with the disease. By the time the epidemic had run its course two weeks later, over a hundred people had become ill and thirty-seven, including eight members of the Martt family had died.

With over a hundred cases in such a small area, the attack rate was extremely high. Anxiety, and indeed panic, must have been rampant. The account in Hardesty's History mentions that many of the victims were buried without coffins and that, in at least one case, five of the victims in the Martt family were buried in a single grave, because manpower to dig separate graves was not available.

Credit for subduing the epidemic was given to a Clay Township farmer, Mr. Middleswarth. Mr. Middleswarth had no medical training, but reportedly had been given a recipe for a cholera cure from a physician in New Orleans. He worked among the stricken, giving nursing care and advice. How much the "cholera cure" helped is not certain. Until the advent of intravenous fluid therapy in the 1900s, there were no treatments for cholera that were ever proven to be effective . . .

Why was Gallipolis spared? Possibly just happenstance, but part of the answer may be in a Gallipolis city ordinance in 1847 that established the Board of Health. The ordinance directed the board to oversee and remove any "building, cellar, or lot or ground vault, or privy, which they may know or believe to be foul, damp or otherwise prejudicial to the public health." Furthermore it directed that property owners would be subject to fines if drainage into street gutters was impeded in any way. They also supervised a system of grading the streets and filling sunken places so that standing water was eliminated. A report on the completion of this project was reported in *The Journal* in April 1849. This may have played an important part in preventing contamination of wells from sewage and runoff from improper outdoor privies.

Source: Elvick Neil. "The 1849 Cholera Epidemic." Gallia County [Ohio] Genealogical Society Available online. URL: http://www.galliagenealogy.org/cholera.htm, Accessed February 5, 2007.

1849 Cholera Epidemic, New York, New York

Social historians sometimes use epidemics to illustrate social or political values at the time and place they occurred, as can be seen in the following account, found on the City University of New York Web site.

Cholera again ravaged Europe in 1848. In December the New York, a ship with three hundred passengers that had been exposed to cholera, was quarantined on Staten Island. Some of the passengers escaped to Manhattan, where cholera cases began to appear before the new year. The freezing winter of 1848–1849 limited the spread of cholera, and few cases were reported during the first months of 1849. But by mid-May, increasing numbers of cholera cases were appearing, and by June the outbreak had reached epidemic proportions.

As in 1832, the center of the outbreak seventeen years later was the Five Points slum district. And, as in 1832, those who could afford to leave the city for the summer did. The economic life of the city once again ground to a halt; even several of the city's churches closed their doors for the summer. For the most part, the city and the nation reacted to cholera's incursion in 1849 in the same ways as they had in 1832—conventional wisdom said it was a scourge of the poor, who had weakened themselves with drink and vice and filth.

At the same time, many pious Americans who had witnessed more than a decade of capitalist expansion and materialist gain and consequently believed that greed had defeated spirituality in the nation's values, interpreted cholera's presence as God's divine judgment. Many clergymen saw greed everywhere—in America's bloody war with Mexico, in the continued existence of slavery, in Sabbath-breaking, and in infidelity. Even President Zachary Taylor responded to the 1849 cholera outbreak by concluding that the nation needed to repent.

The reactions to cholera in 1832 and 1849, in common with responses to most disasters, tended to provide outlets for those promoting certain political or cultural agendas. Clergy, politicians, and elite reformers pointed to the devastation wrought by the disease as proof of how right they were, and how the disease reflected God's support for their respective causes. Disasters often provide the opportunity for national self-examination. In 1849, the meanings that were attached to cholera closely resembled the growing rifts within the nation around the questions of slavery, the direction of the emerging capitalist economy, and the responsibility of the state and elites towards the less fortunate.

Source: City University of New York. "Cholera in Nineteenth Century New York." Available online. URL: http://www.virtualny.cuny.edu/cholera/1849/cholera_1849_set.html. Accessed February 5, 2007.

The National Quarantine, 1893

In response to a renewed cholera epidemic in Europe, and the presence of the disease among some immigrants, the U.S. Congress passed a national quarantine act in 1892. This 1893 article from Harper's Weekly *describes how the law was implemented by U.S. officers both in the ports of departure in Europe and in the ports of arrival in the United States.*

It will be recalled that a year ago there was almost a panic in the United States for fear that cholera would get lodgment on the land through the port of New York, and spread over the country. There seems to be very little fear this year on account of the cholera, though there is probably almost as much cholera in Europe as the year before, and it appears to be spread over a wider area. There are two reasons why there should not be a panic this season. One of these is due to the apprehension that fills nearly every mind as to the business outlook. The other is that the same spectre is powerless to frighten the same community twice. If it were generally known, however, that under the provisions of a bill passed by Congress last February the Supervising Surgeon-General of the United States Marine Hospital Service is empowered to overlook the work of all local quarantine authorities, and to take charge of such work whenever in his discretion he thinks that the quarantine is inefficient, the people of the United states would have another reason for feeling tolerably secure against the invasion of cholera. Last year conditions arose in the port of New York as cannot possibly arise under the regulations now enforced. Ship after ship came into port with cholera on board, and the people were filled with apprehension that the disease would get through the quarantine into the crowded tenement-house section of the metropolis. Fortunately these apprehensions were not well founded. But they resulted in the passage of this national quarantine law, which medical men regard as a very wise measure.

Under this law it is not contemplated that the local authorities, when efficient and thorough in their work, shall be either superseded or interfered with. It is made the duty of the Supervising Surgeon-General of the United States Marine Hospital Service to see that the local authorities are efficient and zealous, and to take charge of the work or supplement it in cases where he deems such a course to be necessary.

The law also empowers Dr. Walter Wyman, the Supervising Surgeon- General, to send assistants abroad to all infected ports, who shall examine all immigrants and passengers about to come to this country, and grant each one a bill of health. Without this a passenger cannot pass the quarantine lines into this country. The bill also gives the President the right to prohibit, in whole or in part, the introduction of persons and property from such countries or places as he shall designate, and for such period of time as it is deemed necessary, whenever, by reason of existence of cholera, or any other infectious or contagious disease in a foreign country, there is serious danger of the introduction of the same into the United States, despite the quarantine defenses. Under the law the Secretary of the Treasury promulgated regulations last spring. These regulations require that in ports infested with cholera passengers of the cabin class must produce evidence as to abode during the four days immediately preceding embarkation, and, if necessary, they and their baggage may be detained, and the baggage subjected to such disinfection as is necessary. Steerage passengers in a cholera-infected port, or from a cholera-infected place must be detained five days under medical observation, and their personal effects and baggage must be disinfected by steam. The regulations further forbid the shipment of certain articles of bedding and clothing from an infected port, also certain articles of merchandise, such as old rags, old jute, and old gunny, during the prevalence of an epidemic, and for thirty days after it has been officially declared at an end. All rags at all times are to be disinfected before shipment to the United States.

The principal ports of embarkation of immigrants to this country are Southampton, Liverpool, Hamburg, Bremen, Rotterdam, Amsterdam, Antwerp, Havre, Marseilles, Genoa, and Naples. A medical officer of the Marine Hospital Service has been detailed to serve in the office of the consul at each of the ports named. These officers have all had experience with ships, and with but two exceptions, Dr. Wyman says, have had actual quarantine experience. They have been at their respective stations for four months past, and their reports show both the necessity of their presence and the good results of their activity. Speaking of this, Dr. Wyman, in an address before the American Medical Association, said: "This is a new departure in quarantine—quarantining in foreign lands—and the ultimate result may be looked for with great interest. Whatever the result may be, certain it is that the presence of these officers in European ports has diminished in a great degree the danger of the introduction of cholera and other diseases from those ports. Their relations in one or two instances with foreign governments were in danger of being strained, but this danger has been averted both by their tact and good judgment, and because of the all-powerful United States law, which practically says to foreign officials that should they object to the official acts of these officers, the alternative is the refusal of the bill of health and the cutting off of all commerce between their ports and the United States."

So as to give these consuls and medical officers at the seaports selected for embarkation full information, the United States consuls in the interior have been instructed by the State Department to notify consuls at ports of the prevalence of any contagious diseases in these interior places, and also when merchandise or passengers are about to leave or have left any section within their respective consulates. At the port of embarkation each immigrant is furnished with an instruction card giving his name, last residence, name of ship, port and date of departure, and a reference number relating to the manifest, which is required by the immigration regulations, and in which is contained further information regarding each immigrant. This card must also bear the stamp of the consulate, and also be stamped or punched at the quarantine at the port of arrival, and again at the immigration depot, and it is to be held by the immigrant until he reaches his final point of destination. These inspection tickets and labels upon the baggage furnish the health officers of the interior States valuable information in regard to immigrants coming within their borders. This provision also ensures care and accuracy on the part of medical officers, and particularly on the part of United States consuls at ports where immigrants do not usually embark for the United States, but which may be sought by them in the hope of avoiding the enforcement of the stringent rules at ports where medical officers have been stationed.

. . . . [The article detailed the cooperative measures taken with Canada to prevent cholera from reaching the northern border.]

The officer charged with the enforcement of the national quarantine keeps a hydrographic map upon which he traces the progress of any contagious disease in any part of the world, taking his facts from reports of consuls and the telegrams in the public press. In this way, bearing in mind the degree of efficiency in dealing with such diseases in the various countries, he is able to anticipate the course of such a disease in any part of the world. It is interesting to know that last summer, when the presence of cholera in Hamburg was still denied by the authorities at that city, Dr. Jenkins, from the quarantine station in New York, compelled the acknowledgement by the authorities that cholera had reached Hamburg. His map showed the course of cholera directly toward that city, and by insisting upon a report from there, through the State Department, the facts were at last given to the public. Dr. Wyman, from his office in Washington, takes careful cognizance of the health of the people all over the world, and is therefore prepared to act with intelligence whenever there is likelihood that any contagious or infectious disease may be imported into this country. American security depends upon the vigilant application of scientific precautions, and there is every reason to believe that such are now being taken.

Source: Harper's Weekly, August 26, 1893. "The National Quarantine." Available online. URL: http://www.fortunecity.com/littleitaly/amalfi/100/quaran93.htm. Accessed August 25, 2006.

Brief History of the Campaign against Tuberculosis in New York City, 1908

Tuberculosis, a chronic and fatal infection of the lungs, was the most common cause of death in 19th-century America. Toward the end of the century local health authorities began devising measures to track and ultimately limit the epidemic. The excerpt below was written by New York City general medical officer Hermann M. Biggs for the catalogue of a tuberculosis exhibit by the city's Department of Health in 1908.

The Campaign against Tuberculosis

The publication in 1882 of the classical researches of Robert Koch on the Etiology of Tuberculosis definitely placed this disease in the group of infectious, communicable and preventable diseases. It then logically became at once the duty of sanitary authorities to adopt, so far as possible, the measures necessary to restrict the prevalence of tuberculosis, but the full significance of the discovery was not at once appreciated, and some years elapsed before any serious attempt was made to apply the demonstrated scientific facts to the practical prevention of this disease.

In 1887, the writer, at that time one of the consulting pathologists of the Department of Health of the City of New York, having felt for several years the primary importance and necessity for administrative action in relation to this disease, urged upon the Board of Health of New York City the immediate enactment of suitable regulations for the sanitary surveillance of the tubercular diseases.

At that time, however, neither the medical profession nor the laity of the City of New York sufficiently appreciated the importance of the matter, and the Board of Health, after seeking advice from various sources, only considered it wise to adopt certain measures designed to extend information among the tenement house population as to the nature and the methods for the prevention of the disease. In 1892 and 1893 the matter was again brought up by the writer for serious discussion, but it was not until early in 1894 that the first definite steps were finally taken by the Board of Health to exercise a genuine surveillance over tuberculous persons.

From the outset the writer has always insisted that a rational campaign for the prevention of tuberculosis (especially pulmonary tuberculosis), must be primarily based on a system providing for the notification and registration of every case of this disease. In accordance with his recommendations, the Board of Health, early in 1894, adopted a series of resolutions providing for a system of notification, partly compulsory and partly voluntary in character. Public institutions of all kinds (hospitals, clinics, dispensaries, etc.) were required to report all cases coming under their supervision within one week, while private physicians were requested to do so. In view of what seemed at that time such a radical procedure as the notification of tuberculosis, it was deemed wiser to at first employ such a compromise scheme.

The original plan (adopted in 1894 by the Board of Health) provided the following:

- First: An educational campaign through the use of specially prepared circulars of information designed to reach different classes of the population (one of which was printed in many different languages), and also the utilization of the public press and lectures for the dissemination of popular information.
- Second: The compulsory notification of cases by public institutions and the request for the notification of private cases with all the data necessary for registration. Proper blanks, postal cards, etc., were provided for these reports.
- Third: The plotting of all reported cases on large maps specially prepared, showing every house lot in the Boroughs of Manhattan and The Bronx (then constituting the City of New York). Each case reported and each death occurring from tuberculosis was plotted by conventional signs showing the month and year that each came under the observation of the Department.
- Fourth: A special corps of medical inspectors was appointed, whose duty consisted in visiting the premises, where cases were reported as existing, and if the patients were not under the care of a private physician, leaving printed and verbal instructions informing the patient and family, what precautions should be taken to prevent the communication of the disease to others.
- Fifth: When premises had been vacated by the death or removal of the consumptive, the inspectors arranged for the removal of bedding, rugs, carpets, clothing, etc., for disinfection by steam, and for the cleaning, disinfection or renovation, as might be required, of the rooms occupied by the consumptive. Where it was considered necessary, the rooms were placarded, forbidding occupation by other persons until the order of the Board of Health, requiring their renovation, had been complied with.
- Sixth: Provision was made for the free bacteriological examination of the sputum from any suspicious case of tuberculosis in the bacteriological laboratory of the Department of Health. (The bacteriological laboratories were first opened in 1892, and were, I believe, the first municipal bacteriological laboratories in the world.)

Facilities were provided for the convenience of physicians desiring to send specimens of sputum by the establishment of depots at convenient points throughout the city, where sputum jars and blanks for recording information could be obtained, and where specimens of sputum for examination could be left. These were collected each day by the collectors of the Department, taken to the laboratory, examined, and a report forwarded to the physician of the results of the examination the following day.

This system of free examination of sputum for diagnosing tuberculosis was in harmony with the policy which the Board of Health adopted in 1892, namely, that "it properly comes within the functions of the sanitary authorities to furnish facilities of all kinds, which are useful or necessary in the diagnosis, specific treatment and prevention of all the diseases which are at the same time infectious, communicable and preventable." It was believed that the free examination of sputum would materially assist in the early diagnosis of tuberculosis, especially among the lower classes, and would encourage physicians to report cases. An early condition was made that no specimens of sputum would be examined, which did not have accompanying them all the data necessary for complete registration of the case.

The result of the first year's work was, on the whole, gratifying. It covered only ten months of the calendar year, and during this time more than four thousand cases of pulmonary tuberculosis were reported, and about five hundred specimens of sputum were sent for examination. As a result of the notification, accurate data as to the chief centers of infection became for the first time available, and thus the Department of Health was enabled to direct its efforts to the best advantage. The very striking existence of tuberculosis in certain localities was demonstrated in a remarkable way by the maps on which were plotted the cases and the deaths from this disease. A number of small sections from these maps were first published in 1892.

Source: University of Michigan Making of America. "Brief History of the Campaign against Tuberculosis in New York City: Catalogue of the Tuberculosis Exhibit of the Department of Health, City of New York, 1908." Available online. URL: http://www.hti.umich.edu/cgi/t/text/text-idx?c=moa;cc=moa;rgn=main;view=text;idno=AGU3214.0001.001. Accessed September 21, 2006.

Letter from Visiting Doctor Reporting Situation to Superintendent, Albuquerque Day School, New Mexico, 1918

The following letter, found in the U.S. National Archives, was written by a doctor during the 1918 influenza epidemic. He had been asked by the Commissioner of Indian Affairs to investigate the flu situation at an Indian boarding school at a pueblo in Albuquerque, New Mexico. Despite his dispassionate, scientific tone, the doctor managed to convey the suffering and fear caused by the epidemic.

Albuquerque, N.M., December 20, 1918

To: P.T.Lonergan, Supt.
From: D.A.Richardson, M.D.
Subject: Influenza Epidemic at Pueblos of Albuquerque Day School Section

It was with a great deal of pleasure that I responded to the urgent request of the Commissioner of Indian Affairs at Denver on the 25th of October, 1918, and with the kindness of the A.T. & S.F. Railway officials at Topeka I was enabled to reach Albuquerque promptly the following day.

From the Agency I was immediately conveyed to Isleta by Mr. Lonergan in person and the same afternoon I arrived in Albuquerque and was able to size up the situation promptly. The following day the deplorable condition at Isleta presented itself in the death of ten Indians. The Pueblo itself, situated in its better portion northward, was in marked contrast to the southerly portion of the Pueblo which was older and presented a mere mass of low ceilinged adobes, small doors, virtually no windows, one pigeon hole leading into another, sometimes in long sections, and in all these it was absolutely impossible for the sun to shine. In these rooms, were, in all stages of the Flu, Indians lying dead or dying or advancing well to the conditions which followed the Flu.

The Flu itself throughout all the pueblos was a matter of primary importance but where directions were carefully followed out, was seldom followed by pneumonia, pleurisy, nephritis, emphysema or aught else of importance. At Isleta, prior to my reaching there, virtually of the Indians has passed through what I am pleased to designate as the influenza proper and the course of the disease is such that I believe it wise in this report to define the origin, course and prognosis of the Flu itself.

The beginning of the Flu is prostration, with headache, coryza, more or less running of the nose, but it is marked by great prostration; the patients, in the case of Indians, literally falling to the floor. You would enter a placito and find all the inmates reclining on thin mattresses with their backs against the cold wall, with hard, racking cough, some sneezing, the children running at the nose, the temperature ranging from 102 to 105, the customary temperature being about 103.5. These patients passed in about five days to what was apparently a normal condition and if they remained within doors, properly care for, would in a majority of instances escape further sequela. These patients were instructed to maintain a horizontal position, to eat nothing but fluid food, to drink abundantly of hot water and to maintain an open toilet. They were to remain thus quiescent at least ten days. I had very little trouble to get the Indians to follow out my instructions where the death rate had begun. The death rate begins immediately upon the advent of pneumonia or other of the rarer complications, such as nephritis, pulmonary aedema etc. Cases of pulmonary aedema were not uncommon.

The pneumonias began sometimes immediately upon the completion of the influenza proper, generally however, a few days intervening between the cessation of the coryza and the beginning of the pneumonia. Almost without exception throughout all the pueblos the pneumonia began as Capillary Bronchitis, with profuse secretion.

The first stage of the pneumonia was marked by a peculiar onset and absence of the subcrepitant rale [wheezing] but with symptoms all over the chest resembling the "creaking hinges" of tubercular fibrosis. In many instances a day would elapse between this demonstration and the appearance of the diagnostic subcrepitant rale of bronchial pneumonia. The respiration would be normal and suddenly increase, in minute number, and in many instances for a few days it would appear as though the prognosis was very favorable, when without warning the positive toxicity of the disease would result in cardiac apoplexy. Many patients would pass through a double pneumonia, be apparently convalescent and suddenly die of pulmonary atelectasis.

Throughout all the pueblos the same cause of death appears and it is due to the ingestion during the progress of this disease of solid food or of sitting up in an erect posture at times, producing thereby hypostatic congestions or exhaustion. The element of fear in all instances among Indians is productive of great harm and should be removed by suggestion or actions as early as possible in the case of Indians.

. . . . [The letter describes the course of the illness in one typical patient, who seemed to recover, and then suddenly worsened and died.]

The average duration of an epidemic of Influenza is six weeks,—two weeks for the Flu—one week for the sequelae and deaths,—and three weeks for the convalescents.

The conditions existed with great similarity at all the pueblos. There have been no relapses at any pueblo after the cessation of the convalescent period. The losses varied with different pueblos from 89 at Isleta to 9 at Tesuque. Smallpox was epidemic at Jemez where I arrived there Nov. 4th and there were no deaths from smallpox, although fully sixty cases presented. A majority of the cases were true varioloid. A small number only of variola.

Complete records of all cases will be delivered at the hands of the various field matrons. Every placita on every pueblo visited was entered—for instance, at Jemez, 380 individuals were cared for at 90 placitas at Jemez. Everywhere all government employes were alive to the situation, earnest of purpose, and extremely efficient and exploited a full, cheerful missionary spirit. The Indians were appreciative of our efforts although at first it was hard for them to willingly accede to our requests, but with death staring them in the face at every corner, they were driven in their fear to accept of our assistance and as success began, appreciation followed.

I am under obligations to the Department for the cooperation everywhere of the employes. I believe this is a fair report of the influenza epidemic at Isleta, San Domingo, Santa Clara, San Juan, Nambe, San Juan Ildefonso, Santa Ana, Zie, Jemez.

Respectfully submitted,
D.A. Richardson, M.D.
[signed]

Source: U.S. National Archives. "Letter from Visiting Doctor Reporting Situation to Superintendent, Albuquerque Day School, New Mexico, December 20, 1918, Bureau of Indian Affairs." Available online. URL: http://www.archives.gov/exhibits/influenza-epidemic/records/visiting-doctor-letter.pdf. Accessed September 19, 2006

1955 Polio Vaccine Trial Announcement

On April 12, 1955, Dr. Thomas Francis, head of the National Foundation for Infantile Paralysis (polio), announced that the polio vaccine, tested on over a million American children, was safe and effective. It was a happy ending for the largest medical field test ever attempted.

ANN ARBOR: The Vaccine Works. It Is Safe, Effective, and Potent.

Dr. Thomas Francis, Jr., UM Director of the Poliomyelitis Vaccine Evaluation Center, told an anxious world of parents that the Salk vaccine has been proved to be up to 80–90 percent effective in preventing paralytic polio.

At a meeting of over 500 scientists and physicians and before the penetrating eyes of cameras and powerful spotlights, Dr. Francis spoke on the effectiveness of the Salk vaccine. The meeting was held at the Rackham

Auditorium in Ann Arbor under the joint sponsorship of the National Foundation for Infantile Paralysis and the University of Michigan.

Dr. Francis declared the vaccine had produced "an extremely successful effect" among bulbar-patients in the areas where vaccine and an inert substance had been tried interchangeably.

Financed by nearly one million dollars worth of dimes which have been donated to the National Foundation, the Francis Report may slow down what has become a double-time march of disease to a snail's pace.

In strong statistical language the historic trial of a vaccine and its subsequent analysis was revealed. Over 113 pages in length, the Report at long last called a halt to speculations and finally re-enforced laboratory findings with concrete field evidence. There can be no doubt now that children can be inoculated successfully against polio.

There can be no doubt that humanity can pull itself up from its own bootstraps and protect its children from the insidious invasion of ultramicroscopic disease.

For one thing what was feared turned out to be unfounded—the vaccine proved incredibly safe. Reactions were nearly negligible. Only 0.4 percent of the vaccinated children suffered minor reactions. An even smaller percent (0.004–0.006) suffered so called "major reactions."

And the persistence of protection appears reasonably good. When good antibody responses were obtained from vaccination, the report said "the effect was maintained with but moderate decline after five months."

Distribution of antibody levels among vaccinated persons was much higher than that in the control population from the same areas.

Out of a total population of 1,829,916 children a total of 1013 cases of polio developed during the study period and were reported to the Center.

In placebo control areas, where vaccine was interchanged with an inert substance, 428 out of 749,236 children contracted the disease.

In the observed control areas where only second graders were inoculated, 585 cases out of 1,080,680 children developed.

Percentages in the placebo areas were: 67.5 paralytic, 17.6 non-paralytic, 7.2 doubtful, and 7.6 not polio. Specifically, 33 inoculated children receiving the complete vaccination series became paralyzed in the placebo areas. This is opposed to 115 uninoculated children. Similarly, in the observed areas there were 38 such children who became paralyzed, as opposed to 330 uninoculated children.

There were four deaths among children who received placebo; none among the vaccinated. In observed areas there were 11 fatalities; none among children receiving the vaccine.

Only one child who had been inoculated with the vaccine died of polio, and this death followed a tonsillectomy two days after the second injection of the vaccine in an area where polio was already prevalent.

The Report also stated that in no area did Type II virus prevail. There was, however, prevalence in certain areas of Types I and III.

Marked sociological differences were noted by the U-M's Survey Research Center among the participating and non-participating children in the study. For example, there was a higher proportion of children participating who had been vaccinated against small-pox, diphtheria, and whooping cough than among the non-participants. Significant auxiliary findings were:

1. The vaccine's effectiveness was more clearly seen when measured against the more severe cases of the disease;
2. Although data were limited, findings in Canada and Finland support the Report in showing a significant effect of the vaccine among cases from whom virus was isolated
3. Vaccination protected against family exposure. Only 1 out of 233 inoculated children developed the disease, while 8 out of 244 children receiving placebo contracted the disease from family contact.
4. In picking the field trial areas, the National Foundation scored a major victory. Although in placebo areas cases were 27 per cent under the 1949–53 average, and 12 per cent less in the observed control areas, it was found that there had been a 26 per cent increase per 100,000 in trial areas as in non-trial areas. This meant that trial areas were appropriately selected for the best testing conditions for the vaccine.

The field trials and the evaluation were made possible by grants totalling $7,500,000 in March of Dimes Funds from the National Foundation for Infantile Paralysis.

Source: University of Michigan School of Public Health. "1955 Polio Vaccine Trial Announcement." Available online. URL:http://www.sph.umich.edu/about/polioannouncement.html. Accessed September 3, 2006

CONTEMPORARY DOCUMENTS

Epidemiologic Notes and Reports: Pneumocystis Pneumonia—Los Angeles, 1981

The HIV virus that causes AIDS emerged in Africa in the first half of the 20th century. However, no patients "presented" with AIDS (showed symptoms of the new disease) until 1980 and 1981, when a few patients appeared in the United States. The following report from the CDC's MMWR (Morbidity and Mortality Weekly Report) *of June 5, 1981, was the first mention in the medical literature of the future pandemic. The five patients discussed in the report suffered from a rare form of pneumonia, and their immune systems were not functioning properly.*

Pneumocystis Pneumonia—Los Angeles

In the period October 1980–May 1981, 5 young men, all active homosexuals, were treated for biopsy-confirmed *Pneumocystis carinii* pneumonia at 3 different hospitals in Los Angeles, California. Two of the patients died. All 5 patients had laboratory-confirmed previous or current cytomegalovirus (CMV) infection and candidal mucosal infection. Case reports of these patients follow.

Patient 1: A previously healthy 33-year-old man developed *P. carinii* pneumonia and oral mucosal candidiasis in March 1981 after a 2-month history of fever associated with elevated liver enzymes, leukopenia, and CMV viruria. The serum complement-fixation CMV titer in October 1980 was 256; in May 1981 it was 32. The patient's condition deteriorated despite courses of treatment with trimethoprim-sulfamethoxazole (TMP/SMX), pentamidine, and acyclovir. He died May 3, and postmortem examination showed residual *P. carinii* and CMV pneumonia, but no evidence of neoplasia.

Patient 2: A previously healthy 30-year-old man developed *p. carinii* pneumonia in April 1981 after a 5-month history of fever each day and of elevated liver-function tests, CMV viruria, and documented seroconversion to CMV, i.e., an acute-phase titer of 16 and a convalescent-phase titer of 28 in anticomplement immunofluorescence tests. Other features of his illness included leukopenia and mucosal candidiasis. His pneumonia responded to a course of intravenous TMP/.SMX, but, as of the latest reports, he continues to have a fever each day.

Patient 3: A 30-year-old man was well until January 1981 when he developed esophageal and oral candidiasis that responded to Amphotericin B treatment. He was hospitalized in February 1981 for *P. carinii* pneumonia that responded to TMP/SMX. His esophageal candidiasis recurred after the pneumonia was diagnosed, and he was again given Amphotericin B. The CMV complement-fixation titer in March 1981 was 8. Material from an esophageal biopsy was positive for CMV.

Patient 4: A 29-year-old man developed *P. carinii* pneumonia in February 1981. He had had Hodgkins disease 3 years earlier, but had been successfully treated with radiation therapy alone. He did not improve after being given intravenous TMP/SMX and corticosteroids and died in March. Postmortem examination showed no evidence of Hodgkins disease, but *P. carinii* and CMV were found in lung tissue.

Patient 5: A previously healthy 36-year-old man with clinically diagnosed CMV infection in September 1980 was seen in April 1981 because of a 4-month history of fever, dyspnea, and cough. On admission he was found to have *P. carinii* pneumonia, oral candidiasis, and CMV retinitis. A complement-fixation CMV titer in April 1981 was 128. The patient has been treated with 2 short courses of TMP/SMX that have been limited because of a sulfa-induced neutropenia. He is being treated for candidiasis with topical nystatin.

The diagnosis of *Pneumocystis* pneumonia was confirmed for all 5 patients antemortem by closed or open lung biopsy. The patients did not know each other and had no known common contacts or knowledge of sexual partners who had had similar illnesses. Two of the 5 reported having frequent homosexual contacts with various partners. All 5 reported using inhalant drugs, and 1 reported parenteral drug abuse. Three patients had profoundly depressed *in vitro* proliferative responses to mitogens and antigens. Lymphocyte studies were not performed on the other 2 patients.

Editorial Note: *Pneumocystis* pneumonia in the United States is almost exclusively limited to severely immunosuppressed patients. The occurrence of pneumocystosis in these 5 previously healthy individuals without a clinically apparent underlying immunodeficiency is unusual. The fact that these patients were all homosexuals suggests an association between some aspect of a homosexual lifestyle or disease acquired through sexual contact and *Pneumocystis* pneumonia in this population. All 5 patients described in this report had laboratory-confirmed CMV disease or virus shedding within 5 months of the diagnosis of *Pneumocystis* pneumonia. CMV infection has been shown to induce transient abnormalities of *in vitro* cellular-immune function in otherwise healthy human hosts. Although all 3 patients tested had abnormal cellular-immune function, no definitive conclusion regarding the role of CMV infection in these 5 cases can be reached because of the lack of published data on cellular-immune function in healthy homosexual males with and without CMV antibody. In 1 report, 7 (3.6%) of 194 patients with pneumocystosis also had CMV infection' 40 (21%) of the same group had at least 1 other major concurrent infection. A high prevalence of CMV infections among homosexual males was recently reported: 179 (94%) had CMV viruria; rates for 101 controls of similar age who were reported to be exclusively heterosexual were 54% for seropositivity and zero fro viruria. In another study of 64 males, 4 (6.3%) had positive tests for CMV in semen, but none had CMV recovered from urine. Two of the 4 reported recent homosexual contacts. These findings suggest not only that virus shedding may be more readily detected in seminal fluid than urine, but also that seminal fluid may be an important vehicle of CMV transmission.

All the above observations suggest the possibility of a cellular-immune dysfunction related to a common exposure that predisposes individuals to opportunistic infections such as pneumocystosis and candidiasis. Although the role of CMV infection in the pathogenesis of pneumocystosis remains unknown, the possibility of *P. carinii* infection must be carefully considered in a differential diagnosis for previously healthy homosexual males with dyspnea and pneumonia.

Source: Morbidity and Mortality Weekly Report, June 5, 1981. "Epidemiologic Notes and Reports: *Pneumocystis* Pneumonia—Los Angeles." Available online. URL:http://www.cdc.gov/mmwr/preview/mmwrhtml/june_5.htm. Accessed September 21, 2006.

Protecting the Nation's Health in an Era of Globalization: CDC's Global Strategy for Addressing Infectious Diseases, 2002

The U.S. Centers for Disease Control and Protection has long been the country's first line of defense against epidemics, whether they be domestic or abroad. As the world grows smaller, international boundaries have become less important in this area. In 2002 the agency issued a "global strategy" report to reflect this fact. The following section details the agency's plans to help protect global public health.

CDC's Role in Promoting Global Public Health

CDC, which is dedicated to the prevention and control of disease and the promotion of health, works by invitation in many different jurisdictions, including U.S. states and cities and other nations. Throughout its history, CDC has provided international leadership in public health, serving as a technical consultant to the World Health Organization (WHO) and ministries of health on projects that address infectious disease problems related to endemic diseases, wars, famines, or other disasters. Many of these projects have been funded and coordinated by the U.S. Agency for International Development (USAID). CDC has also supported research and public health education on diseases of regional or international importance, provided resources and leadership for the smallpox eradication effort, and established long-term collaborative research partnerships with several developing nations. While considerable effort has been devoted to these international activities, CDC's primary focus has remained on domestic health.

In recent years, however, CDC's overseas role has expanded rapidly. *Global polio eradication* and *HIV/AIDS control programs* have led to substantial investments of CDC personnel and financial resources, as have a succession of complex international emergencies. Between 1990 and 2000, CDC provided outbreak assistance on an ad hoc basis to nations in Asia, Africa, Europe, and Latin America to help investigate outbreaks of unknown, highly dangerous, and highly infectious diseases, and provided diagnostic support for hundreds of local investigations around the globe.

Although there are no formal structures and designated resources for international outbreak response, U.S. citizens—as well as foreign governments—have come to rely on CDC to provide outbreak assistance and public health information whenever a new or reemerging disease threat is detected anywhere on the globe. Outbreak assistance by CDC would also be required if an intentionally caused outbreak occurred at home or abroad.

CDC's growing presence overseas presents new opportunities and new challenges. This document—developed in consultation with public and private sector partners, at home and abroad—represents an active effort to further define CDC's evolving global mission. It considers how CDC and its international partners can work together over the long term to improve the capacity to detect, control, and prevent infectious diseases. CDC's ongoing efforts to strengthen U.S. domestic public health infrastructure are critical to the success of these international collaborations.

Protecting the Nation's Health in an Era of Globalization: CDC's Global Strategy for Addressing Infectious Diseases defines CDC's global infectious disease priorities in six areas, selected in consultation with global public health partners. In looking towards the future, CDC envisions increased activity and progress in each area:

1. **International Outbreak Assistance:** An underlying principle of the global strategy is the recognition that international outbreak assistance is an integral function of CDC. Supporting this function will require augmenting, updating, and strengthening CDC's diagnostic facilities, as well as its capacity for epidemiologic investigation overseas. In the future, CDC must also be prepared, as a matter of routine, to offer follow-up assistance after each acute emergency response. Such follow-up will assist host-country ministries of health to maintain control of new pathogens when an outbreak is over.

2. **A Global Approach to Disease Surveillance:** In the years ahead, regional surveillance networks should expand, interact, and evolve into a global "network of networks" that provides early warning of emerging health threats and increased capacity to monitor the effectiveness of public health control measures. CDC will help stimulate this process by providing technical assistance, evaluating regional progress, and working with many partners to strengthen the networks' telecommunications capacities and encourage the use of common software tools and harmonized standards for disease reporting.

3. **Applied Research on Diseases of Global Importance:** A research program on diseases that are of global importance, including some that are uncommon in the United States, is a valuable resource, both for humanitarian reasons and because of the dangers represented by some imported diseases. CDC's laboratorians, epidemiologists, and behavioral scientists will maintain an active research program to develop tools to detect, diagnose, predict, and eliminate diseases of global or regional importance. When a new disease threat is reported anywhere in the world, CDC's laboratorians and field investigators will be available to help answer questions about disease transmission, treatment, control, and prevention.

4. **Application of Proven Public Health Tools:** There is often a long delay between the development of a new public health tool and its widespread use. CDC will intensify efforts to couple applied research with research on ways to promote the use of newly developed tools for disease control ("implementation research"). CDC will help identify the most effective tools and actively encourage their international use, applying expertise and resources in laboratory research, public health policy, program management, and health communications to overcome scientific, financial, and cultural barriers.

5. **Global Initiatives for Disease Control:** CDC will make sustained contributions to global initiatives to reduce the prevalence of HIV/AIDS in young people by 25% and reduce deaths from tuberculosis and malaria by 50% by 2010. CDC will also work with the Global Alliance for Vaccines and Immunization to reduce infant mortality through enhanced delivery and use of new and underutilized vaccines against respiratory illnesses and other childhood diseases. CDC and its partners will also consult on future international priorities for disease control, elimination, and eradication efforts—as well on monitoring for antimicrobial resistance and planning for pandemic influenza—and help evaluate progress through the collection and analysis of disease surveillance data.

6. **Public Health Training and Capacity Building:** CDC will encourage and support the establishment of International Emerging Infections Programs (IEIPs) in developing countries—centers of excellence that integrate disease surveillance, applied research, prevention, and control activities. The IEIP sites will partner with Field Epidemiology Training Programs (FETPs) and other institutions to strengthen national public health capacity and provide hands-on training in public health. Over time, they may help to strengthen capacity in neighboring countries as well as within the host country.

Source: U.S. Centers for Disease Control. "Protecting the Nation's Health in an Era of Globalization: CDC's Global Strategy for Addressing Infectious Diseases." Available online. URL: http://www.cdc.gov/globalidplan/3-exec_summary.htm. Accessed September 5, 2006.

Preventing Flu in Child Care Settings, 2006

Although the public has become concerned about the threat of avian influenza or flu, ordinary seasonal flu continues to take a toll in misery every year, and can sometimes even be fatal, especially among sick people, infants, young children, and the elderly. The Centers for Disease Control issues fact sheets for a variety of work environments about how to limit the damage.

Symptoms

Symptoms of flu include fever, headache, tiredness, cough, sore throat, runny or stuffy nose, and muscle aches. Nausea, vomiting, and diarrhea also can occur, and are much more common among children than adults.

Spread of the Flu

The main way that flu is spread is from person to person through coughs and sneezes. This can happen when people are exposed to droplets from the cough or sneeze of an infected person, or when a person touches droplets, nose drainage or saliva from an infected person, or a soiled object, and then touches one's own (or someone else's) nose or mouth before washing hands.

Preventing Spread of the Flu in Child Care Settings

Vaccination against the flu each fall is the single best way to prevent influenza. Vaccination, along with other measures, also may help to decrease the spread of influenza among children in the child care setting and among care providers.

Recommend influenza vaccination for children and care providers in child care settings.

Influenza vaccine is recommended for:

- all children age 6 months until their 5th birthday
- people who care for children 0–5 years of age
    - Children <6 months old are not eligible for the flu vaccine, but are at high risk of influenza complications. The best way to protect children <6 months of age is to vaccinate everyone around them.
- people of any age who have medical conditions that place them at increased risk for serious influenza-related complications.

Remind children and care providers to wash their hands or use alcohol-based hand rubs, and make sure that supplies are available.

- Encourage care providers and children to use soap and water to wash hands when hands are visibly soiled, or an alcohol-based hand rub when soap and water are not available, and hands are not visibly soiled.
- Encourage care providers to wash their hands to the extent possible between contacts with infants and children, such as before meals or feedings, after wiping the child's nose or mouth, after touching objects such as tissues or surfaces soiled with saliva or nose drainage, after diaper changes, and after assisting a child with toileting.
- Encourage care providers to wash the hands of infants and toddlers when the hands become soiled.

- Encourage children to wash hands when their hands have become soiled. Teach children to wash hands for 15–20 seconds (long enough for children to sing the "Happy Birthday" song twice).
- Oversee the use of alcohol-based hand rubs by children and avoid using these on the sensitive skin of infants and toddlers.
- Rub hands thoroughly until the alcohol has dried, when using alcohol-based hand rub.
- Keep alcohol-based hand rubs out of the reach of children to prevent unsupervised use.
- Ensure that sink locations and restrooms are stocked with soap, paper towels or working hand dryers.
- Ensure that each child care room and diaper changing area is supplied with alcohol-based hand rub when sinks for washing hands are not readily accessible. Alcohol-based hand rubs are not recommended when hands are visibly soiled.

Keep the child care environment clean and make sure that supplies are available.

- Clean frequently touched surfaces, toys, and commonly shared items at least daily and when visibly soiled.
- Use an Environmental Protection Agency (EPA)-registered household disinfectant labeled for activity against bacteria and viruses, an EPA-registered hospital disinfectant, or EPA-registered chlorine bleach/hypochlorite solution. Always follow label instructions when using any EPA-registered disinfectant. If EPA-registered chlorine bleach is not available and a generic (i.e., store brand) chlorine bleach is used, mix ¼ cup chlorine bleach with 1 gallon of cool water.
- Keep disinfectants out of the reach of children.

Remind children and care providers to cover their noses and mouths when sneezing or coughing.

- Advise children and care providers to cover their noses and mouths with a tissue when sneezing or coughing, and to put their used tissue in a waste basket.
- Make sure that tissues are available in all nurseries, child care rooms, and common areas such as reading rooms, classrooms, and rooms where meals are provided.
- Encourage care providers and children to wash their hands or use an alcohol-based hand rub as soon as possible, if they have sneezed or coughed on their hands.

Observe all children for symptoms of respiratory illness, especially when there is increased influenza in the community.

- Observe closely all infants and children for symptoms of respiratory illness. Notify the parent if a child develops a fever (100°F. or higher under the arm, 101°F. orally, or 102°F. rectally) or chills, cough, sore throat, headache, or muscle aches. Send the child home, if possible, and advise the parent to contact the child's doctor.

Encourage parents of sick children to keep their children home. Encourage sick care providers to stay home.

- Encourage parents of sick children to keep the children home and away from the child care setting until the children have been without fever for 24 hours, to prevent spreading illness to others. Similarly, encourage sick care providers to stay home.

Consult your local health department when increases in respiratory illness occur in the child care setting.

- Consult with your local or state health department for recommendations to prevent the spread of respiratory illness.

Source: Centers for Disease Control and Prevention. "Preventing the Spread of Influenza (the Flu) in Child Care Settings: Guidance for Administrators, Care Providers, and Other Staff," November 8, 2006. Available online. URL: http://www.cdc.gov/flu/professionals/infectioncontrol/childcaresettings.htm. Accessed September 15, 2006.

AIDS at 25: An Overview of Major Trends in the U.S. Epidemic, 2006

The year 2006 marked 25 years since the HIV/AIDS epidemic first surfaced in the United States Many government, health, and academic institutions issued summary reports on developments since 1981. The following selection is from the Kaiser Family Foundation of California's report.

Section One:
Overview of Major Trends in the U.S. Epidemic

- HIV incidence in the U.S. rose quickly and steeply in the early years of the epidemic, reaching its peak in the mid-1980s at an estimated 160,000. Since that time, HIV incidence has dropped significantly, largely due to prevention efforts. However, the number of new HIV infections has remained steady for more than a decade, at an estimated 40,000 per year.

- AIDS incidence also increased for the first 15 years of the epidemic. Because AIDS case trends "lag" HIV incidence trends, due to the delay between HIV infection and progression to an AIDS diagnosis, AIDS cases reached their peak in the 1990s, almost a decade later than HIV incidence. New AIDS cases began to drop at this point, primarily due to the introduction of highly active antiretroviral therapy (HAART), which led to significant declines in HIV morbidity and mortality, but also due to prevention efforts that resulted in decreasing HIV incidence in earlier years. Declines in AIDS incidence leveled in recent years and cases have begun to rise again.
- HIV death rates, and deaths among people with AIDS, increased during the first 15 years of the epidemic and were highest in the mid-1990s. Since that time, they have dropped sharply, primarily due to HAART. More recently, however, the decline in deaths has begun to level off.
- Today there are more than one million people estimated to be living with HIV/AIDS in the U.S. including almost half a million with AIDS. HIV/AIDS prevalence is at its highest level ever and continues to rise each year. The only exception to this steady rise was in the mid-1990s, before the advent of HAART, when annual deaths among people with AIDS actually exceeded the number of new HIV infections. Increasing HIV/AIDS prevalence over time is due both to more effective treatments, which have reduced HIV-related morbidity and mortality, and to the continuing number of new HIV infections that occur in the U.S. each year.

Section Two: Major Trends by Population and Other Key Characteristics

- The share of new AIDS cases among Black non-Hispanics has risen significantly over time, surpassing that of whites in 1994. Today, Blacks account for half of all new AIDS cases in the U.S. The share of AIDS cases among Latinos has also risen over time. AIDS case rates per 100,000 are highest among Blacks who, along with American Indian/Alaska Natives, were the only racial/ethnic groups with higher AIDS case rates in 2004 compared to 1990.
- Due to more effective treatments and the drop in HIV incidence from its high level in the 1980s, annual AIDS incidence has fallen over time. However, not all groups have experienced the same rate of

decline—cases among whites dropped the most between 1996 and 2004 (44%). Cases among Blacks dropped by 21% and cases among Latinos dropped by 27%. More recently, cases have started to rise again for all groups.

- While men continue to account for the majority of AIDS cases in the U.S., the share among women has risen over time, from 8% in 1985 to 27% in 2004. In addition, although the number of AIDS cases among men and women has dropped since their peak in the mid 1990s, the decrease has been less pronounced for women (13% for women compared to 35% for men). Cases have recently been on the rise for both men and women.
- HIV transmission patterns have shifted over time, with the share of cases attributable to heterosexual transmission rising from 3% in 1985 to 31% in 2004. Over that same period, the share of cases attributable to sex between men fell from 64% to 42% (although this still represents the single largest transmission category). The share of cases due to injection drug use was 19% in 1985, peaked at 31% in 1993, and was 22% in 2004.
- Although HIV death rates have decreased over time for all racial/ethnic groups, disparities have become more pronounced, particularly for Black men and women (ages 25–44) compared to their white counterparts.

Section Three:
Major Trends by Region, State, and Metropolitan Area

- Over time, there have been regional shifts in the HIV/AIDS epidemic. The share of AIDS cases in the U.S. South has increased, rising from 40% of cases in 1996 to almost half (48%) of cases in 2004. The Northeast and West each accounted for smaller shares in 2004 compared to the earlier period.
- While the number of AIDS cases has declined across all regions, the Western region experienced the greatest percent decline (-43%) and the South experienced the least (-16%). Cases in the Northeast declined by 40% and cases in the Midwest by 25%.
- Despite the growing share of AIDS cases occurring in the South, the Northeast had the highest concentration of AIDS cases, as measured by AIDS case rate per 100,000, in both 1996 and 2004.
- There have also been shifts at the state and local level. Nine of the 10 states accounting for the greatest number of AIDS cases in 1987 remained on the top 10 list in 2004, although their relative order had shifted. There has been a bigger shift by AIDS case rate per 100,000,

with only 6 of the top 10 states in 1987 remaining in the top 10 by 2004.

- Similarly, nine of the 10 metropolitan areas accounting for the greatest number of AIDS cases in 1987 were in the top 10 in 2004; as with states, their relative order has shifted over time. Only 3 metropolitan areas with the top 10 highest AIDS case rates per 100,000 in 1987 remained in the top 10 in 2004.

Section Four:
Major Trends in Federal Funding for HIV/AIDS

- Federal funding to address the newly emerging AIDS epidemic began soon after the first cases of AIDS were reported, with $8 million allocated in FY 1982. Funding has increased significantly over time, reaching $1.6 billion by 1988, $10 billion by 1998, and $22 billion by FY 2006.
- Federal funding for HIV/AIDS has shifted by category over the course of the epidemic. In the earliest years, most funding was for HIV research, as scientists sought to identify the causal agent of the new disease, and develop diagnostic and therapeutic options. Funding for care and treatment quickly began to rise and, by 1990, represented the same share as research. Funding for the global epidemic first began in the late 1980s and was at 3% in 1990. By 2006, domestic care and treatment accounted for the majority of federal funding for HIV/AIDS (58%). Global funding accounted for the next largest share (15%). Domestic prevention funding accounted for the smallest share (4%).
- Funding for HIV research has risen significantly over time, and is now at just over $2 billion, although its rate of increase has slowed recently. Funding for domestic HIV prevention at the Centers for Disease Control and Prevention, which accounts for the bulk of federal funding for domestic prevention efforts, has also risen over time but it too has slowed in recent years, and decreased between FY 2005 and FY 2006.
- Spending by federal Medicaid on care and treatment for people with HIV/AIDS in the U.S. represents the greatest share of HIV/AIDS care funding, and has risen significantly and steadily over time. Medicare accounts for the second largest share, and has also risen steadily over time.
- Funding for the Ryan White CARE Act, first enacted in 1990, now accounts for the third largest share of federal care funding. It has not

risen as steeply as Medicaid and Medicare spending and, in recent years, has remained relatively flat.

Source: The Henry J. Kaiser Family Foundation, May 31, 2006. "AIDS at 25: An Overview of Major Trends in the U.S. Epidemic" (#7525). Available online. URL: http://www.kff.org/hivaids/7525.cfm. Accessed September 5, 2006. This information was reprinted with permission from the Henry J. Kaiser Family Foundation. The Kaiser Family Foundation, based in Menlo Park, California, is a nonprofit, private operating foundation focusing on the major health care issues facing the nation and is not associated with Kaiser Permanente or Kaiser Industries.

The Lyme Controversy

Doctors and public health workers agree that Lyme disease is a growing problem in many areas of the United States However, there are major differences of opinion within these groups about just how widespread and serious the problem is. This has caused serious legal and financial disputes among state health and legal authorities, insurance companies, doctors, and hospitals. The following two sets of guidelines show some of these differences of opinion.

IDSA Guidelines, 2006

The Infectious Diseases Society of America (IDSA) issued new diagnosis and treatment guidelines for Lyme disease in 2006. They probably represent the mainstream opinion within the medical community nationwide. The IDSA, as can be seen, does not recommend routine use of antibiotics ("antimicrobial prophylaxis") for most people with tick bites. In addition, the IDSA seems to be skeptical about the existence of a post-Lyme syndrome when there is no longer clear proof that a patient is infected with the disease bacteria.

Tick Bites and Prophylaxis of Lyme Disease

For prevention of Lyme disease after a recognized tick bite, routine use of antimicrobial prophylaxis or serologic testing is not recommended. A single dose of doxycycline may be offered to adult patients (200 mg dose) and to children ≥8 years of age (4 mg/kg up to a maximum dose of 200 mg) when *all* of the following circumstances exist: (a) the attached tick can be reliably identified as an adult or nymphal *I. scapularis* tick that is estimated to have been attached for ≥36 h on the basis of the degree of engorgement of the tick with blood or of certainty about the time of exposure to the tick; (b) prophylaxis can be started within 72 h of the time that the tick was removed; (c) ecologic information indicates that the local rate of infection of these ticks with *B. burgdorferi* is≥20%; *and* (d) doxycycline treatment is not contraindicated. The time limit of 72 h is suggested because of the absence of data on the efficacy of chemoprophylaxis for tick bites following tick removal after longer time intervals. Infection of ≥20% of ticks with *B. burgdorferi* generally occurs in parts of New England, in parts of the mid-Atlantic States, and in parts of Minnesota and Wisconsin, but not in most other locations in the United States. Whether use of antibiotic prophylaxis after a tick bite will reduce the incidence of HGA or babesiosis is unknown.

Doxycycline is relatively contraindicated in pregnant women and children <8 years old. The panel does not believe that amoxicillin should be substituted for doxycycline in persons for whom doxycycline prophylaxis is contraindicated because of the absence of data on an effective short-course regimen for prophylaxis, the likely need for a multiday regimen (and its associated adverse effects), the excellent efficacy of antibiotic treatment of Lyme disease if infection were to develop, and the extremely low risk that a person with a recognized bite will develop a serious complication of Lyme disease.

Prophylaxis after *I. pacificus* bites is generally not necessary, because rates of infection with *B. burgdorferi* in these ticks are low in almost the entire region in which the tick is endemic. However, if a higher infection rate were documented in specific local areas (≥20%), prophylaxis with single-dose doxycycline would be justified if the other criteria mentioned above are met.

To prescribe antibiotic prophylaxis selectively to prevent Lyme disease, health care practitioners in areas of endemicity should learn to identify *I. scapularis* ticks, including its stages (*figure 1*), and to differentiate ticks that are at least partially engorged with blood (*figure 2A* and *2B*) (A-III). Testing of ticks for tickborne infectious agents is not recommended, except in research studies.

* *** *

Post–Lyme Disease Syndromes

There is no well-accepted definition of post–Lyme disease syndrome. This has contributed to confusion and controversy and to a lack of firm data on its incidence, prevalence, and pathogenesis. In an attempt to provide a framework for future research on this subject and to reduce diagnostic ambiguity in study populations, a definition for post–Lyme disease syndrome is proposed in these guidelines. Whatever definition is eventually adopted, having once had objective evidence of *B. burgdorferi* infection must be a condition sine qua non. Furthermore, when laboratory testing is done to support the original diagnosis of Lyme disease, it is essential that it be performed by well-qualified and reputable laboratories that use recommended and appropriately validated testing methods and interpretive criteria. Unvalidated test methods (such as urine antigen tests or blood microscopy for *Borrelia* species) should not be used.

There is no convincing biologic evidence for the existence of symptomatic chronic *B. burgdorferi* infection among patients after receipt of recommended treatment regimens for Lyme disease. Antibiotic therapy has not proven to be useful and is not recommended for patients with chronic (≥6 months) subjective symptoms after recommended treatment regimens for Lyme disease.

Source: University of Chicago. "ISDA Guidelines." *Clinical Infectious Diseases* 43(2006): 1089–1134, August 2006. Available online. URL:http://www.journals.uchicago.edu/CID/journal/issues/v43n9/40897/40897.html?erFrom = -3587796628356696720Guest. Accessed September 12, 2006.

ILADS Guidelines for the Management of Lyme Disease, 2003

The International Lyme and Associated Diseases Society (ILADS) is a professional medical society whose members are involved in treating Lyme disease. This selection from the society's treatment guidelines, released in November 2003, shows that the group disagrees with the approach taken by the IDSA in the previous selection. ILADS believes that many cases of chronic Lyme disease are misdiagnosed as other diseases, causing patients to suffer needlessly. They favor the use of antibiotics in many cases where the IDSA would not.

Chronic Lyme disease: a growing epidemic

The Centers for Disease Control and Prevention (CDC) consider Lyme disease the fastest growing vector-borne disease in the USA. By conservative estimate, the number of new Lyme disease infections per year may be ten times higher than the 17,730 cases reported to the CDC during 2000. The prevalence of chronic Lyme disease ranges from 34% in a population-based, retrospective cohort study to 62% in a specialty clinic located in an area endemic for Lyme disease. Clinic patients presented with arthralgia, arthritis, cardiac and neurologic symptoms.

* *** *

The need for new guidelines

Guidelines of the Infectious Disease Society of America (IDSA) fall short of meeting the needs for diagnosis and treatment of individuals with chronic Lyme disease. The latest IDSA Guidelines (2000) fail to take into account the compelling, peer-reviewed, published evidence confirming persistent, recurrent and refractory Lyme disease and, in fact, deny its existence.

The IDSA's symptomatic approaches to Lyme disease are limited and exclude many individuals with persisting clinical and laboratory evidence of active *B. burgdorferi* infection. In addition, physicians treating individuals with Lyme and other tick-borne infections recognize the need for new guidelines to better serve the patient population.

* *** *

Competency and training

The appropriateness of treatment hinges on the clinician's experience in treating Lyme disease. Competence requires diagnostic and treatment skills heretofore not offered in medical school or postresidency training.

Clinicians more practiced in treating Lyme disease achieve better outcomes and encounter fewer complications because of an enhanced ability to interpret clinical data, the prompt prescription of antibiotics and the use of measures to reduce adverse events, e.g., employing acidophilus to replace normal intestinal flora that is depleted by antibiotics.

* *** *

Highlights of guidelines

- Since there is currently no definitive test for Lyme disease, laboratory results should not be used to exclude an individual from treatment
- Lyme disease is a clinical diagnosis and tests should be used to support rather than supersede the physician's judgment
- The early use of antibiotics can prevent persistent, recurrent and refractory Lyme disease
- The duration of therapy should be guided by clinical response, rather than by an arbitrary (i.e., 30 day) treatment course

- The practice of stopping antibiotics to allow for delayed recovery is not recommended for persistent Lyme disease. In these cases, it is reasonable to continue treatment for several months after clinical and laboratory abnormalities have begun to resolve and symptoms have disappeared

* *** *

Symptomatic presentation

Variable symptomatic presentations have been increasingly documented in Lyme disease, with the best example being encephalopathy. Encephalopathic presentations were described in an initial cohort of 27 patients as a symptom complex including memory loss (81%), fatigue (74%), headache (48%), depression (37%), sleep disturbance (30%) and irritability (26%), often without objective markers. Only two of the 27 patients presented with objective findings on lumbar puncture: one had pleocytosis (seven cells) and a second had an antibody index of greater than one.

Neuropsychiatric presentations in acute and chronic Lyme disease have been increasingly recognized and can include depression, anxiety and rage. These are presumably related to persistent infection and are potentially reversible with antibiotics. Neuropsychiatric symptoms may reflect additional psychosocial processes including the stress of coping with a chronic illness.

Asch and colleagues found that more than half of 215 patients in a Lyme-endemic region had symptomatic presentations of chronic Lyme disease. The patients presented with chronic fatigue, headaches and joint pain (but not headaches alone) in this retrospective cohort study.

Increasing evidence of persistent infection

Persistent, recurrent and refractory presentations from ongoing infection are the most feared of the long-term complications of Lyme disease.

Laboratory culture of *B. burgdorferi* has documented persistent infection in chronic Lyme disease patients, but the yields are quite low by current methods. In fact, there is no reliable, commercially available culture assay that can confirm the eradication of the organism. Using experimental techniques, however, *B. burgdorferi* has been detected in virtually every organ in the body, and the spirochete has a strong predilection for the central nervous system. Oral antibiotic levels in the central nervous system are low, and this fact may necessitate the addition of drugs with good penetration across the blood–brain barrier, such as intravenous ceftriaxone or cefotaxime.

Most studies demonstrate a beneficial effect of antibiotics in the management of chronic Lyme disease, but the extent of optimal treatment is still uncertain. Recent clinical trials questioning the benefits of antibiotics have been criticized for enrolling patients with refractory Lyme disease who were sick for a mean of 4.7 years despite an average of three courses of antibiotics, and for relying only on one treatment protocol (1 month of i.v. ceftriaxone followed by 2 months of low-dose oral doxycycline). In view of these methodological problems, persistent infection remains a continued concern for physicians.

Source: International Lyme and Associated Diseases Society. "Evidence-based Guidelines for the Management of Lyme Disease," November 2003. Available online. URL: http://www.ilads.org/files/ILADS_Guidelines.pdf. Accessed September 23, 2006.

Executive Order Relating to the Immunization of Young Women from the Cancer-Causing Human Papillomavirus, 2007

The Food and Drug Administration (FDA) in 2006 approved a new vaccine to protect people against the human papilloma virus. This virus, which can cause cervical cancer in women, has become very common in recent years. Some religious groups announced their opposition to mass vaccination. They feared it might send a subtle message that girls were expected to have sex before marriage. In early 2007, however, the conservative governor of Texas issued an executive order making his state the first to require HPV vaccination, covering young schoolgirls. As Governor Perry noted, "Young women who have abstained from sex until marriage have contracted HPV from their husbands and faced the difficult task of defeating cervical cancer." Governor Perry's order was overturned by the Texas legislature in April 2007.

Austin, Texas, February 2, 2007

WHEREAS, immunization from vaccine-preventable diseases such as Human Papillomavirus (HPV) protects individuals who receive the vaccine; and

WHEREAS, HPV is the most common sexually transmitted infection-causing cancer in females in the United States; and

WHEREAS, the United States Food and Drug Administration estimates there are 9,710 new cases of cervical cancer, many of which are caused by HPV, and 3,700 deaths from cervical cancer each year in the United States; and

WHEREAS, the Texas Cancer Registry estimates there were 1,169 new cases and 391 deaths from cervical cancer in Texas in 2006; and

WHEREAS, research has shown that the HPV vaccine is highly effective in preventing the infections that are the cause of many of the cervical cancers; and

WHEREAS, HPV vaccine is only effective if administered before infection occurs; and

WHEREAS, the newly approved HPV vaccine is a great advance in the protection of women's health; and

WHEREAS, the Advisory Committee on Immunization Practices and Centers for Disease Control and Prevention recommend the HPV vaccine for females who are nine years through 26 years of age;

NOW THEREFORE, I, RICK PERRY, Governor of Texas, by virtue of the power and authority vested in me by the Constitution and laws of the State of Texas as the Chief Executive Officer, do hereby order the following:

Vaccine. The Department of State Health Services shall make the HPV vaccine available through the Texas Vaccines for Children program for eligible young females up to age 18, and the Health and Human Services Commission shall make the vaccine available to Medicaid-eligible young females from age 19 to 21.

Rules. The Health and Human Services Executive Commissioner shall adopt rules that mandate the age appropriate vaccination of all female children for HPV prior to admission to the sixth grade.

Availability. The Department of State Health Services and the Health and Human Services Commission will move expeditiously to make the vaccine available as soon as possible.

Public Information. The Department of State Health Services will implement a public awareness campaign to educate the public of the importance of vaccination, the availability of the vaccine, and the subsequent requirements under the rules that will be adopted.

Parents' Rights. The Department of State Health Services will, in order to protect the right of parents to be the final authority on their children's health care, modify the current process in order to allow parents to submit a request for a conscientious objection affidavit form via the Internet while maintaining privacy safeguards under current law.

This executive order supersedes all previous orders on this matter that are in conflict or inconsistent with its terms and this order shall remain in effect and in full force until modified, amended, rescinded, or superseded by me or by a succeeding governor.

Source: State of Texas. "Executive Order RP65—February 2, 2007." Available online. URL: http://www.governor.state.tx.us/divisions/press/exorders/rp65. Accessed February 10, 2007.

DOCUMENTS REGARDING POSSIBLE FUTURE EVENTS

National Strategy for Pandemic Influenza, Implementation Plan, 2006

The U.S. Homeland Security Council, a body within the Office of the President, was set up after September 11, 2001, to coordinate national policy in response to both terror and natural disasters, such as epidemic disease. In May 2006 the council published a 234-page implementation plan, which outlines the respective responsibilities of federal, state, local, and nongovernmental bodies for dealing with the threat of avian flu and other potential new influenzas. The selection below is from the "Executive Summary."

Chapter 2—U.S. Government Planning for a Pandemic

The President announced the *National Strategy for Pandemic Influenza (Strategy)* on November 1, 2005. The Strategy provides a high-level overview of the approach that the Federal Government will take to prepare for and respond to a pandemic, and articulates expectations of non-Federal entities to prepare themselves and their communities. The Strategy contains three pillars: (1) preparedness and communication; (2) surveillance and detection; and (3) response and containment.

Preparedness for a pandemic requires the establishment of infrastructure and capacity, a process that can take years. For this reason, significant steps must be taken now. The Strategy affirms that the Federal Government will use all instruments of national power to address the pandemic threat. The Federal Government will collaborate fully with international partners to attempt containment of a potential pandemic wherever sustained and efficient human-to-human transmission is documented, and will make every reasonable effort to delay the introduction of a pandemic virus to the United States. If these efforts fail, responding effectively to an uncontained pandemic domestically will require the full participation of all levels of government and all segments of society. The Implementation Plan (Plan) for the *Strategy* makes it clear that every segment of society must prepare for a pandemic and will be a part of the response. The Plan further recognizes that the Federal Government must provide clear criteria and decision tools to inform State, local, and private sector planning and response actions, and that Federal agencies must be prepared to supplement and support State and local efforts where necessary and feasible.

The *Strategy* must be translated into tangible action that fully engages the breadth of the Federal Government. This Plan provides a common frame of reference for understanding the pandemic threat and summarizes key planning considerations for all partners. It also proposes that Federal departments and agencies take specific, coordinated steps to achieve the goals of the *Strategy* and outlines expectations of non-Federal stakeholders in the United States and abroad. Joint and integrated planning across all levels of government and the private sector is essential to ensure that available national capabilities and authorities produce detailed plans and response actions that are complementary, compatible, and coordinated.

The Federal Government has already taken a historic series of actions, domestically and internationally, to address the pandemic threat. The actions include the development of a promising human vaccine against the H5N1 avian influenza virus, the submission of a $7.1 billion budget request over several years to support pandemic preparedness, the establishment of the International Partnership on Avian and Pandemic Influenza, and the first Cabinet-level exercise to assess the Federal Government response to a naturally occurring threat.

Chapter 3—Federal Government Response to a Pandemic

The goals of the Federal Government response to a pandemic are to: (1) stop, slow, or otherwise limit the spread of a pandemic to the United States; (2) limit the domestic spread of a pandemic, and mitigate disease, suffering and death; and (3) sustain infrastructure and mitigate impact to the economy and the functioning of society (see *Stages of Federal Government Response* between Chapters 5 and 6).

Unlike geographically and temporally bounded disasters, a pandemic will spread across the globe over the course of months or over a year, possibly in waves, and will affect communities of all sizes and compositions. In terms of its scope, the impact of a severe pandemic may be more comparable to that of war or a widespread economic crisis than a hurricane, earthquake, or act of terrorism. In addition to coordinating a comprehensive and timely national response, the Federal Government will bear primary responsibility for certain critical functions, including: (1) the support of containment efforts overseas and limitation of the arrival of a pandemic to our shores; (2) guidance related to protective measures that should be taken; (3) modifications to the law and regulations to facilitate the national pandemic response; (4) modifications to monetary policy to mitigate the economic impact of a pandemic on communities and the Nation; (5) procurement and distribution of vaccine and antiviral medications; and (6) the acceleration of research and development of vaccines and therapies during the outbreak.

The center of gravity of the pandemic response, however, will be in communities. The distributed nature of a pandemic, as well as the sheer burden of disease across the Nation over a period of months or longer, means that the Federal Government's support to any particular State, Tribal Nation, or community will be limited in comparison to the aid it mobilizes for disasters such as earthquakes or hurricanes, which strike a more confined geographic area over a shorter period of time. Local communities will have to address the medical and non-medical effects of the pandemic with available resources. This means that it is essential for communities, tribes, States, and regions to have plans in place to support the full spectrum of their needs over the course of weeks or months, and for the Federal Government to provide clear guidance on the manner in which these needs can be met.

Command, Control, and Coordination of the Federal Response during a Pandemic

It is important that the Federal Government have a defined mechanism for coordination of its response. The *National Response Plan* (NRP) is the primary mechanism for coordination of the Federal Government's response to Incidents of National Significance, and will guide the Federal pandemic response. It defines Federal departmental responsibilities for sector-specific responses, and provides the structure and mechanisms for effective coordination among Federal, State, local, and tribal authorities, the private sector, and non-governmental organizations (NGOs). Pursuant to the NRP and Homeland Security Presidential Directive 5 (HSPD-5), the Secretary of Homeland Security is responsible for coordination of Federal operations and resources, establishment of reporting requirements, and conduct of ongoing communications with Federal, State, local, and tribal governments, the private sector, and NGOs.

A pandemic will present unique challenges to the coordination of the Federal response. First and foremost, the types of support that the Federal Government will provide to the Nation are of a different kind and character than those it traditionally provides to communities damaged by natural disasters.

Second, although it may occur in discrete waves in any one locale, the national impact of a pandemic could last for many months. Finally, a pandemic is a sustained public health and medical emergency that will have sustained and profound consequences for the operation of critical infrastructure, the mobility of people and freight, and the global economy. Health and medical considerations will affect foreign policy, international trade and travel, domestic disease containment efforts, continuity of operations within the Federal Government, and many other aspects of the Federal response.

Pursuant to the NRP, as the primary agency and coordinator for Emergency Support Function #8 (Public Health and Medical Services), the Secretary of Health and Human Services will lead Federal health and medical response efforts and will be the principal Federal spokesperson for public health issues, coordinating closely with DHS on public messaging pertaining to the pandemic. Pursuant to HSPD-5, as the principal Federal official for domestic incident management, the Secretary of Homeland Security will provide coordination for Federal operations and resources, establish reporting requirements, and conduct ongoing communications with Federal, State, local, and tribal governments, the private sector, and NGOs. In the context of response to a pandemic, the Secretary of Homeland Security will coordinate overall non-medical support and response actions, and ensure necessary support to the Secretary of Health and Human Services' coordination of public health and medical emergency response efforts.

The NRP stipulates mechanisms for coordination of the Federal response, but sustaining these mechanisms for several months to over a year will present unique challenges. Day-to-day situational monitoring will occur through the national operations center, and strategic policy development and coordination on domestic pandemic response issues will be accomplished through an interagency body composed of senior decision-makers from across the government and chaired by the White House. These and other considerations applicable to response to a pandemic will be incorporated in the NRP review process and will inform recommendations on revisions and improvements to the NRP and associated annexes.

Pursuant to the NRP, policy issues that cannot be resolved at the department level will be addressed through the Homeland Security Council/National Security Council (HSC/NSC)-led policy coordination process.

Source: Homeland Security Council. *National Strategy for Pandemic Influenza: Implementation Plan*, May, 2006. Available online. URL: http://www.whitehouse.gov/homeland/nspi_implementation.pdf. Accessed September 24, 2007

Pandemic Influenza Plan, 2006

In February 2006 the New York State Department of Health published an influenza plan, in line with its responsibilities under the federal Pandemic Influenza Plan issued the previous year. It outlined the duties and rights of state and local bodies to prepare for and deal with a possible deadly flu epidemic. The section extracted below deals with contact tracing, an important public health tool.

Appendix 8-B—Contact Identification and Management

Surveillance of contacts of cases infected with a novel influenza virus may be helpful in *early* control efforts. Through rapid identification, evaluation, and monitoring of exposed contacts, further transmission of disease may be prevented or reduced. Contacts who are found to be clinically ill can be quickly isolated to avoid further novel influenza virus transmission. When contact identification and management is indicated, surveillance of contacts will be conducted by LHDs [local health department], with assistance from NYSDOH as needed. NYSDOH, in consultation with CDC [U.S. Centers for Disease Control) and LHDs, will provide guidance regarding if and when contact tracing should be conducted.

- **Definitions**
  - **Close Contact**: A person who cared for or lived with a person with a novel influenza virus or who had a high likelihood of direct contact with respiratory secretions and/or body fluids of a person with a novel influenza virus (during encounters with the patient or through contact with materials contaminated by the patient), during the period of 24 hours prior to the patient's onset to 14 days

after onset of symptoms (*note: the definition of the infectious period is under discussion with the CDC*). Examples of close contact include kissing or embracing, sharing eating or drinking utensils, close conversation (< 3 feet), physical examination, and any other direct physical contact between persons. Close contact does not include activities such as walking by a person or sitting across a waiting room or office for a brief time.

- **Infectious Period**: Period of time from the 24 hours prior to onset symptoms to up to 14 days after the onset of symptoms (*note: the definition of the infectious period is under discussion with the CDC*).

- **Contact Identification and Tracing**
  - Determine the time period in which the case was infectious.
  - Initiate identification of a case's contacts as soon as possible after a diagnosis of probable or confirmed infection with a novel influenza virus.
    - Obtain information about the case and all contacts from the case, next of kin, workplace representatives, or others with appropriate knowledge of the case-patient's recent whereabouts and activities.
  - Attempt to locate and contact all close contacts within 12 hours of the case/contact report.
    - Use work and school contact numbers, telephone directories, voting lists, neighborhood interviews, site visits, etc. to trace contacts when locating information is unknown or incomplete.
    - If having difficulty locating a contact, consult with STD and/or TB staff who have contact tracing experience.
  - If the contact has left the county and/or state, notify the NYSDOH Regional Epidemiologist.

- **Contact Evaluation and Monitoring**
  - Alert contacts of their potential exposure to a novel influenza virus.
  - Verify exposures.
  - Verify exposure to index case during the period of infectiousness.
  - Verify the type of exposure.
  - If initial contact is made at a home or workplace visit, the appropriate personal protective equipment (PPE) should be utilized since the contact's health status will be unknown.
  - Evaluate contact's health status using the Pandemic Influenza Contact Record Form (Appendix 8-C).

- Ensure prophylaxis is provided, if indicated.
- Identify any additional contacts who may not have been listed by the index case.
- Enter data from the Contact Record Form on the HIN.
- Consider quarantine of contacts based on the level of influenza activity:

- **Ill Contacts**
  - If the contact is febrile or has respiratory symptoms, make arrangements for a medical evaluation by a healthcare provider.
    - Ensure that the medical facility staff are informed and prepared to handle a suspect novel influenza virus case.
    - Ensure that the contact does not take public transportation en route to their medical evaluation.
    - Advise the contact to remain at home and use respiratory precautions until they are evaluated by a healthcare provider.
  - Ill contacts should be counseled, interviewed, and reported as a suspected novel influenza virus case using the Pandemic Influenza Case Reporting Form (see Section 2: Surveillance and Laboratory Testing), and his/her contacts should be identified using the Pandemic Influenza Contact Record Form

- **Well Contacts**
  - Initiate plans for ongoing symptom monitoring for 10 days after their last exposure to a novel influenza virus case. Monitoring of contacts may be active (e.g., regular workplace body temperature monitoring by a supervisor) or passive (e.g., self monitoring of symptoms and temperature by the contact with reporting to the local health department at least once a day).
    - Determine the time period in which the contact must be monitored (10 days after last exposure).
    - Provide thermometers to any contacts who do not have and are not willing to purchase one.
    - Provide contact with a daily temperature/symptom log (Appendix 8-D).
    - Complete the Pandemic Influenza Contact Daily Temperature Log Tracking Form (Appendix 8-E). Update the form each day.
    - Enter contact monitoring/symptom data on the HIN.

- Provide information on seeking medical care should the contact develop fever and/or respiratory symptoms while they are being monitored.
    - Immediately notify the LHD.
    - Seek medical evaluation by a healthcare provider.
    - Ensure the medical facility is informed and prepared to handle a suspect novel influenza virus case.
    - Ensure the contact does not take public transportation en route to their medical evaluation.
    - Advise the contact to remain at home and use respiratory precautions until they are evaluated by a healthcare provider.

Modify, as needed, existing procedures for locating contacts who are lost to follow-up during the monitoring period.

Source: New York State Department of Health. *Pandemic Influenza Plan,* February 2006. Available online. URL: http://www.health.state.ny.us/diseases/communicable/influenza/pandemic/docs/pandemic_influenza_plan.pdf#search=%22new%20york%20state%20pandemic%20influenza%20plan%22. Accessed May 17, 2006

It's Not Flu as Usual: What Businesses Need to Know about Pandemic Flu Planning, 2005

The Trust for America's Health is a nonprofit organization in Washington, D.C., interested in disease prevention programs. This brochure is designed to encourage businesses to plan and prepare for a flu pandemic.

What a Pandemic Flu Could Mean to Your Business

Each winter, the flu kills approximately 36,000–40,000 Americans, hospitalizes more than 200,000, and costs the U. S. economy over $10 billion in lost productivity and direct medical expenses.

Bad as that is, health experts are now warning about a far more lethal kind of flu—a pandemic flu that could kill over half a million in the U.S., hospitalize more than 2 million, and cost our economy a staggering $70-$160 billion.

A pandemic flu will spread rapidly and easily from person to person, affecting all age groups. It will cause illness in a high proportion of those infected. Health officials are concerned that the avian "bird flu" emanating from Asia could mutate to a new strain of flu that humans have no natural immunity against—the World Health Organization has said that a bird flu pandemic could infect 25–30 percent of the world's population.

With that much of the population and workforce affected, a pandemic flu could disrupt your business—perhaps even force it to close down for a time.

What to Do in the Event of an Outbreak

If a pandemic flu strikes, government health officials will issue information and warnings and work with the media to disseminate advice on how to avoid becoming ill. Your company's managers, human resources department, and employees should pay close attention to the guidance provided by local and state health departments and the U.S. Centers for Disease Control and Prevention (www.cdc.gov.). Other organizations that provide assistance in public health emergencies include the American Red Cross (www.redcross.org), and the World Health Organization (www.who.org).

In a worst-case scenario, "business as usual" may cease. Government health officials may have to implement dramatic measures, including shutting down certain businesses that involve high levels of interaction with the public, such as restaurants and theatres. Health officials may also have to restrict travel, cancel public events such as concerts or sports, and close schools.

Plan Now to Keep Your Business in Business

"Business continuity" means ensuring that essential business functions can survive a natural disaster, technological failure, human error, or other disruption. In recent times, assuring business continuity has also meant planning for terrorist-related biological, chemical, or nuclear attacks.

Many existing business continuity plans anticipate disruptions such as fires, earthquakes, and floods; these events are restricted to a certain geographic area, and the time frames are fairly well defined and limited. Pandemic flu, however, demands a different set of continuity assumptions since it will be widely dispersed geographically and potentially arrive in waves that could last several months at a time.

Depending on the flu strain and based on previous pandemics, public health officials project **cumulative absentee rates of 25–30 percent over three to four months.** Absentees will include sick employees, and those who must care for others who are sick. Fear will also impact rates of absenteeism.

11 STEPS YOUR BUSINESS CAN TAKE

- Check that existing contingency plans are applicable to a pandemic.
- In particular, check to see that core business activities can be sustained over several weeks.
- Plan accordingly for interruptions of essential governmental services like sanitation, water, power, and disruptions to the food supply.
- Identify your company's essential functions and the individuals who perform them. The absence of these individuals could seriously impair business continuity.
- Build in the training redundancy necessary to ensure that their work can be done in the event of an absentee rate of 25–30 percent.
- Maintain a healthy work environment by ensuring adequate air circulation and posting tips on how to stop the spread of germs at work. Promote hand and respiratory hygiene. Ensure wide and easy availability of alcohol-based hand sanitizer products.
- Determine which outside activities are critical to maintaining operations and develop alternatives in case they cannot function normally. For example, what transportation systems are needed to provide essential materials? Does the business operate on "just in time" inventory or is there typically some reserve?
- Establish or expand policies and tools that enable employees to work from home with appropriate security and network access to applications.
- Expand online and self-service options for customers and business partners.
- Tell the workforce about the threat of pandemic flu and the steps the company is taking to prepare for it. In emergencies, employees demonstrate an increased tendency to listen to their employer, so clear and frequent communication is essential.
- Update sick leave and family and medical leave policies and communicate with employees about the importance of staying away from the workplace if they become ill. Concern about lost wages is the largest deterrent to self-quarantine.

Protecting Employees' Health

Flu is caused by viruses that infect the nose, throat, and lungs, and is generally spread from person to person when an infected person coughs or sneezes. An effective vaccine, when available, will be the best safeguard against pandemic flu.

In addition, the following simple, common-sense precautions can also help. Recommended by the Centers for Disease Control and Prevention, these precautions should be communicated to the workforce and posted in common areas:

- **Avoid close contact with people who are sick.** If you are sick, keep your distance from others to protect them from getting sick, too.
- **Stay home when you're sick or have flu symptoms.** Get plenty of rest and check with a health care provider as needed.
- **Cover your mouth and nose with a tissue when coughing or sneezing.** It may prevent those around you from getting sick.
- **Clean your hands.** Washing your hands often will help protect you against germs. When soap and water are not available, use alcohol-based disposable hand wipes or gel sanitizers.
- **Avoid touching your eyes, nose, or mouth.** Germs are often spread when a person touches something that is contaminated with germs and then touches his or her eyes, nose or mouth.
- **Practice other good health habits.** Get plenty of sleep, be physically active, manage stress, drink plenty of fluids, eat nutritious foods, and avoid smoking, which may increase the risk of serious consequences if you do contract the flu.

Source: Trust for America's Health. "It's Not Flu as Usual: What Businesses Need to Know about Pandemic Flu Planning." Available online. URL: http://healthyamericans.org/reports/flu/brochures/FluBrochure.pdf, Accessed 2005.

NIAID Biodefense Research Agenda for CDC Category A Agents: 2006 Progress Report

Following the September 11, 2001, terrorist attacks on New York City and Washington, and the subsequent anthrax attacks through the mail, the federal government began to ramp up research on infectious disease agents that could be used in bioterrorism, focused at the National Institute of Allergy and Infectious Diseases (NIAID). NIAID's 2006 progress report on "Category A agents" (the most deadly microbes) paints a rather rosy picture of rapid advances in understanding potential weapons such as anthrax, smallpox, plague, botulism, tularemia, and viral hemorrhagic fevers (Ebola and others).

Introduction

In 2002, the National Institute of Allergy and Infectious Diseases (NIAID), part of the National Institutes of Health (NIH), convened a Blue Ribbon

Panel on Bioterrorism and Its Implications for Biomedical Research. This panel of experts came together to provide guidance on the Institute's biodefense research agenda, which was published soon afterward. The panel included researchers from academia, industry, government, civilian agencies, and the military.

In 2003, NIAID released its first progress report on accomplishments toward the goals outlined in the Research Agenda. Since that time, extraordinary progress has been made to advance scientific knowledge of these potentially deadly pathogens. To demonstrate the enormity of the research efforts conducted over the last several years, the 2006 progress report details many examples of scientific accomplishments organized according to the areas of emphasis specified in the Research Agenda: biology of the microbe, host response, vaccines, diagnostics, and therapeutics. The achievements made meet all of the immediate goals outlined in the Research Agenda.

* *** *

While this report focuses on specific pathogens, NIAID's biodefense research is generating scientific discoveries, new technologies, and expanded resources with broader applications for improving global public health. Studies of microbial biology and the pathogenesis of organisms with bioterror potential will lead to a better understanding of other more common and naturally occurring infectious diseases. For instance, advances in biodefense research are likely to have an enormous positive impact on our ability to diagnose, treat, and prevent major infectious killers such as malaria, tuberculosis, and HIV/AIDS. Furthermore, NIAID biodefense research promises to enhance the understanding of molecular and cellular mechanisms of the immune system, which may help in the search for new ways to treat and prevent immune mediated diseases such as diabetes and rheumatoid arthritis.

New insights into the mechanisms of regulation of the human immune system will advance research on cancer, neurologic diseases, and allergic and hypersensitivity diseases.

While it is impossible to capture the true breadth of the NIAID biodefense research portfolio and accomplishments therein, the activities cited in this report most clearly demonstrate the determination and steadfastness of the Institute toward achieving the goal of developing new therapies, diagnostic tests, and vaccines.

Progress on General Recommendations of the Blue Ribbon Panel

Recommendation: Develop Regional Centers of Excellence for Bioterrorism and Emerging Infectious Diseases Research

The National Institute of Allergy and Infectious Diseases (NIAID) completed a national network of 10 Regional Centers of Excellence for Biodefense and Emerging Infectious Diseases (RCEs) in 2005. Each Center comprises a consortium of universities and complementary research institutions serving a specific geographical region. The Centers, located throughout the United States, will build and maintain a strong scientific infrastructure supporting multifaceted research and development activities that promote scientific discovery and translational research capacity required to create the next generation of therapeutics, vaccines, and diagnostics for biodefense and emerging infectious diseases. In the event of a national biodefense emergency, the RCEs will provide facilities and support to first-line responders.

Recommendation: Expand the capacity to conduct Phase I, II, and III evaluations of candidate vaccines and treatments for agents of bioterrorism.

- The NIAID Vaccine Research Center (VRC) has completed the first human clinical trial of a DNA vaccine designed to prevent Ebola infection. The vaccine, composed of three DNA plasmids, was well tolerated and elicited both humoral and cellular immune responses at all doses. In parallel, nonhuman primate challenge studies have refined the design of the final Ebola vaccine products. The DNA plasmid and recombinant adenovirus (rAd) products are currently being manufactured for clinical testing.
- The VRC has evaluated modified vaccinia Ankara (MVA) as an alternative smallpox vaccine. Two Phase I clinical trials directly testing the capacity of MVA to protect against a vaccinia (Dryvax®) challenge were performed in both vaccinia-naïve and vaccinia-immune subjects. Injection of two or more doses of MVA was shown to attenuate the clinical reaction to Dryvax and improve the vaccinia-specific immune responses. (*Dryvax® is a registered trademark of Wyeth.)
- NIAID intramural scientists have continued to develop and test vaccine formulations for each dengue subtype, and to improve formula-

tions based on clinical data. The goal is to combine the best formulation for each subtype into a tetravalent dengue vaccine. Through a contract with the Johns Hopkins Bloomberg School of Public Health Center for Immunization Research, these dengue vaccine formulations are being evaluated in clinical trials. Vaccine candidates against West Nile virus and tick-borne viral encephalitis are also being tested.

- Between 2003 and 2006, NIAID Vaccine and Treatment Evaluation Units (VTEUs) conducted 14 Phase I and II clinical trials of vaccines and therapeutics for several Category A agents, including anthrax, smallpox, and tularemia.
- NIAID physician researchers initiated a clinical protocol in 2002 to study the natural history of anthrax. The goal is to look at the infectious disease process over time, from initial infection through the clinical course and beyond recovery. A small number of anthrax survivors from the 2001 attacks have enrolled. Because the medical literature on anthrax does not include any findings regarding long-term complications in survivors, information gained in this study will be valuable to patients and doctors.
- NIAID has established the Food and Waterborne Diseases Integrated Research Network (FWDIRN) to support multidisciplinary research to facilitate development and preclinical evaluation of products to rapidly identify, prevent, and treat food and waterborne diseases that threaten public health.
- NIAID has established the Respiratory Pathogens Research Network to develop a focused and coordinated basic and clinical human respiratory pathogens research program under which preclinical research activities and Phase I clinical trials can be conducted. The network consists of a Viral Respiratory Pathogens Research Unit, a Bacterial Respiratory Pathogens Research Unit, and a Bacterial Respiratory Pathogens Reference Laboratory. Research themes include understanding microbial pathogenesis and host/pathogen interactions and identifying correlates of protection and genetic factors that may influence susceptibility to infection.
- NIAID has expanded the Collaborative Antiviral Study Group (CASG) by approximately 20 percent. A clinical protocol has been developed for the treatment of smallpox with cidofovir in the event of an outbreak or release. A Phase I clinical trial to assess initial safety, tolerability, and pharmacokinetics of a new oral derivative of cidofovir in people infected with cytomegalovirus or adenovirus is planned to begin in 2006–2007.

- In order to support increased clinical research activities, NIAID has expanded contracts for regulatory support, assay development, immunology quality assurance and quality control, and clinical trial management.

Source: "NIAID Biodefense Research Agenda for CDC Category A Agents: *2006 Progress Report*," U. S. Department of Health and Human Services, National Institutes of Health Publication No. 06-5883, January 2007.

5

International Documents

The primary sources reproduced in this chapter are from official reports, laws, firsthand accounts, or scholarly articles. The documents are divided into four sections: governmental strategies, firsthand accounts, scientific statements and findings, and regulations and guidelines. Within these sections, documents are arranged in chronological order. All documents have been excerpted. Follow the references below each excerpt to check out an entire document or article.

GOVERNMENTAL STRATEGIES

1970s: Smallpox and Its Eradication

One of the most impressive achievements of modern civilization was the eradication of smallpox in the 1970s, less than 200 years after vaccination became an accepted scientific technique. The program, supervised by the World Health Organization, was successful thanks to tireless and creative work on the part of hundreds of government agencies and thousands of determined individuals around the world. The following excerpts, concerning Indonesia, describe how difficult it was to get a handle on the problem to begin with, and how tenaciously the disease held on until its final defeat.

Estimates of the Completeness of Case Notification

It was common knowledge that many cases of smallpox were not reported to the health authorities but the general belief was that the true figure was not more than perhaps 2-3 times the number of recorded cases. The fact that 10,067 cases were known in 1967 to have occurred that year was of concern to health officials but it was not cause for real alarm. Dr. Keja suspected that underreporting was a much more serious problem and performed a number of simple calculations to estimate its magnitude.

The 1968 survey teams had found that 69 out of 8,636 children under one year of age had the characteristic facial pockmarks and thus had contracted smallpox during the preceding year, 1967. Extrapolating from this rate of 4.5 cases per 1,000 to the entire population of children under one year (2,457,000), Dr. Keja arrived at a figure of 11,056 cases. However, since Indonesian data showed that 40% in this age group died of smallpox, he reasoned that the actual number who had had smallpox was 1.67 times larger. Making further corrections to allow for the fact that at least 10 percent survived without recognizable pockmarks, and calculating that those under one year of age accounted for not more than one-fifth of all smallpox cases, he estimated that at least 100,000 cases of smallpox had occurred during 1967 in Java alone, or ten times more than the number recorded.

The numbers in the survey were small and the methods of estimation, although unsophisticated in technical terms, were understandable to nontechnical people. The Minister of Health was incredulous and asked other statisticians to examine the data.

All of Dr. Keja's assumptions served to understate the magnitude of the problem. Case-fatality rates among infants under one year were nearer 50 percent than 40 percent; the proportion of those surviving without recognizable pockmarks was closer to 35 percent than 10 percent; and the proportion of cases in Indonesia among those under one year were 14 percent rather than 20 percent. Finally, Dr. Keja had made no effort to correct the estimate to reflect the fact that the children who were examined were all less than one year of age and thus, on average, had actually been exposed to smallpox only over a six-month period.

His decision to develop a conservative but understandable estimate had been deliberate. The figure of 100,000 cases was impressive in itself. When Indonesian statisticians independently made their own estimates, they calculated that the number of cases had more likely been in the range of 200,000–500,000. The Minister was persuaded that smallpox was indeed a problem of high priority in Indonesia.

Indonesia's Last Outbreak, 1971

After the last cases occurred in Sulawesi in November 1971, four weeks elapsed during which no smallpox cases were reported in Indonesia. It appeared that transmission had been interrupted, but on 14 December 1971, the Director of the Smallpox Eradication Programme received a report from Tangerang Regency (one of the 24 regencies/municipalities in West Java) of 45 cases and six deaths in Sepatan Subdistrict, only 28 kilometers from

Jakarta. Tangerang (population, 1 million) had recorded its last cases in February 1971, fully 10 months earlier. A village-by-village search had been conducted in West Java between June and August 1971 in the subdistricts which had reported cases during 1970–71; lack of personnel had precluded a search in all subdistricts. Sepatan Subdistrict had not reported cases during this period and thus had not been searched.

On investigation, it was found that as early as December 1970, a whole year earlier, many cases in Sepatan had begun to be reported to the health center by the subdistrict's vaccinator. The medical officer of the health center periodically organized ineffectual mass vaccination campaigns to control the outbreaks but deliberately suppressed the reports of smallpox, fearing that he might be punished for incompetence. In mid-December 1971, a provincial mobile surveillance and supervisory team visited the area on routine tour and was informed of the outbreaks by the local staff.

Search and containment activities were immediately instituted. In the realization that the suppression of reports might be widely prevalent, the decision was made to offer a transistor radio to any person who reported an active case of smallpox. This, so far as is known, was the first occasion in the Intensified Programme when a reward was offered for case reporting. It proved to be highly effective. Numerous suspected cases with illnesses of all types were reported by people throughout the area. Eventually, 160 smallpox cases with 15 deaths were confirmed in 3 villages (total population, 7982) of Sepatan Subdistrict; nearly one-third were unprotected when containment vaccination had begun.

The outbreak had started in Sarakan village in December 1970, one year previously, as a result of an importation from West Jakarta. Smallpox spread slowly, only 14 cases occurring between December 1970 and May 1971. Eventually, the outbreak was contained by a local vaccinator. Meanwhile the disease had spread to Sangiang village in May 1971 and, in September, numerous cases began to occur. In all, 131 persons eventually developed smallpox in this village of 3106 persons. At the end of November the disease was reintroduced into Sarakan village and, in December, it spread to nearby Gaga village. Finally, late in December, an outbreak of cases developed in a village 80 kilometers distant. The last two known cases in Indonesia occurred on 23 January 1972, one of them in Gaga village, and the other in Kapshandap village.

Concerned that other hidden foci might be present elsewhere in Indonesia, the programme staff decided in May 1972 to offer a reward of 5000 rupiah

($12) to anyone reporting a case. This was widely publicized. The following month, teams from throughout Indonesia began an active search programme. Numerous rumors were investigated and many specimens were examined, but no further cases were found.

Source: F. Fenner, et al., *Smallpox and Its Eradication,* Geneva, World Health Organization, 1988, pp. n636, 654–55. Available online. URL:http://whqlibdoc.who.int/smallpox/9241561106.pdf. Accessed August 23, 2007.

1990s: Report of the BSE Inquiry

When "mad cow" disease (bovine spongiform encephalitis or BSE) began spreading through the cattle herds of the United Kingdom in the 1980s, the British government repeatedly assured its citizens that they were under no risk of contracting the disease. Then, starting in the early 1990s more than 170 people contracted "variant Creutzfeld-Jakob disease," the human form of the disease, apparently after eating British beef. The news caused a major panic in Britain and around the world, forcing the government to undertake an inquiry. Some of the inquiry committee's conclusions are printed below. Among other things, the commission called for greater openness by the government in matters of public health, even when the government lacks complete information.

Executive Summary of the Report of the Inquiry Key conclusions

- BSE has caused a harrowing fatal disease for humans. As we sign this Report the number of people dead and thought to be dying stands at over 80, most of them young. They and their families have suffered terribly. Families all over the UK have been left wondering whether the same fate awaits them.
- A vital industry has been dealt a body blow, inflicting misery on tens of thousands for whom livestock farming is their way of life. They have seen over 170,000 of their animals dying or having to be destroyed, and the precautionary slaughter and destruction within the United Kingdom of very many more.
- BSE developed into an epidemic as a consequence of an intensive farming practice—the recycling of animal protein in ruminant feed. This practice, unchallenged over decades, proved a recipe for disaster.
- In the years up to March 1996 most of those responsible for responding to the challenge posed by BSE emerge with credit. However, there were a number of shortcomings in the way things were done.

- At the heart of the BSE story lie questions of how to handle hazard—a known hazard to cattle and an unknown hazard to humans. The Government took measures to address both hazards. They were sensible measures, but they were not always timely nor adequately implemented and enforced.
- The rigour with which policy measures were implemented for the protection of human health was affected by the belief of many prior to early 1996 that BSE was not a potential threat to human life.
- The Government was anxious to act in the best interests of human and animal health. To this end it sought and followed the advice of independent scientific experts—sometimes when decisions could have been reached more swiftly and satisfactorily within government.
- In dealing with BSE, it was not MAFF's policy to lean in favour of the agricultural producers to the detriment of the consumer.
- At times officials showed a lack of rigour in considering how policy should be turned into practice, to the detriment of the efficacy of the measures taken.
- At times bureaucratic processes resulted in unacceptable delay in giving effect to policy.
- The Government introduced measures to guard against the risk that BSE might be a matter of life and death not merely for cattle but also for humans, but the possibility of a risk to humans was not communicated to the public or to those whose job it was to implement and enforce the precautionary measures.
- The Government did not lie to the public about BSE. It believed that the risks posed by BSE to humans were remote. The Government was preoccupied with preventing an alarmist over-reaction to BSE because it believed that the risk was remote. It is now clear that this campaign of reassurance was a mistake. When on 20 March 1996 the Government announced that BSE had probably been transmitted to humans, the public felt that they had been betrayed. Confidence in government pronouncements about risk was a further casualty of BSE.
- Cases of a new variant of CJD (vCJD) were identified by the CJD Surveillance Unit and the conclusion that they were probably linked to BSE was reached as early as was reasonably possible. The link between BSE and vCJD is now clearly established, though the manner of infection is not clear.

* *** *

Dealing with uncertainty and the communication of risk

* *** *

The problem is not an easy one. The public are anxious to understand the basis upon which the Government's decisions on risk management are taken. The Government does not set out to achieve zero risk, but to reduce risk to a level which should be acceptable to the reasonable consumer. The individual consumer wishes to be satisfied that the Government has drawn the line in the right place. How can the Government best satisfy the public that this aim has been achieved? We discussed this question with a number of witnesses.

Throughout the BSE story, the approach to communication of risk was shaped by a consuming fear of provoking an irrational public scare. This applied not merely to the Government, but to advisory committees, to those responsible for the safety of medicines, to Chief Medical Officers and to the Meat and Livestock Commission. All witnesses agreed that information should not be withheld from the public, but some spoke of the need to control the manner of its release. Mr Meldrum spoke of the desirability of releasing information 'in an orderly fashion'—of ensuring that the whole package of information was put together, taking care in the process not to 'rock the boat'.

Mr Brian Dickinson, who was a member of MAFF's Food Safety Group, put the matter in this way: "Given the strength of public debate on the matter at the time one was aware of slightly leaning into the wind. You could not just stand upright and give a totally impartial, objective view of what was the situation. There was a stronger danger of being misinterpreted one way rather than the other, and we tended to make more reassuring sounding statements than might ideally have been said."

We felt that this was an accurate description of the general approach to risk communication. We have seen that it provoked increasing scepticism and, on 20 March 1996, the reaction that the Government had been deceiving the public.

* *** *

Everyone agreed that the Government had a problem with credibility. A number of Government Ministers told us that they had lost credibility with the public, so that it was necessary to get independent experts to lend credibility to public pronouncements about risk. Mrs Bottomley spoke of the need for the public to receive information free of 'political overtones'. She told us that she did all that she could to promote the Chief Medical Officer as an independent expert who could be trusted by the nation.

Our experience over this lengthy Inquiry has led us to the firm conclusion that a policy of openness is the correct approach. When responding to public or media demand for advice, the Government must resist the temptation of attempting to appear to have all the answers in a situation of uncertainty. We believe that food scares and vaccine scares thrive on a belief that the Government is withholding information. If doubts are openly expressed and publicly explored, the public are capable of responding rationally and are more likely to accept reassurance and advice if and when it comes. We note, by way of example, that SEAC and MAFF have made public the fact that an investigation is being carried out into the question of whether BSE has passed into sheep. We do not understand that this has led to a boycott of lamb.

Source: BSE Inquiry. Available online. URL: http://www.bseinquiry.gov.uk/report/index.htm. Accessed August 23, 2006.

1993: Asian SARS Outbreak Challenged International and National Responses

The General Accounting Office (since renamed the Government Accountability Office) is an agency of the U. S. Congress that conducts audits and investigations of federal government programs. Below are excerpts from its report to Congress on the international and U.S. response to the Severe Acute Respiratory Syndrome (SARS) epidemic of 1993.

Why GAO Did This Study

Severe acute respiratory syndrome (SARS) emerged in southern China in November 2002 and spread rapidly along international air routes in early 2003. Asian countries had the most cases (7,782) and deaths (729). SARS challenged Asian health care systems, disrupted Asian economies, and tested the effectiveness of the International Health Regulations. GAO was asked to examine the roles of the World Health Organization (WHO), the U.S. government, and Asian governments (China, Hong Kong, and Taiwan) in responding to SARS; the estimated economic impact of SARS in Asia; and efforts to update the International Health Regulations.

What GAO Recommends

GAO is recommending that the Secretaries of Health and Human Services (HHS) and State work with WHO and other member states to strengthen WHO's global infectious disease network. GAO is also recommending that the Secretary of HHS complete steps to ensure that the agency can obtain passenger contact information in a timely manner, including, if necessary, the promulgation of specific regulations; and that the Secretary of State work with other relevant agencies to develop procedures for arranging medical evacuations during an airborne infectious disease outbreak. HHS, State, and WHO generally concurred with the report's content and its recommendations.

[Omitted sections discuss the roles of the WHO and the U.S. government in the SARS epidemic, the initially poor communication and secrecy within the Chinese government, and deficiencies in disease surveillance and public health in all the countries involved.]

Basic Public Health Strategies Eventually Worked to Control SARS Outbreak

The SARS outbreak was ultimately brought under control by a more coordinated response that included the implementation of basic public health strategies. Measures such as improved screening and reporting of cases, rapid isolation of SARS patients, enhanced hospital infection control practices, and quarantine of close contacts were the most effective ways to break the chain of person-to-person transmission.

Improved Screening and Reporting

Screening of patients with symptoms of SARS permitted the early identification of suspect cases during the early phase of illness. Furthermore, because SARS is transmitted when individuals have symptoms of the disease, detecting symptomatic patients was considered critical to stopping its spread. For example, in Beijing, fever clinics were established to screen people with fevers before presentation to hospitals or other health care providers to limit exposure to SARS. Between May 7 and June 9, 2003, there were 65,321 fever clinic visits. Through this effort, 47 probable SARS cases were identified, representing only 0.1 percent of all fever clinic visits but 84 percent of all probable cases hospitalized during that period. In addition, policies were implemented requiring daily reports from all areas regardless of whether any SARS cases were found. In Hong Kong, designated medical centers were established to conduct medical monitoring of close contacts of SARS patients to ensure early detection of secondary cases. In Taiwan, hospital staff and other individuals who had contact with SARS patients in hospitals were monitored on a daily basis to detect SARS symptoms.

Rapid Isolation and Contact Tracing

The identification of patients with suspect and probable cases of SARS and their close contacts reduced the rate of contact between SARS patients and healthy individuals in both community and hospital settings. For example, toward the end of the outbreak, one Chinese province decreased the average time between onset of SARS symptoms to hospitalization from 4 days to 1, and the time to trace contacts of these patients from 1 day to less than half a day. These declines in the time for hospitalization and contact tracing generally coincided with a decrease in the number of new cases. In Hong Kong, officials facilitated tracing by linking a SARS database used by public health officials with police databases to track and verify the addresses of relatives and other close contacts of SARS patients. To limit the spread of SARS in the hospital system, specific hospitals were designated to treat suspected SARS patients in all SARS-affected areas. Another strategy in SARS-affected areas was the cancellation of school, large public gatherings, and holiday activities. For example, in China the weeklong May Day celebration was shortened.

Enhanced Hospital Infection Control

The widespread use of personal protective equipment helped contain the spread of SARS in hospitals. For example, in China, when hospital infection control measures were instituted toward the end of the outbreak in a 1,000-bed hospital constructed exclusively for SARS patients, there were no further cases of SARS transmission in health care workers. Similarly in Hong Kong and Taiwan, these measures led to a decline in the number of infections in health care workers. In addition, in all these affected areas, guidelines were ultimately established for the use of personal protective equipment in outbreak situations.

Quarantine Measures

China, Taiwan, and Hong Kong implemented quarantine measures to isolate potentially infected individuals from the larger community, which, when restricted to close contacts of SARS patients, proved to be an efficient and effective public health strategy. In Hong Kong, for example, close contacts of SARS patients and people in high-risk areas were isolated for 10 days in designated medical centers or at home to ensure early detection of secondary cases. However, more wide-scale quarantine took place in

Taiwan, where 131,000 individuals who had any form of contact with a SARS patient or traveled to SARS-affected areas were placed under quarantine, and in Beijing, where more than 30,000 people were quarantined. Analysis of data from these areas indicated that the quarantine of individuals with no close contact to SARS patients was not an effective use of resources. For example, among the 133 probable and suspect cases identified in Taiwan, most were found to have had direct contact with a SARS patient. ("Use of Quarantine to Prevent Transmission of Severe Acute Respiratory Syndrome—Taiwan 2003," *MMWR*, vol. 52, no. 29 [July 25, 2003].) Similarly, researchers found that in Beijing, limiting quarantine to close contacts of actively ill patients would have been a more efficient strategy and a better use of resources. ("Efficiency of Quarantine during an Epidemic of Severe Acute Respiratory Syndrome—Beijing, China 2003," *MMWR*, vol. 52, no. 43 [Oct. 31, 2003].)

[The report included a final section on "Efforts Under Way to Build Public Health Capacity for Future Outbreaks" in Asian countries.]

Source: General Accounting Office (GAO). "Asian SARS Outbreak Challenged International and National Responses," April 2004. Available online. URL: http://www.gao.gov/new.items/d04564.pdf. Accessed

President Yoweri Museveni, Uganda Address on World AIDS Day, 2003

Uganda was one of the first sub-Saharan African countries to face up to the threat of AIDS with a frank national education program. President Yoweri Museveni summed up the philosophy of his country's approach in this address, delivered on World AIDS Day in 2003.

Fellow Ugandans,

This year's World Aids Day is of special significance for us. We have been joined by the Big Brother Housemates and they have been accompanied by young people living with AIDS from their respective countries. You are all welcome.

The main theme of their Youth-focused mission is "Celebrate Youth, Celebrate Life—Africa United Against Stigma and Discrimination."

For three months earlier this year the Big Brother Housemates kept our youth and the not so young glued to their TV sets around Africa. You have lots of fans and you emerged from your seclusion as celebrities. You are, therefore, very well placed to work in partnership with African leaders and the people living with HIV/AIDS to put an end to the stigma and discrimination and to involve the youth in the crusade against this deadly disease. With your help, I hope, there will be greater involvement of the youth in this crucial campaign.

These last two years, 2002/2003 the HIV/AIDS campaign around the world has focused on Stigma, Discrimination and Human Rights issues. This theme is central to the HIV/AIDS crusade. Stigma and discrimination undermine prevention, care and treatment efforts and increase the impact of the epidemic on individual's families, communities and nations.

HIV/AIDS related stigma and discrimination prevail worldwide and are a reality in our country. People living with HIV/AIDS are stigmatized and discriminated against in various ways—at work, by health care providers, in religious circles, in schools by teachers and fellow students, even in families.

Blaming and abusing people living with HIV/AIDS forces the epidemic underground and creates ideal conditions for its spread. Consequently stigma and discrimination lead to the violation of human rights of people infected and affected by the epidemic.

Here in Uganda when we started our crusade against HIV/AIDS in 1986, individuals, entire communities and even countries kept silent about it. The fear was stigma and discrimination.

We decided to break this silence and gave HIV/AIDS a face because a faceless enemy is a very dangerous enemy. Denial and concealment, we realized, would not get rid of the disease, but only make it worse.

Our messages to the people were simple and to the point. "This is how HIV/AIDS is contracted; this is how it can be prevented. We made it very clear that there is no cure. There has never been any finger pointing, stigmatization or discrimination in our campaigns.

After the infection of 2 million people and the death of 1 million Ugandans over the last 20 years is there a single family or a single community here that has not been affected by HIV/AIDS? And if there is none we are all in the same boat. In our situation stigmatization and discrimination do not make any sense at all.

And let me salute all those who have cared for people living with HIV/AIDS these last twenty years; those children who have taken charge of families and looked after their young siblings, those elderly men and women who have looked after the children orphaned by their sons and daughters; the numerous NGOs, both local and foreign, that have done what they can to fight HIV/AIDS; and those living with HIV/AIDS for their courage.

Last October Uganda hosted the 11th International Conference for People Living with HIV/AIDS. They came from all over the world and to me each one of them is a profile in courage. They have conquered stigma because they came out in the open to have their meetings and did not care who was watching. These are clearly not the problem but part of the solution to the HIV/AIDS pandemic. They are not weighed down by self-pity and do not solicit pity from any quarter.

Let us be honest. The difference between those who declare their HIV/AIDS status and those who do not is a difference in courage. It does not mean that if you have not found out your status then you are HIV/AIDS negative and can stigmatise and discriminate against those who have the courage to find out what their status is. It also means that while those who know their status can get help and plan their lives those who do not live in darkness.

People in a free country like ours cannot be forced to find out or declare their HIV/AIDS statuses. This would be a serious violation of the right to privacy. Nevertheless it is for your own good if you know what your status is as early as possible so that if you are infected you can get help.

In Uganda, I believe, we have overcome the silence and that is why the sero-prevalence rates have dramatically declined from over 30 percent in 1992 to 6 percent today. We must realize that HIV/AIDS can neither be denied nor concealed forever. It eventually shows and by the time it does one is beyond help. It is the fear of stigma and discrimination that leads to this state of affairs but is stigma and discrimination worse than death?

As a leader my main duty is to ensure that people live. Under my watch one million people have died from AIDS. And this is not because I as a leader or as leaders we have lacked the will and courage to confront HIV/AIDS; we have done what we can. As you all know I am an optimist and once I set myself a task I follow it through to the end. We shall not lose the battle against HIV/AIDS.

Out of an estimated 42 million people living with HIV/AIDS in the world 29 million are in sub-Saharan Africa. Therefore, HIV/AIDS is an overwhelmingly African disease. Poverty and ignorance are very closely linked with the distribution of HIV/AIDS. But the world as a whole has the resources to defeat HIV/AIDS; only the will is lacking.

At the UN 2000 General Assembly Special Session on HIV/AIDS there was a declaration of commitment on HIV/AIDS adopted to make every effort to provide universal sustainable treatment for HIV/AIDS, including the prevention and treatment of opportunistic infections and the provision of antiretroviral treatment.

In Brazil antiretroviral therapy has reduced mortality by a whopping 80 percent. Unfortunately in sub-Saharan Africa only 1 percent of the 4.1 million people who need antiretroviral therapy have access to it. However at the recent International Conference on HIV/AIDS in Barcelona, Spain, it was agreed that sub-Saharan Africa should reach a target of 3 million people accessing antiretroviral therapy by the year 2005. Presently only about 200,000 are doing so. Today 9,000 in Uganda have access to antiretroviral therapy. If the Barcelona target is realized 100,000 Ugandans should have access to antiretroviral therapy by 2005.

But we should aim at universal access to antiretroviral therapy by all who need it and this is possible.

Two years ago African leaders agreed to devote 15 percent of their national budgets to health, far greater than many African Countries had ever devoted to health before, largely because of the HIV/AIDS pandemic. Globally, Aids has given rise to a Global Fund for HIV/AIDS, Tuberculosis and Malaria.

The UNAIDS Executive Director recently revealed that he has at his disposal US $ 4.7 billion including funds from the Global Fund to fight AIDS, TB and Malaria, as well as from the World Bank. However, the minimum required "to mount an effective, comprehensive response in low and middle-income countries is US$ 10 billion per annum."

Surely for a committed world and a world which came up with a declaration at the UN on sustainable treatment for HIV/AIDS not so long ago US$ 10 billion is small beer. Let me give you an example. If the farmers of the Quad countries—USA, European Union, Canada and Japan—forgo their subsidies for only 10 days in a year they would raise US$ 10 billion—what we need to stop the 3 million people dying from AIDS every year around the world.

So it is a matter of will not resources. Whatever the rest of the world does or does not do it is our responsibility to roll back the HIV/AIDS pandemic. We, therefore, need a new partnership of leaders, the youth and the people with HIV/AIDS to confront the challenges of HIV/AIDS. I know that our will alone cannot get rid of HIV/AIDS but it can substantially reduce it.

No one should take advantage of the people living with HIV/AIDS. To do so is immoral. I therefore, appeal to those health managers in charge of resources to make sure that the intended beneficiaries derive maximum benefit from the resources available. HIV/AIDS should not be turned into an industry for the benefit of those whom we entrust with the resources and care of the suffering.

Thank you.

Source: Uganda National Web site. "H.E.'s Address on World AIDS Day, December 1, 2003." Available online. URL: http://www.statehouse.go.ug/news.detail.php?newsId=21&category=News%20Release. Accessed December 2, 2007.

The Uganda HIV/AIDS Status Report, July 2004–June 2005

In June 2005 the Ugandan government issued a national status report on the AIDS epidemic. The following section deals with prevention strategies.

National Response to the HIV/AIDS Epidemic
1.0 Prevention
Overview

Prevention strategies are covered under goal one of the Revised National Strategic Framework 2003/4-2005/5; which is to reduce HIV prevalence by 25%.

The objectives related to this goal include:

a) To promote safe sexual behavior among particular population categories, especially young people aged 15–24 years.

b) To reduce the current 2–4% (Yr 2000) risk of blood borne transmission by at least 50%.

c) To reduce prevalence of sexually transmitted infections, other than HIV, by 25%.

d) To reduce the current 15–25% risk of mother to child HIV transmission (MTCT) by 30%.

A number of interventions are currently being implemented to achieve the above stated objectives. These include;

- Promotion of safe sexual behaviors among particular populations,
- Reduction of the risk of blood borne HIV transmission,
- Reduction of prevalence of STIs other than HIV and reduction of the current risk of mother to child HIV transmission.

Situation and Challenges as of June 2004

Over the last 3 years HIV Sero-prevalence had stagnated between 6–6.5%. However recent estimates from a country wide Sero-behavioral survey indicate that the prevalence now stands at 7.1%.

The ABC comprehensive strategy [Abstention, Be faithful, use Condoms] has been discussed by the stake holders and plans to develop it further are currently ongoing. Although district coverage of 100% has been achieved in the last year, sub-county coverage stands at 31% *(Mapping report 2005).*

PMTCT services [prevention of mother-to-child transmission] are now also available in all districts up from 49 districts in the past year. However coverage at the HC III level [Health Center III stands at a paltry 4.4%. HIV seroprevalence for donated blood has reduced to 1.9% from 2.1% and there has been a 10% increase in the number of blood units collected for transfusion, over the past year.

Condom use with last non regular partner among youth aged 15–24 years is still less than 60% for both sexes.

In pursuit of the goal and objectives pertinent to the prevention thematic area, the 3rd Uganda AIDS partnership forum made the following undertakings for the period July 2004–June 2005:

- Develop comprehensive communication strategy for HIV prevention, care and treatment
- Provide comprehensive HIV prevention information to young people in and out of school
- Revise the VCT [voluntary counseling and testing] package to have elements like material, medical and psychosocial support
- Ensure quality supply of VCT kits
- Ensure quality and adequate supply of condoms.
- Establish HIV programmes in emergency settings
- Develop HIV programmes for fishing communities

Achievements against the Aide Memoire 2004 Undertakings

[The report includes two tables showing degrees of progress toward specific prevention goals, such as public knowledge about HIV/AIDS and how to prevent it, the availability of clinics and condoms, and regional differences in accomplishment.]

Constraints/Challenges

Knowledge and Behaviour

- Peer education training as well as implementation of other preventive strategies is posing a big challenge in the internally displaced communities
- Knowledge on ways of prevention of HIV is still lower among the young females compared to their male counterparts
- The percentage of young men aged 15 to 24 years having sex with non regular partners is twice that of their female peers.

Condom Use

- Disparities in free condom distribution still exist at the sub-county level
- Social marketing programmes are currently not present in six districts.
- The national target of 8 condoms per sexually active person per year was not achieved
- The country also experienced some unforeseen shortage of condoms due to quality problems with one of the batch of condoms imported

Voluntary Counseling and Testing

- VCT kits still fell short of the requirements for the year

Blood Transfusion Services

- The ratio of districts to blood bank centers to district improved from 1:6.2 to 1:4.7. These centers are however still restricted to a regional level
- There is lack of Information on eligible persons getting PEP

Prevention of Mother-to-Child Transmission (PMTCT)

- All the districts in the country now have some level of PMTCT services as compared to 49 districts previously, however in almost half (22) the districts coverage ranges from <25% to 50%
- TOTs for health workers on the different PMTCT strategies has been conducted
- Twenty two percent (22%) of the women who attended ANC were not offered HIV counseling
- Thirty seven percent (37%) of the mothers who were counseled did not accept to test for HIV

- Ninety percent of the HIV positive mothers did not receive a complete course of ARVs for PMTCT
- There is no data available on the proportion of HIV positive mothers who are aware of alternatives to breast feeding

Recommended actions

Knowledge and Behaviour

- To strengthen and improve the coordination mechanisms of the existing IEC delivery channels to ensure that they complement each other
- To ensure operationalisation of peer education activities by the trained facilitators in order to reduce the mis-match between training and coverage indices
- There is need to rapidly scale up the training of teachers in life skill based HIV/AIDS education

Condom Use

- The need to adopt national distribution strategies that will ensure more even coverage of condom services at the sub county level.
- Social marketing should be scaled up to embrace all the districts
- On the average social marketing, free services and private services should procure/provide about 79,200,000 per year to achieve the national target of required condoms
- Quality control measures for condoms imported need to be further strengthened

Voluntary Counseling

- Scale up VCT to the remaining two-thirds of the sub counties through both facility and non facility based services options
- HIV prevention services should be further scaled up in the emergency areas

Blood transfusion services

- There should be a progressive increase in the number of blood centers to meet the national target of 100% districts
- There is need to strengthen client recruitment mechanisms in order to further reduce the prevalence of HIV positive donors

Prevention of Mother-to-Child Transmission (PMTCT)

- The need to scale up PMTCT services with particular focus on districts with a coverage of less than 50%.

- Health education and counseling services during ANC needs to be further strengthened to ensure that all women attending ANC access the full services.
- There is need to collect baseline information on mothers knowledge regarding PMTCT infant feeding interventions.
- There is need to collect information on pre and in service health workers sensitized as well as that for policy makers lobbied for promotion of PMTCT.
- There is also need to put in place mechanisms to ensure adequate supplies of PMTCT drugs, test kits, supplies and alternative feeds.
- There is need for mechanisms to increase involvement of men in PMTCT services.

Source: AIDS Uganda. "The Uganda Hiv/Aids Status Report, July 2004–June 2005." Available online. URL:http://www.aidsuganda.org/texbits/THE%20UGANDA%20HIV-AIDS%20STATUS%20REPORT%202005.FINAL%20VERSION.pdf. Accessed August 17, 2006

India: Overview of Malaria Control Activities and Programme Progress, 2005

Since independence in 1947, India has made it an important priority to control, and then to eradicate malaria, a disease that has killed millions of its citizens and disabled millions more. The disease incidence is far lower than in the past, but complete eradication has yet to be achieved. The following is from the Roll Back Malaria Web site.

Overview of malaria control activities and programme progress

Areas of India that are highly endemic for malaria include the north-eastern region and tribal forested and hilly areas of several states including Maharashtra, and selected non-tribal districts. Nearly one quarter of all reported cases are from Orissa State, and 80% of reported cases originate from 20% of the population. During 1995–1996, malaria outbreaks and deaths caused by malaria were reported from tribal parts of Maharashtra State. Nationwide, the reported incidence of laboratory-confirmed cases has declined from 3.0 million in 1996 to 2.1 million in 2001 to 1.78 million in 2003 during a time when there were no changes in laboratory diagnostic or reporting procedures. Around 47% of cases are caused by P. falciparum, with some fluctuation but no consistent trend over time. About 1000 deaths are reported annually, but these figures do not include cases treated in private and not-for-profit health facilities. CQ-resistant P. falciparum and insecticide-resistant malaria vectors are prevalent in some areas.

The NMCP operates under the National Vector-Borne Disease Control Programme in 5-year strategic plans (current plan 2002–2007) and coordinates strategic decisions with the National Technical Advisory Committee on Malaria and with state health authorities. The National Health Policy of 2002 reinforced the commitment to malaria control and set as goals the reduction of malaria mortality by 50% by 2010 and the efficient control of malaria morbidity. Malaria control in India relies heavily on active case detection: every year nearly 100 million blood smears are taken from fever cases identified in the home, and patients are treated promptly if a diagnosis of malaria is confirmed. Access to prompt diagnosis and treatment and education is further provided through village health workers, drug distribution depots and fever treatment depots. In selected areas, there is targeted vector control through IRS, larviciding and ITNs.

Malaria is currently under control in vast areas of India, covering almost 80% of the population despite increasing population density and aggregation, rapid and unplanned urbanization and increased migration. However, developmental activities, expansion of agriculture and deforestation have the potential for increasing anopheline mosquito breeding sites. A survey in Orissa State in 2003 demonstrated coverage with the drug distribution depots and fever treatment depots of 98.7% of villages. About half of fever cases sought treatment at the drug distribution depots and fever treatment depots, about 36% from a health worker or primary health centre, and only about 13% from other sources such as private medical practitioners. This represents a considerable increase in the proportion of people with fever seeking treatment from government sources compared with observations in the National Sample Survey in 1995–1996. Following the 1995–1996 malaria outbreak, Maharashtra State introduced intensified active surveillance, prompt radical treatment, selective IRS with pyrethroids and larviciding in high-risk areas. ITNs were distributed in areas of medium transmission.

Under the MoH's Enhanced Malaria Control Project, which aims to control malaria in eight states including Gujarat, Andra Pradesh and Maharashtra, malaria morbidity dropped in the project's districts by 46% compared to 1997. Before 2004, approximately 1.8 million ITNs had been distributed and an additional 3.8 million ITNs are being procured. Over the same period, the population covered by IRS decreased by more than 50%.

The Ministry of Finance allocates funds to the Ministry of Health and Family Welfare for the various national health programmes, including malaria, a portion of which is released to state governments. Over US$ 49 million was allocated to malaria control from the MoH in 2003. In addition, many states allocate significant budgets for malaria control activities from state resources. The World Bank has supported the MoH's Enhanced Malaria Control Project since 1997, disbursing approximately US$ 140 million to date; however, the project is expected to close in October 2005. Starting in 2005, the GFATM will provide an additional US$ 30 million for malaria control activities for 2 years in states that are not covered by the Enhanced Malaria Control Project, which are primarily in the north-eastern part of the country. In addition, the Government of India has recently requested funding from the World Bank for a Vector Borne Disease Control Project that is proposed to begin mid-2006 and is expected to significantly expand the number of states covered.

Source: Roll Back Malaria. "India Country Profile." *World Malaria Report 2005.* April 28, 2005. Available online. URL: http://www.rbm.who.int/wmr2005/profiles/india.pdf. Accessed August 23, 2007.

South African National HIV Prevalence, HIV Incidence, Behaviour and Communication Survey, 2005

In November 2005 the Human Sciences Research Council of South Africa, a government agency, issued a 156-page report on their HIV "household survey," which was conducted all across the country. Over 23,000 individuals were questioned, and nearly 16,000 took an HIV test. The excerpt below includes the council's recommendations for education and prevention.

Chapter 4.2 Recommendations

The HIV prevalence in South Africa among persons aged 2 years and older at 10.8 percent translates to 4.8 million (95% CI: 4.2–5.3 million) people living with HIV/AIDS in 2005.

False sense of security

Factors underpinning continued high HIV prevalence are partly illustrated by the finding that half of the respondents in this study who were found to be HIV positive did not think they were at risk of HIV infection. Put another way, over two million people who are HIV positive in South Africa do not think they are at risk. This means they may be unaware of their risk of potentially infecting others. For this reason it is also recommended that HIV/AIDS campaigns and programmes address this false sense of security in the general population, with a particular emphasis on finding out one's

HIV status. Counselling and other services need to be expanded to provide additional support to persons who find out that they are HIV positive.

Stigmatising attitudes are decreasing

The survey showed that nearly half of South Africans aged 15 years and older think it is acceptable to marry a person with HIV and also that a similar proportion would not have a problem having protected sex with an HIV-positive person. These results suggest that South Africans are accepting HIV/AIDS as a reality in South Africa. It is critical that service providers capitalise on this window of opportunity to encourage disclosure of HIV status.

Integration of family planning and HIV/AIDS services is vital

In view of the high prevalence and incidence of HIV amongst pregnant women and women in the child-bearing age group, it is critical that the government targets this group and strengthens family planning programmes. This is important, given that one in five South African women of reproductive age are not using any contraceptive method. For those who use injectable contraceptives and contraceptive pills, it is important to emphasise consistent use of condoms with regular and non-regular partners as long as they are not certain of their own, or their sexual partner's HIV status.

The high risks of HIV transmission from mother to baby before, during, and after pregnancy, and including the risk of becoming HIV positive late in pregnancy or during the period of breastfeeding, need to be noted as important areas of risk. Teenage females have been underemphasised as a target group, although pregnancy levels are high in this age group. We recommend that urgent action on a national scale be taken to make women aware of the risks of HIV infection during pregnancy so they can make informed choices about how best to protect themselves and their offspring, from becoming infected. HIV/AIDS campaigns should also target would be parents to encourage them to (a) plan the pregnancy, (b) each get tested for HIV before trying to conceive and disclose the results to each other. Prospective parents should also be informed that women run a greater risk of being infected with HIV towards the end of pregnancy.

Periodic HIV testing is crucial

South Africa appears to have a well-established VCT [voluntary counseling and testing] system, and most respondents know of a place to get tested. However, many respondents found to be HIV positive in this survey had not been tested. Knowledge of HIV status is a critical aspect of prevention as it is linked to motivation to address HIV prevention risk to others. It also serves as an entrée into seeking a treatment for opportunistic infects and ARV [anti-retroviral drugs] (in the case of advanced HIV infection).

Periodic HIV testing should be encouraged for men and women in stable partnerships and especially when planning to have a child. Should one of the partners be HIV positive, he/she should be counseled to discuss the advisability of conception. The current environment is conducive to discussing the matter of HIV sero-discordance and the need to prevent transmission to the uninfected partner. This is important because the couple needs to be aware that the HIV-negative partner is at risk of becoming infected with HIV.

The extremely high HIV incidence in females aged 15–24 years (six times higher than males of the same age) is a source of concern. Since half of those who are HIV positive do not know their HIV status, we recommend that HIV/AIDS campaigns and programmes should sensitise this young female group to the fact that the risk of HIV is real. They should be strongly encouraged to know their HIV status through the VCT sites that are available and accessible. Annual testing, particularly amongst young females, is recommended.

It is also recommended that VCT services continue to be promoted, but that routine testing also be considered for persons seeking healthcare for other reasons—particularly, as recommended by UNAIDS/WHO, STI [sexually-transmitted infection] patients and patients with diseases associated with HIV infection.

Young people should be encouraged to delay sexual debut

Data from this study shows clearly that the more sex one has, the greater the chances of acquiring HIV. Sexually active persons had an HIV prevalence that was four times higher than that of those who said they had not had sex and 75% higher than that of those who had abstained from sex in the past 12 months. When controlling for age of the participant, the relationship remained strong for the youth. For this reason, it is critical that young people be encouraged to delay sexual debut.

Avoid high partner turnover and concurrent sexual partnerships

Frequent partner turnover and concurrent sexual partnerships partly contribute to high HIV prevalence among men and women. Clearly there is a need for prevention campaigns and programmes to emphasise this aspect of risk. To reduce HIV risk, it is recommended that sexually active persons should: (a) avoid engaging in unprotected sex with any person whose HIV status they do not know; (b) access and consistently use condoms from the government or other sources to protect themselves in every sexual encounter; and (c) avoid frequent partner turnover and concurrent sexual partnerships.

Sexual partners amongst youth should be within a five-year age range

What distinguishes HIV risk between young females and young males is the age group with which each has sex. The study found that young females are more likely to have male partners who are five years older than themselves (females: 15–19=2% and 20–24=28.4%) versus (males: 15–19=2% and 20–24=1%). Older male sexual partners have a higher HIV prevalence than younger male partners. Although the young males have very high rates of multiple partners, they tend to use condoms more than older males. Although this study did not measure consistency of condom use, the fact that the HIV incidence among young males aged 15–24 years is just 1.1% suggests that they are partly protecting themselves against HIV. Young females who have sexual partners who are at least five years older than themselves increase their chances of being with a sexual partner who is already HIV positive.

Inform women that they are more at risk and encourage self-protection

Women are biologically susceptible to HIV infection and men are more efficient at transmitting HIV. In addition to social factors that increase vulnerability to HIV, biological factors increase susceptibility to HIV among women. While men are more efficient at transmitting HIV, females are more susceptible to HIV infection. It is recommended that women ensure that they use condoms to prevent themselves from becoming infected.

Get treated for STIs and abstain from sex when one has STIs

Sexually transmitted infections increase susceptibility to HIV infection. This study found a strong association between having a history of STI and being HIV positive. For this reason, we recommend that the risks of HIV infection with concurrent STI infection need to continue to be emphasized in prevention programmes. Those who have signs or symptoms of STIs should immediately seek treatment and also not have sex when symptoms are present.

[The report went on to discuss the risks of HIV among older people, and among children. It also supported educational programs being tested in African countries called "Healthy Relationships" and "Options for Health."]

Source: S.A. Human Sciences Research Council. "South African National HIV Prevalence, HIV Incidence, Behaviour and Communication Survey, 2005." Available online. URL: http://www.hsrcpress.co.za/freedownload.asp?id=2134. Accessed September 1, 2006

European Union: Final Exercise Report, 2006

The European Union government is trying to play a wider coordinating role in health issues affecting its 27 members. For example, it has staged exercises using fictitious disease events, so that members can better coordinate their response to pandemic threats. The following excerpts are from the final report following one such exercise based on a possible future flu pandemic.

Executive Summary

Introduction

Exercise COMMON GROUND was conducted by the UK's Health Protection Agency (HPA) as a Command Post Exercise (CPX) over a two-day period on 23 to 24 November 2005. This exercise was the second of two European Union exercises commissioned by the European Commission (EC) to evaluate the ability and capabilities of Member States to respond to a health-related crisis, in this case an influenza pandemic.

Conduct of the Exercise

The conduct of this exercise as a CPX provided scope for hundreds of players at two levels of response—national and international—to react to a series of fictitious events as they would have to do in the event of a real emergency. Players in the exercise included the EC, European Centre for Disease Control (ECDC), the 25 Member States, European Economic Area (EEA) States, Switzerland, European Agency for the Evaluation of Medicinal Products (EMEA), European Vaccine Manufacturers (EVM), pharmaceutical companies and the World Health Organisation (WHO). The exercise was intended, amongst other objectives, to provide the players with an opportunity to explore international coordination with the EC's Health Emergency Operations Facility and was based on a realistic model of an influenza pandemic developed by the modelers at the HPA.

Issues Identified

The experience served to heighten the issues identified on Exercise NEW WATCHMAN, which was conducted along similar lines in October 2005. The main issues identified during Exercise COMMON GROUND were that:

- There seems to be some variability as to what extent Member States, EEA States and Switzerland have included an international dimension in their Pandemic Influenza Plans; it was noted that many focused on national issues rather than international affairs during the early stage of the exercise.
- The EC should consider further developing their generic plan taking into account the international dimension of the national plans of Member States to include a checklist of appropriate measures that have to be taken by Member States and the Community applicable to each phase / alert level.
- The roles and responsibilities of the WHO, the EC, and the ECDC during a crisis response need to be better understood by the Member States.
- Existing communication tools in the Commission will have to be enhanced and adapted:
    - The Early Warning Response System (EWRS) is a robust system for the purpose for which it was intended. However, it was used as a decision support tool during the exercise, which it was not designed for. The system needs to be used strictly for the purpose it is intended under EC law (Decision 2119) i.e. notification of cases, information, consultation and coordination of public health measures.
    - A restricted web site for crisis management and situational awareness (Health Emergency and Diseases Information System—HEDIS) which is currently under development needs further enhancement.
    - The system needs to be extended to include adequate decision support capacity and analytical tools.
- Teleconferences during a crisis posed some difficulties.
- Member States EEA States and Switzerland need to have adequate command and control centers with good liaison systems (audio and video conference tools, adequately equipped crisis rooms) with other States, the Commission and partner agencies as well as international organizations, in particular the WHO.

Responding to the Crisis

There were some obvious examples of coordination efforts by the EC and ECDC during the exercise, particularly the holding of audio-conferences with detailed agenda and attention points which helped immediate issues. Also, the setting up by the ECDC of a helpful website, which provided a good overview of the situation and reporting forms for surveillance purposes. Additionally, the EC provided reporting forms for the Member States to feed-back on public health measures taken. These initiatives would be useful in a real crisis.

There were also a number of examples of good, coordinated cooperation on the development of media responses between Member States but overall it appears that most responses to media requests were provided at the national level without reference to or consultation with others. Although not required by Community law, there was no EC coordination on messages to the public. It is desirable that such coordination takes place. Cooperation in providing common, coordinated media themes could be enhanced.

Expanding and improving the capability of the EC to coordinate a response to a crisis is highly desirable. The issues identified in Exercise COMMON GROUND are complex and their resolution will not be easy. However, the value of an exercise is that authorities and organisations are able to learn from their experiences and they have an opportunity to enhance their capabilities so that responses to real crises are improved. The recommendations can be found in part 6 of this document.

Source: European Union. "Exercise Common Ground: Final Exercise Report." March 27, 2006. Available online. URL: http://ec.europa.eu/health/ph_threats/com/common.pdf. Accessed June 15, 2006

FIRSTHAND ACCOUNTS

Thucydides, *The History of the Plague of Athens,* 1857

The historian Thucydides, one of the most famous writers of ancient Greece, is today admired for his attention to factual detail and his sharp powers of observation. His essay on the epidemic that devastated Athens during the Peloponnesian War remains as vivid today as it was 2,500 years ago.

Chapter 47

* *** *

At the very commencement of the next summer, the Lacedaemonians and their allies, still under the command of Archidamas, invaded Attica with two-thirds of their forces, as on the former occasion; and after encamping, they laid waste the country. But they had not been many days in Attica before the epidemic, which is the immediate topic of this essay, first began to appear among the Athenians; although, if rumor might be credited, it had previously shown itself in Lemnos and the adjoining territory. And such a pestilence as this, and such destruction of life as followed in its train had never happened before. Physicians at first, from unacquaintance with its nature, were unsuccessful in their treatment of it, and, indeed, they themselves, from their attendance upon the sick, died in a far greater proportion than others; nor was any other human art of any avail. So, too, all the resources of religion, whether supplications in the temple, or divinations, or other like means, were equally inefficacious, and, at length, overcome by the infliction, men came to lay even these aside.

Chapter 48

The disease was said to have begun in that part of Ethiopia which is above Egypt, to have come down into Egypt and Libya, and, thence, to have invaded a great part of the Persian dominions; and it had been heard of about Lemnos and its neighborhood before it reached the Pyraeus, whence it soon spread, with increased violence, to the upper city of Athens. And as the Pyraeus, where it first broke out, is without springs, the people were for a time disposed to attribute this deadly malady to poison which the Peloponnesians had thrown into their water-tanks or reservoirs. Let every one, whether or not professionally acquainted with medicine, speak, after his own knowledge, concerning it; let him show from what source it was likely to have arisen; and what the cause which he thinks adequate to account for the change thus suddenly wrought from health to sickness. As to myself, I shall describe it such as it was; and so explain its symptoms, both from having suffered under it and having witnessed it in others, that every one, should it ever reappear, may, by reference to this record, being forewarned, be prepared for its reception.

Chapter 49

It was universally admitted that the year in which it broke out, was peculiarly free from ordinary disorders; as also that if any individual were suffering under any previous illness, the symptoms of that illness assumed, eventually, the character of those of the prevalent malady. When, however, it was established, persons in full health were seized suddenly, without any ostensible cause, with hot flushes about the head, redness and turgescence of the eyes, while the parts within, both the pharynx and the tongue, became, at once, blood red, and the breath was extremely fetid;

and in succession to these symptoms, followed sneezing and hoarseness. Shortly afterwards the disorder descended into the chest, occasioning a violent cough, and, settling on the heart, it caused both a reversion of the heart and every kind of bilious evacuation which has ever been designated by physicians; and these were accompanied by great distress, that is, to use medical terms, were accompanied to tormina and tenesmus. A hollow hiccup came on in most cases, giving rise to a violent spasm, which, in some instances, ceased soon, and in others only after a considerable interval. The surface of the body was neither very hot to the touch, nor was it pale, but reddish, livid, and covered with small vesicles and sores; while, inwardly, it was so burnt up that the sufferers were impatient of garments of the lightest tissue or covering of the finest linen; their only desire, in fact, was to lie naked. Thus, they longed for nothing so much as to cast themselves into cold water; and many, who were not well attended to, urged by an unquenchable thirst, actually did so, by plunging into the cisterns; and yet, whether they drank much or little, it was all the same. The distress caused by restlessness (by jactitation, that is, to use professional language), and want of sleep, pressed heavily upon the sufferers throughout; and yet, so long as the disease was at its height, the body was not sensibly emaciated. On the contrary, it resisted this accumulated suffering so far beyond expectation, that most of those who perished by that internal heat, within the seventh or ninth day of the disease, retained to the last somewhat of their natural strength. Very many, however, of those who survived those critical days, were eventually carried off by the debility and exhaustion which ensued from the disease passing down into the abdomen, and there causing extensive ulceration together with profuse diarrhea. For the disease, which had its first seat in the head, beginning from above, passed through the whole body, and if any one did get safely through its most dangerous stages, he had yet to endure a seizure of the extremities, which left traces of its virulence behind. The malady, in fact, lighted upon, or rather, to speak medically, it was, by a process of metastasis, resumed in the pudenda, the fingers, and toes, with such violence, that many of those who recovered were not only deprived of those parts, but some of them also lost their eyes; while others, at the commencement of their recovery, had so completely lost their memory as to have no recollection either of their friends or themselves.

Chapter 50

The character of the disease, in fine, was violent beyond description, and while, in other respects, it attacked individuals with a severity beyond what human nature could well endure, in this it showed itself to be something different from other maladies, that the birds and beast which prey on human bodies, of which many lay unburied, either did not approach them or died after having tasted them. As proof of which, there was a manifest scarcity of birds of that kind; none indeed were to be seen either in the neighborhood or about the dead, but the dogs, from being domesticated with men, afforded better evidence of the result alluded to.

Chapter 51

. . . It seemed to matter little for the safety of those who were attacked whether they were attended to or not, as some perished amid neglect, and some died notwithstanding all the advantages of nursing and treatment. For there was no settled remedy which could be relief on, as that which, seemingly, did good to one was harmful to another; and no constitution of body, whether strong or weak, appeared to be proof against it, as all alike, even such as had previously been dietetically treated, yielded to its influence. But the most terrible part of the whole infliction was the despondency which took possession of the mind as soon as any one felt that he was sickening; for the sufferers, losing at once all hope and offering no moral resistance, rather gave themselves up to than were subdued by the malady; and being, moreover, charged with infection, from attending on one another, they died like sheep. This was, it may be added, the cause of the greatest mortality, as they, who, through fear, were unwilling to maintain their wonted intercourse, were so completely deserted that whole households were swept away, from the want of attendants; while most of those who would still visit their friends were seized by the pestilence.

Source: Thucydides, trans. C. Collier, *The History of the Plague of Athens* (Oxford, England: Oxford University Press, 1857), pp.22–28.

The Black Death

A pandemic spread throughout the civilized world in the 14th century, probably a combination of bubonic and pneumonic plague. In Europe, where perhaps a third of the population died, it was called the Black Death. A disaster on such a scale inevitably brought social, economic, and political changes, as these excerpts show.

Ibn Khaldoun, *Muqaddimah*, 1377

Ibn Khaldoun is considered one of the greatest pre-modern historians. He is known for his attempts to clarify the causes of historical change. One of those causes is surely pandemic disease. In this passage from his famous Muqaddimah, *Khaldoun tells of the impact in the Muslim world of the mid 14th-century pandemic known in Europe as the Black Death. The plague first struck when he was about 15 years old.*

> This was the situation until, in the middle of the eighth [fourteenth] century, civilization both in the East and the West was visited by a destructive plague which devastated nations and caused populations to vanish. It swallowed up many of the good things of civilization and wiped them out. It overtook the dynasties at the time of their senility, when they had reached the limit of their duration. It lessened their power and curtailed their influence. It weakened their authority. Their situation approached the point of annihilation and dissolution.
>
> Civilization decreased with the decrease of mankind. Cities and buildings were laid waste, roads and way signs were obliterated, settlements and mansions became empty, dynasties and tribes grew weak. The entire inhabited world changed. The East, it seems, was similarly visited, though in accordance with and in proportion to (the East's more affluent) civilization. It was as if the voice of existence in the world had called out for oblivion and restriction, and the world had responded to its call. God inherits the earth and whomever is upon it.
>
> When there is a general change of conditions, it is as if the entire creation had changed and the whole world been altered, as if it were a new and repeated creation, a world brought into existence anew.

Source: Ibn Khaldoun, *The Muqaddimah: An Introduction to History,* ed. by N. J. Dawood, trans. by Franz Rosenthal (Princeton, N.J.: Princeton University Press, 1969).

Giovanni Boccaccio, *The Decameron*, ca. 1348–1353

The Italian writer Giovanni Boccaccio was a keen observer of the plague in Florence in 1348. His eyewitness account, included in the first chapter of his Decameron, *gives some sense of the horror most people would have felt.*

> The symptoms were not the same as in the East, where a gush of blood from the nose was the plain sign of inevitable death; but it began both in men and women with certain swellings in the groin or under the armpit. They grew to the size of a small apple or an egg, more or less, and were vulgarly called tumors. In a short space of time these tumors spread from the two parts

named all over the body. Soon after this the symptoms changed and black or purple spots appeared on the arms or thighs or any other part of the body, sometimes a few large ones, sometimes many little ones. These spots were a certain sign of death, just as the original tumor had been and still remained.

No doctor's advice, no medicine could overcome or alleviate this disease, An enormous number of ignorant men and women set up as doctors in addition to those who were trained. Either the disease was such that no treatment was possible or the doctors were so ignorant that they did not know what caused it, and consequently could not administer the proper remedy. In any case very few recovered; most people died within about three days of the appearance of the tumors described above, most of them without any fever or other symptoms.

The violence of this disease was such that the sick communicated it to the healthy who came near them, just as a fire catches anything dry or oily near it. And it even went further. To speak to or go near the sick brought infection and a common death to the living; and moreover, to touch the clothes or anything else the sick had touched or worn gave the disease to the person touching.

* *** *

Others again held a still more cruel opinion, which they thought would keep them safe. They said that the only medicine against the plague-stricken was to go right away from them. Men and women, convinced of this and caring about nothing but themselves, abandoned their own city, their own houses, their dwellings, their relatives, their property, and went abroad or at least to the country round Florence, as if God's wrath in punishing men's wickedness with this plague would not follow them but strike only those who remained within the walls of the city, or as if they thought nobody in the city would remain alive and that its last hour had come.

* *** *

Thus, a multitude of sick men and women were left without any care, except from the charity of friends (but these were few), or the greed of servants, though not many of these could be had even for high wages, Moreover, most of them were coarse-minded men and women, who did little more than bring the sick what they asked for or watch over them when they were dying. And very often these servants lost their lives and their earnings. Since the sick were thus abandoned by neighbors, relatives and friends, while servants were scarce, a habit sprang up which had never been heard of before. Beautiful and noble women, when they fell sick, did not scruple to take a young or old man-servant, whoever he might be, and with no sort of shame, expose every part of their bodies to these men as if they had been women, for they were compelled by the necessity of their sickness to do so. This, perhaps, was a cause of looser morals in those women who survived.

The plight of the lower and most of the middle classes was even more pitiful to behold. Most of them remained in their houses, either through poverty or in hopes of safety, and fell sick by thousands. Since they received no care and attention, almost all of them died. Many ended their lives in the streets both at night and during the day; and many others who died in their houses were only known to be dead because the neighbors smelled their decaying bodies. Dead bodies filled every corner. Most of them were treated in the same manner by the survivors, who were more concerned to get rid of their rotting bodies than moved by charity towards the dead. With the aid of porters, if they could get them, they carried the bodies out of the houses and laid them at the door; where every morning quantities of the dead might be seen. They then were laid on biers or, as these were often lacking, on tables.

Such was the multitude of corpses brought to the churches every day and almost every hour that there was not enough consecrated ground to give them burial, especially since they wanted to bury each person in the family grave, according to the old custom. Although the cemeteries were full they were forced to dig huge trenches, where they buried the bodies by hundreds. Here they stowed them away like bales in the hold of a ship and covered them with a little earth, until the whole trench was full.

Source: Giovanni Boccaccio. *The Decameron*, vol. I, trans. Richard Aldington (London: G.P. Putnam, 1930).

SCIENTIFIC STATEMENTS AND FINDINGS

University of Illinois at Chicago, "Paleopathology/ Disease in the Past," 1999

Historical records go back through several thousand years of the human story, but modern humans existed for thousands of years before then. Scientists have been able to make many interesting deductions about health, nutrition, and disease using the evidence of ancient skeletal remains found at archaeological digs. The following 1999 summary from the University of Illinois at Chicago online course Web site shows some of their techniques.

(1) Wear on teeth and analysis of dental caries. High rates of dental caries are invariably associated with soft, sticky foods as with agricultural diets. The rate of wear and incidence of decay go up with the adoption of agriculture. The rate of wear in many agricultural people is often a result of grit from grinding stones.

(2) Iron deficiency causes anemia. When prolonged, perotic hyperostosis occurs—a distinctive porosity seen in the cranial vault or the eye sockets. The anemia itself can be caused by parasites or a variety of infections.

(3) Vitamin D deficiency causes legs to grow bent.

(4) Malnutrition or under-nutrition is inferred from skeletal measurements. A decline of stature of historic populations has been used to indicate nutritional status. Deciduous teeth in particular seem to be sensitive to nutrition.

(5) Certain infections leave specific traces in the skeleton. Tuberculosis leaves characteristic traces on the ribs and tends to destroy the bodies of the lumbar vertebrae. Infections from the treponema spirochete in yaws or syphilis can produce either local or widespread skeletal damage. When syphilis is congenital, it can leave the characteristic 'Hutchinson's incisor' defect. Leprosy is characterized by damage to the bones of the face, fingers, and toes.

(6) Various cancers are identifiable in the skeleton. Primary bone cancer is rare, but the skeleton is a common site for the secondary spread of cancerous growth from other tissues. Studies of rates of bone cancers in prehistoric populations suggest that they are extremely rare—even when the relative scarcity of elderly people is taken into account.

(7) Trauma in skeletons is clearly evident in bone fractures, especially when they have not healed successfully. It is often possible to distinguish between traumas resulting from a fall and a blow such as sustained in violence. Studies of Neanderthal skeletons reveals that the pattern of fractures correlates well with those seen in contemporary rodeo riders. This implies close contact "of the dangerous kind" with large animals.

(8) The individual workload leaves traces in the skeleton. High rates of physical labor can appear as degenerative joint disease. Muscular development results in increasing size of muscle attachment areas on bone. Women who spend a lot of time grinding corn develop deltoid tuberosities similar to those that develop among modern bodybuilders.

(9) Growth-disrupting and growth-retarding stresses during childhood will leave transverse lines of dense bone visible in radiographs of

long bones of the body. These are the so-called Harris lines. The formation of tooth enamel is also vulnerable to stress. When those are grossly visible to the naked eye, they are known as enamel hypoplasias. When visible only as lines in microscopic cross sections they are known as Wilson bands. Markers such as hypoplasia, Wilson bands, and Harris lines can be produced in the skeleton by a variety of stressors, including starvation, severe malnutrition and severe infection.

(10) The age of an individual at death can be determined based on the development and eruption of teeth (both deciduous and permanent) providing a fairly precise indicator of age up to fifteen years. Adult ages are harder to determine, since environment can also influence the rate of degeneration. Signs of degeneration include patterns of wear and other changes to the teeth; changes in the sutures of the skull bones, changes in the articular surfaces of the pelvis and changes in the microscopic structure of bone.

Source: Online course OSCI 590, University of Illinois at Chicago, 1999. "Paleopathology/Disease in the Past." Available online. URL: http://www.uic.edu/classes/osci/osci590/4_4PaleopathologyDiseaseInThePast.txt.htm. Accessed September 13, 2006.

A Declaration by Scientists and Physicians Affirming HIV is the Cause of AIDS, 2001

At the 2000 International AIDS Conference in Durban, South Africa, 5,000 scientists from around the world signed a statement reaffirming that the HIV virus was the cause of AIDS. They were responding to statements by South African president Thabo Mbeki questioning that fact. The scientists were concerned that such doubts might get in the way of antiviral treatments, the only proven therapy for the disease.

Durban Declaration

Seventeen years after the discovery of the human immunodeficiency virus (HIV), thousands of people from around the world are gathered in Durban, South Africa to attend the XIII International AIDS Conference. At the turn of the millennium, an estimated 34 million people worldwide are living with HIV or AIDS, 24 million of them in sub-Saharan Africa. Last year alone, 2.6 million people died of AIDS, the highest rate since the start of the epidemic. If current trends continue, Southern and South-East Asia, South America and regions of the former Soviet Union will also bear a heavy burden in the next two decades.

Like many other diseases, such as tuberculosis and malaria that cause illness and death in underprivileged and impoverished communities, AIDS spreads by infection. HIV-1, the retrovirus that is responsible for the AIDS pandemic, is closely related to a simian immunodeficiency virus (SIV) which infects chimpanzees.

HIV-2, which is prevalent in West Africa and has spread to Europe and India, is almost indistinguishable from an SIV that infects sooty mangabey monkeys. Although HIV-1 and HIV-2 first arose as infections transmitted from animals to humans, or zoonoses, both are now spread among humans through sexual contact, from mother to infant and via contaminated blood.

An animal source for a new infection is not unique to HIV. The plague came from rodents. Influenza and the new Nipah virus in South-East Asia reached humans via pigs. Variant Creutzfeldt-Jakob disease in the United Kingdom came from 'mad cows'. Once HIV became established in humans, it soon followed human habits and movements. Like other viruses, HIV recognizes no social, political or geographic boundaries.

The evidence that AIDS is caused by HIV-1 or HIV-2 is clear-cut, exhaustive and unambiguous. This evidence meets the highest standards of science. The data fulfill exactly the same criteria as for other viral diseases, such as poliomyelitis, measles and smallpox:

- Patients with acquired immune deficiency syndrome, regardless of where they live, are infected with HIV.
- If not treated, most people with HIV infection show signs of AIDS within 5–10 years. HIV infection is identified in blood by detecting antibodies, gene sequences or viral isolation. These tests are as reliable as any used for detecting other virus infections.
- Persons who received HIV-contaminated blood or blood products develop AIDS, whereas those who received untainted or screened blood do not.
- Most children who develop AIDS are born to HIV-infected mothers. The higher the viral load in the mother the greater the risk of the child becoming infected.
- In the laboratory HIV infects the exact type of white blood cell (CD4 lymphocytes) that becomes depleted in persons with AIDS.
- Drugs that block HIV replication in the test tube also reduce viral load and delay progression to AIDS. Where available, treatment has reduced AIDS mortality by more than 80%.

- Monkeys inoculated with cloned SIV DNA become infected and develop AIDS.

Further compelling data are available. HIV causes AIDS. It is unfortunate that a few vocal people continue to deny the evidence. This position will cost countless lives.

In different regions of the world HIV/AIDS shows altered patterns of spread and symptoms. In Africa, for example, HIV-infected persons are 11 times more likely to die within 5 years, and over 100 times more likely than uninfected persons to develop Kaposi's sarcoma, a cancer linked to yet another virus.

As with any other chronic infection, various co-factors play a role in determining the risk of disease. Persons who are malnourished, who already suffer other infections or who are older, tend to be more susceptible to the rapid development of AIDS following HIV infection. However, none of these factors weaken the scientific evidence that HIV is the sole cause of AIDS.

In this global emergency, prevention of HIV infection must be our greatest worldwide public health priority.

The knowledge and tools to prevent infection exist. The sexual spread of HIV can be prevented by monogamy, abstinence or by using condoms. Blood transmission can be stopped by screening blood products and by not re-using needles. Mother-to-child transmission can be reduced by half or more by short courses of antiviral drugs.

Limited resources and the crushing burden of poverty in many parts of the world constitute formidable challenges to the control of HIV infection. People already infected can be helped by treatment with life-saving drugs, but high cost puts these treatments out of reach for most. It is crucial to develop new antiviral drugs that are easier to take, have fewer side effects and are much less expensive, so that millions more can benefit from them.

There are many ways to communicate the vital information about HIV/AIDS. What works best in one country may not be appropriate in another. But to tackle the disease, everyone must first understand that HIV is the enemy. Research, not myths, will lead to the development of more effective and cheaper treatments, and hopefully a vaccine. But for now, emphasis must be placed on preventing sexual transmission.

There is no end in sight to the AIDS pandemic. By working together, we have the power to reverse the tide of this epidemic. Science will one day triumph over AIDS, just as it did over smallpox. Curbing the spread of HIV will be the first step. Until then, reason, solidarity, political will and courage must be our partners.

Source: Canadian AIDS Society. "HIV Causes AIDS—How to Respond to Denialist Arguments." May 2001. Available online. URL: http://www.cdnaids.ca/web/setup.nsf/(ActiveFiles)/PS_HIV_Causes_AIDS/$file/Responding_to_HIV_Denialists_En_Red.pdf. Accessed August 18, 2006

Meissner, Strebel, Orenstein, "Measles Vaccines and the Potential for Worldwide Eradication of Measles," 2004

The goal of eliminating measles from the world is definitely reachable, according to a 2004 article in the journal Pediatrics. *The article, by Doctors H. Cody Meissner, Peter M. Strebel, and Walter A. Orenstein, recounted the success of the measles vaccine in developed countries, and defended its safety. In this excerpt, the authors call for a global effort to eliminate the disease, an important cause of childhood suffering and death.*

Global Eradication of Measles

Is it possible that measles can reach the same degree of disease control (viz, worldwide eradication) as has occurred with smallpox and soon may be achieved with polio? Several conditions must be satisfied before any vaccine-based eradication program can be successful. First, there must be no reservoir for the virus apart from humans. This is the case for measles virus, and chronic shedding of measles virus (i.e., >2 months after rash onset) has not been documented. Subacute sclerosing panencephalitis is caused by a persistent infection with a defective measles virus; however, this condition is not infectious. Measles virus cannot survive in the environment for more than a few hours apart from human infection or growth in tissue culture. Second, there must be an adequate test for rapid diagnosis. A sensitive and specific enzyme-linked immunosorbent assay for measles immunoglobulin M is often positive on the first day of rash and is widely available for surveillance, rapid diagnosis, and identification of measles cases. Third, a safe and effective form of intervention must be available. Although the nucleotide sequences of certain measles genes show evolutionary drift, there is only a single strain of antigenically stable measles virus, and the measles virus vaccine elicits an immune response that is active against all known isolates. Finally, evidence of a prolonged period of interruption and elimination of endogenous transmission has been demonstrated in a number of countries. On September 22, 2003, the Pan American Health Organization announced that the western hemisphere had been free of endemic measles for 10 consecutive months. Thus, it seems that measles satisfies the conditions needed for eradication.

Recently, the threat from bioterrorism has been raised as an obstacle to the possibility of global measles eradication. The existence of measles virus in laboratories throughout the world will serve as a reservoir of virus making it unlikely that measles immunization programs could be discontinued. However, inability to eliminate the threat from reintroduction of measles is not a sufficient basis to forgo the opportunity to eliminate the suffering caused by continued circulation of measles at the present time. In addition, the potential cost savings from global measles eradication represents an incentive to both industrialized and developing countries. The United States currently spends at least $45 million annually for the measles component of the MMR vaccine, and it has been estimated that >$1.5 billion is spent annually on prevention and treatment of measles worldwide. If measles were no longer circulating on a global basis, then it would be feasible to replace the 2-dose MMR vaccine schedule with either a single MMR immunization or a single MMR followed by a mumps-rubella vaccine. A recent estimate of the cumulative cost savings to 7 industrialized countries from this change projected yearly savings of between $69 and $623 million.

Conclusion

Measles infection continues to account for nearly 50% of the 1.6 million deaths caused each year by vaccine-preventable diseases of childhood. In view that a safe and effective vaccine has been available for 40 years, which obstacles account for the failure to make greater progress in worldwide measles control? An important factor is the lack of appreciation of disease severity, particularly in developed countries, where measles rates are low and disease is seldom encountered. A political commitment to control measles is necessary not only in developing countries with a limited public health infrastructure, where most of the estimated yearly 31 million cases of measles occur, but also in industrialized countries, where measles is no longer a high health priority. Second, unscientific and erroneous accusations regarding a risk between measles vaccine and neurologic disorders must not be permitted to undermine the success of measles control programs. Estimates from mathematical models indicate that for industrialized countries such as the United States, herd immunity may be lost and endemic transmission of measles may be reestablished if measles immunity falls below 93% to 95%. Finally, measles is more severe in human immunodeficiency virus–infected individuals, and the burgeoning acquired immune deficiency syndrome epidemic provides an increased susceptibility to measles among increasing numbers of people. To eradicate one of humankind's great scourges is a challenge that is not easily met. Before global eradication of measles can be achieved, additional work is needed to address operational barriers (eg, injection safety), to build political and financial commitments, and to develop effective partnerships. As has been learned from the Polio Eradication Initiative, the availability of effective vaccination strategies alone is not sufficient to ensure that eradication can be achieved.

Source: "Measles Vaccines and the Potential for Worldwide Eradication of Measles." *Pediatrics* 114, no. 4 (October 2004): 1065–1069 (doi:10.1542/peds.2004-0440).

REGULATIONS AND GUIDELINES

African Program for Onchocerciasis Control, "Practical Guide for Trainers of Community-Directed Distributors," 2005

The African Program for Onchocerciasis Control was founded in 1995 and is headquartered in Burkina Faso in West Africa. It faces the difficult challenge of defeating an endemic parasitic disease in countries with limited health care systems. It puts great emphasis on community-based programs. This guideline was designed for staff members who distribute the drug ivermectin to villages.

Summary Of Steps In Community-Directed Treatment With Ivermectin (CDTI)

Step 1 Health worker pays a visit to community chief; secures appointment date for a meeting between CDTI facilitation team and community leaders. (It is advisable for the health worker to obtain an estimate from the district office of the population likely to be covered by the CDTI project, so that the required number of tablets will be available when the community decides to implement CDTI).

Step 2 Meeting of community chief/leaders and the facilitation team. Set date for meeting with entire community.

Step 3 Meeting of facilitation team and entire community. Selection of CDDs may be take place at this meeting.

Step 4 Allow community time to select distributors (CDDs) from their own rank based on their own criteria. Community informs health worker and trainer (facilitation team) about community's preferred date for training CDDs.

Step 4a If the facilitation team has information on the total population figure of the community, it should take an estimated number of tablets likely to be required for distribution to the community on the day of training.

Step 5 Training of CDD

Step 5a In cases where the facilitation team does deliver tablets during the training session, CDDs should begin distributing ivermectin as soon as possible after completing their training.

Step 6 CDDs conduct census, record in notebook, and keep a copy in home of village/community leader.

Step 7 Community decides on month and dates of ivermectin distribution.

Step 8 CDD informs health worker/facilitation team about chosen date of distribution. If possible, CDD should collect ivermectin during the same meeting.

Step 9 If the ivermectin has not already been collected, CDDs should collect ivermectin tablets from the health post on a date previously agreed with health workers.

Step 10 Distribution of ivermectin by CDDs

Step 11 CDDs monitor adverse reactions, treat cases of minor reactions where possible, and refer cases of severe adverse reactions to nearest health facility.

Step 12 Complete the treatment record notebooks/forms and return a copy to the post from which ivermectin is collected.

Step 12a CDDs keep ivermectin tablets and treat, at a later date, those community members who did not receive treatment due to absenteeism, sickness, etc., making careful note of any such treatment.

Step 12b Health worker during any future visit to the village monitors the CDDs treatment record notebooks and updates the health post record accordingly.

Source: APOC. "Practical Guide for Trainers of Community-Directed Distributors." January 25, 2005. Available online. URL: http://www.apoc.bf/en/cdti_PracticalGuide.htm. Accessed July 5, 2006.

WHO, International Health Regulations, 2005

In May 2005 the World Health Assembly of the WHO approved a new set of International Health Regulations, after many years of discussion. They went into effect in June 2007. The new rules include some of the old specifics concerning ships, planes, and ports of entry (as in the 1951 regulations below), but there is a new focus on surveillance and communication in order to fight new outbreaks before they can become pandemics—as indicated in the following selection.

PART II – INFORMATION AND PUBLIC HEALTH RESPONSE

Article 5

Surveillance

1. Each State Party shall develop, strengthen and maintain, as soon as possible but no later than five years from the entry into force of these Regulations for that State Party, the capacity to detect, assess, notify and report events in accordance with these Regulations, as specified in Annex 1.

2. Following the assessment referred to in paragraph 2, Part A of Annex 1, a State Party may report to WHO on the basis of a justified need and an implementation plan and, in so doing, obtain an extension of two years in which to fulfill the obligation in paragraph 1 of this Article. In exceptional circumstances, and supported by a new implementation plan, the State Party may request a further extension not exceeding two years from the Director-General, who shall make the decision, taking into account the technical advice of the Committee established under Article 50 (hereinafter the "Review Committee"). After the period mentioned in paragraph 1 of this Article, the State Party that has obtained an extension shall report annually to WHO on progress made towards the full implementation.

3. WHO shall assist States Parties, upon request, to develop, strengthen and maintain the capacities referred to in paragraph 1 of this Article.

4. WHO shall collect information regarding events through its surveillance activities and assess their potential to cause international disease spread and possible interference with international traffic. Information received by WHO under this paragraph shall be handled in accordance with Articles 11 and 45 where appropriate.

Article 6
Notification

1. Each State Party shall assess events occurring within its territory by using the decision instrument in Annex 2. Each State Party shall notify WHO, by the most efficient means of communication available, by way of the National IHR Focal Point, and within 24 hours of assessment of public health information, of all events which may constitute a public health emergency of international concern within its territory in accordance with the decision instrument, as well as any health measure implemented in response to those events. If the notification received by WHO involves the competency of the International Atomic Energy Agency (IAEA), WHO shall immediately notify the IAEA.

2. Following a notification, a State Party shall continue to communicate to WHO timely, accurate and sufficiently detailed public health information available to it on the notified event, where possible including case definitions, laboratory results, source and type of the risk, number of cases and deaths, conditions affecting the spread of the disease and the health measures employed; and report, when necessary, the difficulties faced and support needed in responding to the potential public health emergency of international concern.

Article 7
Information-sharing during unexpected or unusual public health events

If a State Party has evidence of an unexpected or unusual public health event within its territory, irrespective of origin or source, which may constitute a public health emergency of international concern, it shall provide to WHO all relevant public health information. In such a case, the provisions of Article 6 shall apply in full.

Article 8

Consultation

In the case of events occurring within its territory not requiring notification as provided in Article 6, in particular those events for which there is insufficient information available to complete the decision instrument, a State Party may nevertheless keep WHO advised thereof through the National IHR Focal Point and consult with WHO on appropriate health measures. Such communications shall be treated in accordance with paragraphs 2 to 4 of Article 11. The State Party in whose territory the event has occurred may request WHO assistance to assess any epidemiological evidence obtained by that State Party.

Article 9

Other reports

1. WHO may take into account reports from sources other than notifications or consultations and shall assess these reports according to established epidemiological principles and then communicate information on the event to the State Party in whose territory the event is allegedly occurring. Before taking any action based on such reports, WHO shall consult with and attempt to obtain verification from the State Party in whose territory the event is allegedly occurring in accordance with the procedure set forth in Article 10. To this end, WHO shall make the information received available to the States Parties and only where it is duly justified may WHO maintain the confidentiality of the source. This information will be used in accordance with the procedure set forth in Article 11.

2. States Parties shall, as far as practicable, inform WHO within 24 hours of receipt of evidence of a public health risk identified outside their territory that may cause international disease spread, as manifested by exported or imported:

(a) human cases;

(b) vectors which carry infection or contamination; or

(c) goods that are contaminated.

Article 10

Verification

1. WHO shall request, in accordance with Article 9, verification from a State Party of reports from sources other than notifications or consultations of events which may constitute a public health emergency of international concern allegedly occurring in the State's territory. In such cases,

WHO shall inform the State Party concerned regarding the reports it is seeking to verify.

2. Pursuant to the foregoing paragraph and to Article 9, each State Party, when requested by WHO, shall verify and provide:

(a) within 24 hours, an initial reply to, or acknowledgement of, the request from WHO;

(b) within 24 hours, available public health information on the status of events referred to in WHO's request; and

(c) information to WHO in the context of an assessment under Article 6, including relevant information as described in that Article.

3. When WHO receives information of an event that may constitute a public health emergency of international concern, it shall offer to collaborate with the State Party concerned in assessing the potential for international disease spread, possible interference with international traffic and the adequacy of control measures. Such activities may include collaboration with other standard-setting organizations and the offer to mobilize international assistance in order to support the national authorities in conducting and coordinating on-site assessments. When requested by the State Party, WHO shall provide information supporting such an offer.

4. If the State Party does not accept the offer of collaboration, WHO may, when justified by the magnitude of the public health risk, share with other States Parties the information available to it, whilst encouraging the State Party to accept the offer of collaboration by WHO, taking into account the views of the State Party concerned.

Article 11
Provision of information by WHO

1. Subject to paragraph 2 of this Article, WHO shall send to all States Parties and, as appropriate, to relevant intergovernmental organizations, as soon as possible and by the most efficient means available, in confidence, such public health information which it has received under Articles 5 to 10 inclusive and which is necessary to enable States Parties to respond to a public health risk. WHO should communicate information to other States Parties that might help them in preventing the occurrence of similar incidents.

2. WHO shall use information received under Articles 6 and 8 and paragraph 2 of Article 9 for verification, assessment and assistance purposes

under these Regulations and, unless otherwise agreed with the States Parties referred to in those provisions, shall not make this information generally available to other States Parties, until such time as:

(a) the event is determined to constitute a public health emergency of international concern in accordance with Article 12; or

(b) information evidencing the international spread of the infection or contamination has been confirmed by WHO in accordance with established epidemiological principles; or

(c) there is evidence that:

(i) control measures against the international spread are unlikely to succeed because of the nature of the contamination, disease agent, vector or reservoir; or

(ii) the State Party lacks sufficient operational capacity to carry out necessary measures to prevent further spread of disease; or

(d) the nature and scope of the international movement of travellers, baggage, cargo, containers, conveyances, goods or postal parcels that may be affected by the infection or contamination requires the immediate application of international control measures.

3. WHO shall consult with the State Party in whose territory the event is occurring as to its intent to make information available under this Article.

4. When information received by WHO under paragraph 2 of this Article is made available to States Parties in accordance with these Regulations, WHO may also make it available to the public if other information about the same event has already become publicly available and there is a need for the dissemination of authoritative and independent information.

Article 12
Determination of a public health emergency of international concern

1. The Director-General shall determine, on the basis of the information received, in particular from the State Party within whose territory an event is occurring, whether an event constitutes a public health emergency of international concern in accordance with the criteria and the procedure set out in these Regulations.

2. If the Director-General considers, based on an assessment under these Regulations, that a public health emergency of international concern is occurring, the Director-General shall consult with the State Party in whose territory the event arises regarding this preliminary determination. If the

Director-General and the State Party are in agreement regarding this determination, the Director-General shall, in accordance with the procedure set forth in Article 49, seek the views of the Committee established under Article 48 (hereinafter the "Emergency Committee") on appropriate temporary recommendations.

3. If, following the consultation in paragraph 2 above, the Director-General and the State Party in whose territory the event arises do not come to a consensus within 48 hours on whether the event constitutes a public health emergency of international concern, a determination shall be made in accordance with the procedure set forth in Article 49.

4. In determining whether an event constitutes a public health emergency of international concern, the Director-General shall consider:

(a) information provided by the State Party;

(b) the decision instrument contained in Annex 2;

(c) the advice of the Emergency Committee;

(d) scientific principles as well as the available scientific evidence and other relevant information; and

(e) an assessment of the risk to human health, of the risk of international spread of disease and of the risk of interference with international traffic.

5. If the Director-General, following consultations with the State Party within whose territory the public health emergency of international concern has occurred, considers that a public health emergency of international concern has ended, the Director-General shall take a decision in accordance with the procedure set out in Article 49.

Source: World Health Organization. WHA58.3, Documents of the 58th World Health Assembly. Available online. May 23, 2005. URL: http://www.who.int/gb/ebwha/pdf_files/WHA58/WHA58_3-en.pdf. November 3, 2006.

United Nations, International Sanitary Regulations, 1951

In 1882 the first International Sanitary Convention was signed, to help prevent the spread of epidemics through travel and trade across borders. After several revisions, the convention was replaced in 1951 by a set of similar International Sanitary Regulations approved by the members of the United Nations at the Fourth World Health Assembly. A major revision was approved in 2005 and was implemented in June 2007.

Part IV—Sanitary Measures and Procedure

Chapter I—General Provisions

Article 23

The sanitary measures permitted by these Regulations are the maximum measures applicable to international traffic, which a State may require for the protection of its territory against the quarantinable diseases.

Article 24

Sanitary measures and health formalities shall be initiated forthwith, completed without delay, and applied without discrimination.

Article 25

1. Disinfection, disinsecting, deratting, and other sanitary operations shall be so carried out as—

a. not to cause undue discomfort to any person, or injury to his health;

b. not to produce any deleterious effect on the structure of a ship, an aircraft, or a vehicle, or on its operating equipment;

c. to avoid all risk of fire.

2. In carrying out such operations on goods, baggage, and other articles, every precaution shall be taken to avoid any damage.

Article 26

1. A health authority shall, when so requested, issue free of charge to the carrier a certificate specifying the measures applied to a ship, or an aircraft, or a railway carriage, wagon, or road vehicle, the parts thereof treated, the methods employed, and the reasons why the measures have been applied. In the case of an aircraft this information shall, on request, be entered instead in the General Declaration.

2. Similarly, a health authority shall, when so requested, issue free of charge—

a. to any traveler a certificate specifying the date of his arrival or departure and the measures applied to him and his baggage;

b. to the consigner, the consignee, and the carrier, or their respective agents, a certificate specifying the measures applied to any goods.

Article 27

1. A person under surveillance shall not be isolated and shall be permitted to move about freely. The health authority may require him to report to it, if necessary, at specified intervals during the period of surveillance. Except as limited by the provisions of Article 69, the health authority may also

subject such a person to medical investigation and make any inquiries which are necessary for ascertaining his state of health.

2. When a person under surveillance departs for another place, within or without the same territory, he shall inform the health authority, which shall immediately notify the health authority for the place to which the person is proceeding. On arrival the person shall report to that health authority which may apply the measure provided for in paragraph 1 of the Article.

Article 28

Except in case of an emergency constituting grave danger to public health, a ship or an aircraft, which is not infected or suspected of being infected with a quarantinable disease, shall not on account of any other epidemic disease be prevented by the health authority for a port or an airport from discharging or loading cargo or stores, or taking on fuel or water.

Article 29

A health authority may take all practicable measures to control the discharge from any ship of sewage and refuse which might contaminate the waters of a port, river, or canal.

Chapter II – Sanitary Measures on Departure

Article 30

1. The health authority for a port or an airport or for the local area in which a frontier post is situated may, when it considers it necessary, medically examine any person before his departure on an international voyage. The time and place of this examination shall be arranged to take into account the customs examination and other formalities, so as to facilitate his departure and to avoid delay.

2. The health authority referred to in paragraph 1 of this Article shall take all practicable measure—

a. to prevent the departure of any infected person or suspect;

b. to prevent the introduction on board a ship, an aircraft, a train, or a road vehicle of possible agents of infection or vectors of a quarantinable disease.

3. Notwithstanding the provisions of sub-paragraph (a) of paragraph 2 of this Article, a person on an international voyage who on arrival is placed under surveillance may be allowed to continue his voyage. If he is doing so

by air, the health authority for the airport shall record the fact on the General Declaration.

Chapter III—Sanitary Measures Applicable between Ports or Airports of Departure and Arrival

Article 31

No matter capable of causing any epidemic disease shall be thrown or allowed to fall from an aircraft when it is in flight.

Article 32

1. No sanitary measure shall be applied by a State to any ship which passes through its territorial waters without calling at a port or on the coast.

2. If for any reason such a call is made, the sanitary laws and regulations in force in the territory may be applied without exceeding, however, the provisions of these Regulations.

Article 33

1. No sanitary measure, other than medical examination, shall be applied to a healthy ship, as specified in Part V, which passes through a maritime canal or waterway in the territory of a State on its way to a port in the territory of another State, unless such ship comes from an infected local area or has on board any person coming from an infected local area, within the incubation period of the disease with which the local area is infected.

2. The only measure which may be applied to such a ship coming from such an area or having such a person on board is the stationing on board, if necessary, of a sanitary guard to prevent all unauthorized contact between the ship and the shore, and to supervise the application of Article 29.

3. A health authority shall permit any such ship to take on, under its control, fuel, water, and stores.

4. An infected or suspected ship which passes through a maritime canal or waterway may be treated as if it were calling at a port in the same territory.

Article 34

Notwithstanding any provision to the contrary in these Regulations except Article 75, no sanitary measure, other than medical examination, shall be applied to—

a) passengers and crew on board a healthy ship from which they do not disembark;

b) passengers and crew from a healthy aircraft who are in transit through a territory and who remain in a direct transit areas of an airport of that territory, or, if the airport is not yet provided with such an area, who submit to the measures for segregation prescribed by the health authority in order to prevent the spread of disease; if such persons are obliged to leave the airport at which they disembark solely in order to continue their voyage from another airport in the vicinity of the first airport, no such measure shall be applied to them if the transfer is made under the control of the health authority or authorities.

[The section concluded with a list of similar provisions applicable when a ship or plane arrives at a port, and applicable on goods or mail shipped between countries.]

Source: International Sanitary Regulations: World Health Organization Regulation No. 2. World Health Organization Library. Available online. URL: http://whqlibdoc.who.int/trs/WHO_TRS_41.pdf. Accessed May 3, 2006.

PART III

Research Tools

6

How to Research Pandemics and Global Health

CHOOSING A TOPIC

The field of epidemic disease and global health offers a large variety of topics suitable for student research projects. Even a beginner with little background will be able to pick out a subject area that can be summarized meaningfully in a brief report, with some good hard data to back up the main points. More ambitious students can find a wealth of material at all levels of difficulty to complete a term paper.

Students who have not studied much science might be a bit intimidated at first. They need not worry: Unlike such current events topics as the causes of war or the globalization of the job market, you will not have to fight your way through a mass of contradictory opinions before you can even narrow down your topic. In most cases you will find basic agreement on the main facts, such as the cause of AIDS. Once you have mastered the facts you can, if you wish, deal with such controversies as how best to educate young people on the dangers of unsafe sex, how to strengthen the health care delivery system in rich and in poor countries, or how to pay for drug research and production.

When looking for a topic, try writing about a specific infectious disease. A student might choose to write about one of the big current killers such as malaria, tuberculosis, HIV/AIDS, or infant diarrhea; historic pandemics such as smallpox or bubonic plague; diseases that are now being effectively fought such as polio or measles; or possible future scourges such as avian flu or Ebola. One can report on the disease itself, such as its causes, its short-term symptoms and long-term effects, and its treatments and cures, if there are any. Or, one can cover the epidemic nature of the disease, such as where it usually occurs, how it spreads, how many people have been affected or are currently suffering, and its possible course in the future.

Other students might choose to focus on ways of combating epidemics, from the technical perspective (for example, malaria can be fought with bednets, with antilarva pesticides, and with antiparasite medicines), or from the perspective of the world community (for example, how should the fight against malaria be organized and paid for?). Closer to home, students may want to explore how their own class, school, or community could help promote better world health through education, volunteering, and/or fundraising.

Different countries or regions and different areas of the United States have their own stories waiting to be told about specific diseases and epidemics or about health and health care in general. A student who has lived in a foreign country, or has visited one, may choose to use his or her knowledge to explore health-related topics pertaining to that country.

History buffs can find many interesting research topics in this field. Epidemics have been documented from ancient times to the recent past. One can report on the bare facts, or join in the speculation as to when and how the disease first emerged or how and why it spread in different historical eras. The way different societies and cultures responded to particular diseases and epidemics is another fascinating topic, touching on religion and anthropology as well as history. One might even want to read and report on fictional accounts of infectious disease. Famous examples include Daniel Defoe's *Journal of a Plague Year,* a fictional account of the Great Plague of London of 1665, Albert Camus's novel *The Plague*, set in the author's native Algeria, or Thomas Mann's novella *Death in Venice*.

Of course, anyone considering a career in medicine, nursing, biology, chemistry, or public health might well be motivated to explore more deeply the latest developments in disease detection and control. Scientists are constantly making progress in understanding how diseases work on the molecular level; how genetics plays a role (as the disease microbe evolves or as a person's genetic profile comes into play); and how different vaccines or medicines work and how they can be made better or cheaper. This activity is reported and disseminated faster than ever before, often in forms that lay people can understand. An adventurous student who is willing to spend time working through more difficult sources can now access a vast treasury of information never before available to the ordinary individual.

FINDING INFORMATION

For most students, finding information will not be hard. If anything, it may be difficult to choose from the large variety of available resources.

A teacher or a librarian—at a school or at a local public library—can help with getting started. They should be able to point a student's way to find the best material for his or her purposes. They might even help refine a topic based on available books or Web sites. The two major categories available to today's students are printed books and online Web sites.

Books

Despite promises of a wired, interactive future, books have so far remained an essential source for anyone looking for in-depth information. And most books (especially newer ones) are not yet fully available online.

Books have many advantages over the Internet. They can bring together in one place many different aspects of a topic. Even if readers only skim the chapters they do not use, at least they are aware of these other aspects and are thus better able to understand the material. Books have the space—and authors expect readers to devote the time—to cover topics in detail and in depth. Students may find that what they thought they knew about a topic, based on brief news reports, was really incomplete or misleading.

Good authors will expose their readers to different points of view, a very important feature when dealing with matters of public policy. Most books in this field have footnotes or bibliographies or both, which point readers to still more sources of information. Furthermore, books almost always provide the author's name and qualifications, and the date and place of publication. They usually also provide an author's preface or introduction explaining why and how the book was written. This information helps smart readers understand a book's point of view and any possible bias that could distort the information. By contrast, a great many Web articles are unsigned, or are copied from site to site, until the important identifying information completely disappears.

Among the disadvantages of books is that they can never be as up-to-date as the latest newspaper headline. Even a book that has just been published may be based mostly on information gathered a year or two in the past. If a student's topic is very current, he or she should always use the Internet to supplement what is learned from books.

A final practical disadvantage to books is that few high school or local branch libraries can carry more than a small selection on any given topic, especially among more recent titles. If a student lives in a large city, however, he or she should become familiar with central or regional library branches, which usually have many more books to choose from. In addition, some college libraries make their resources available to serious high school students in their community; it is always worthwhile to ask.

FINDING THE RIGHT BOOKS

The first place to start is the annotated bibliography in this book—and in the bibliographies *within* those books. Even if some of the books turn out to be unavailable, looking for them will get students into the library or into online catalogues which contain other books that may be within reach.

The largest online catalogue is that of the Library of Congress, one of the largest repositories of data in human history—the library owns over 30 million books and tens of millions of other items of interest. Check its home page at http://www.loc.gov, not just for information on how to use the catalogue, but also for helpful tips on doing research. One can send e-mail queries, or even chat online with a librarian during weekday afternoons.

Catalogues for many other major collections can be accessed online as well. Serious researchers might be able to borrow books via interlibrary loan or even purchase photocopies, but even if not, it can be exciting and educational just to browse through these catalogues. For example, try the Harvard University libraries home page at http://lib.harvard.edu, or the New York Public Library research libraries' catalogue at http://catnyp.nypl.org.

Of course, a great many of the materials listed in such major catalogues will be specialized or scientific works, outdated books, or titles written in a variety of foreign languages. For popular, recent English language books, one can try searching on Amazon.com, Barnesandnoble.com, Books.google.com, or other commercial sites. These sites provide a wealth of information about the books, often including reviews by experts and/or ordinary readers. Further information can often be found on the Web site of the book's publisher. Many publishers have made their books available for limited online browsing via Amazon and Google Books. Sometimes this is all one needs to get an important nugget of information; other times this peek will inspire a student to seek the book at a library, or even to buy it.

Newspapers and Magazines

For anyone who wants to be an informed citizen, there is probably no substitute for reading a good newspaper every day—whether a hard copy or online; most daily newspapers cover far more stories each day than a television or radio news broadcast could possibly manage. The major national or regional newspapers, such as *USA Today* or the *Washington Post*, can usually be counted on to keep an eye on the latest developments in this field. Even smaller local papers will cover topics such as the major current or future pandemics, often using news service articles.

The established newsmagazines, such as *Time*, *Newsweek*, and *US News & World Report*, also pride themselves on health and science coverage, though they impose a high degree of selection, editing, and condensation on the raw news material. Science magazines for the general reader, like *Popular Science,* will often cover issues of global health as well.

Online Resources

Unless a topic is purely historical, one will not be able to complete his or her research in the fields of pandemics and global health without devoting time on the Internet. One can start, for fun, by plugging a few keywords into a favorite search engine, but there is no guarantee that whatever sites come up on page one will be accurate and unbiased. Sooner or later, it would help to use the following types of resources, which at least aim for objectivity and completeness. Once the basics are known, one can explore more intelligently through the vast sea of online sites.

GOVERNMENT SITES

The U.S. Government sponsors a number of very informative sites that cover a huge variety of topics relating to health and medicine. The information is up-to-date and the tone is serious yet readable. These sites reflect the consensus point of view of the medical profession. Links are often provided to other reliable government or nongovernment sites.

The Centers for Disease Control and Prevention home page bills itself as "your online source for credible health information," and it certainly is *one* of the best all-around sites (http://www.cdc.gov). Users can search for information using keywords, select from the CDC's catalogue of "Health and Safety Topics," find statistics and charts to illustrate and enhance their projects, or learn about the agency itself. Within each major topic one can investigate further; for example, there is a home page for each major disease, with links to pages covering every aspect of the topic, such as its biology, diagnosis and treatment, and epidemiology. There are also links to the CDC's free scholarly journal, *Emerging Infectious Diseases.*

Another excellent source is the MedlinePlus site of the National Institutes of Health (NIH); the home page can be found at http://medlineplus.gov. It is a vast compendium of information, designed mostly for nonprofessionals. Apart from its many service features including news summaries, directories of doctors, information on clinical trials, and links to local resources, the site covers 740 health topics in laypeople's terms and has a complete illustrated medical encyclopedia (a bit more technical). One can even see videos of common surgical procedures.

Many other government bodies around the world have put a great deal of medical information on the Web as well. They can be excellent sources of information about the individual countries and regions; it is always interesting to see how the same topic is treated from a different perspective. Health Canada, for example, at http://www.hc-sc.gc.ca, can be a rich source of information. The government of India Web site (http://india.gov.in/citizen/health.php), whose default language is English, has many links to epidemic control programs and other matters relating to public health. A careful reader will detect the influence of local culture on how the site treats health issues—for example, the Indian site gives prominence to "alternative" or traditional systems of medicine.

Agencies of the United Nations, especially the World Health Organization, maintain many informative sites. They focus on UN activities, but also serve as clearinghouses of information, especially about pandemics and about health and medicine in the developing world. The WHO home page (http://www.who.int/en/) is a good place to start.

NEWSPAPERS, JOURNALS, AND MAGAZINES

In recent years nearly every important print periodical, from tabloid newspapers to the most specialized scientific journal, has established itself on the Internet. Access is often free, and even paying sites usually offer some free material. A school or public library may well have institutional subscriptions to many of the periodicals a student is likely to use.

One excellent source for science news for laypeople is the *New York Times* (http://www.nytimes.com), which keeps all articles going back to 1851 online. *Discover* magazine goes back to 1992 online, and is well worth a visit sometime during a student's research (http://www.discovermagazine.com).

Several professionally oriented magazines and scientific journals offer a selection of free articles and news items, and maintain archives going back as far as 20 years. Check in when preparing to research—a last-minute news item can add some immediacy and credibility to a student's work. Try, among others, *New Scientist* (http://www.newscientist.com), *Nature* (http://www. nature.com/news), and *Scientific American* (http://www.sciam.com). The Science Daily site (http://www.sciencedaily.com/news/plants-animals/nature/) is a very rich treasury of science and medical news; bear in mind, however, that most of its stories are in fact press releases from university research departments, pharmaceutical companies, or other parties who may exaggerate the importance of their discoveries.

Most articles in medical journals are quite technical, but students might want to check anyway to get a flavor of what scientists do. The journals included in the Public Library of Science (PLoS; http://www.plos.org) are available free to read online, and can be used freely as long as the source is credited. Most other journals require a subscription, but the important ones can usually be accessed via public or college libraries.

Nongovernmental Organizations

Most of the growing ranks of nongovernmental organizations that deal with global health issues have informational Web sites, often beautifully designed and with multimedia features. The "Organizations" section in this book, which lists 25 such groups, would be a good place to start. Most of them include links to other organizations and Web sites.

Bear in mind that every nongovernmental organization has interests and viewpoints of its own, even though most of them are not-for-profit and were founded and are supported by charitable individuals. On the other hand, such groups can sometimes afford to highlight unpleasant truths and policy failures without the political restraints of a government or UN agency. The best guarantee of accurate, unbiased information is to use a variety of different types of sources.

Some universities, medical schools, or schools of public health maintain useful Web sites. For example, Harvard University School of Public Health has a site with links to stories on recent world health news; it is updated weekly.

Encyclopedias

Most popular general encyclopedias, such as *Encyclopaedia Britannica,* can now be found on the Internet, although a library subscription is often necessary to unlock most of the articles. McGraw Hill's *AccessScience* online service, available from many libraries, includes a well-written, up-to-date encyclopedia and dictionary. The *Gale Encyclopedia of Medicine* is another useful source accessible from many libraries.

Wikipedia, the Free Encyclopedia, has become one of the most popular Web sites in the world. Almost every subject in the field of infectious disease and public health is covered, often in some detail. In many subject areas, such as politics and history, Wikipedia articles must be used with caution. Since anyone can edit and change them, errors and biases often crop up until the volunteer editors can clean them up. However, this does not seem to be as much a problem in the sciences. In late 2005 the prestigious British journal *Nature* conducted a peer review of scientific entries on *Wikipedia* as compared with parallel articles in *Britannica.* Although the *Wikipedia* articles were often found to be poorly constructed, they stood up to the comparison in terms of accuracy.

Some commercially supported Web sites include reliable encyclopedic information in the medical field. For example, eMedicine (http://www.emedicine.com) provides an extensive database of clinical information written by doctors. It covers all the major infectious diseases thoroughly, but due to its clinical focus, it does not have much information on epidemiology or public health. InteliHealth (http://www.intelihealth.com), a partnership between the health insurer Aetna and the Harvard Medical School's Consumer Health Information, tends to have a similar clinical focus. MedicineNet is another, similar site (http://medicinenet.com).

Clash of Opinions

Once students have learned some basic facts, they might want to check out the blogs—weblogs that record the personal opinions of everyone from informed, dispassionate experts to patients or health professionals on the front line of the fight against epidemics to angry individuals with personal or institutional axes to grind. Many blogs also include breaking news from the media or from personal sources.

There are few signposts in the vast sea of millions of blogs. To get started, use a favorite search engine and plug in the terms "blog" and either a disease name or a topic name such as "pandemics" or "global health." Each site will provide links to many others. Students should try to avoid the pitfall of staying with blogs whose views they agree with. Seek out others with different perspectives. Some interesting bloggers will write about aspects of the topic that can often be overlooked, such as the experiences of various minority groups, or the impact of religion or culture on health and disease.

7

Facts and Figures

1. "SPANISH FLU" HIT YOUNG ADULTS HARD

1.1 Spanish Flu Cases in the United States, 1918

Young people were more likely to be stricken with Spanish flu than the elderly. About one out of every three people aged 30 or less in the United States took ill.

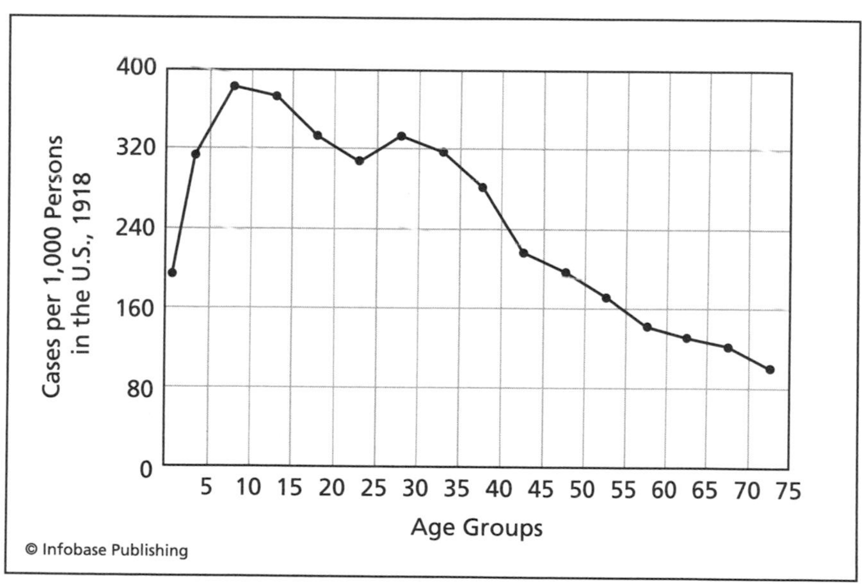

Source: Jeffrey Taubenberger and David M. Morens. "1918 Influenza, the Mother of All Pandemics." *Emerging Infectious Diseases* 12, no. 1 (January 2006).

1.2 Deaths among Persons Ill with Pneumonia and Flu

Influenza combined with pneumonia is often deadly for older men and women and for infants—as shown by the dotted line, showing mortality in the ordinary winter of 1928–29. But the 1918 Spanish flu epidemic was unusually deadly to men and women in the 20 to 40 age group, as shown by the solid line. For every 1,000 patients aged 27, for example, about 30 died in 1918–19, compared with about 1 in a normal year.

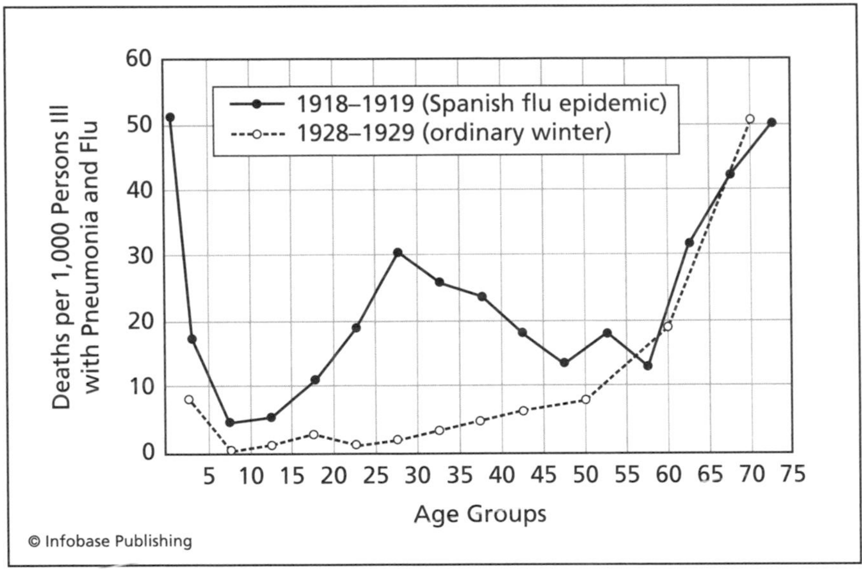

Source: Jeffrey Taubenberger and David M. Morens. "1918 Influenza, the Mother of All Pandemics." *Emerging Infectious Diseases* 12, no. 1 (January 2006).

1.3 Deaths in 1918, by Age Group

Since more young people took ill, and young patients were often hit hardest, total deaths were greatest for that age group. Out of every 1,000 people aged 27, 10 died.

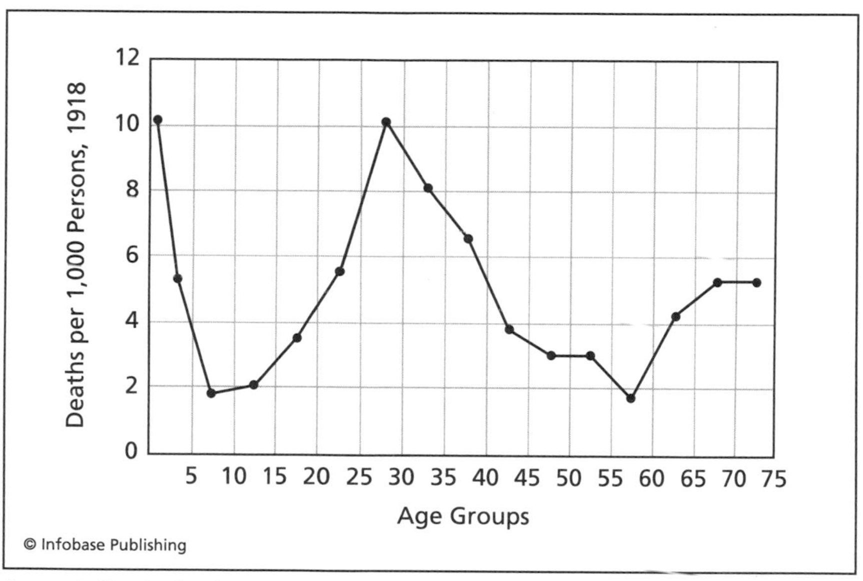

Source: Jeffrey Taubenberger and David M. Morens. "1918 Influenza, the Mother of All Pandemics." *Emerging Infectious Diseases* 12, no. 1 (January 2006).

2. GLOBAL HIV EPIDEMIC, 1990–2007

The world-wide epidemic of HIV (which causes AIDS) continues to claim new victims every year. By the end of 2007, over 33 million people were infected—apart from the many millions who had already died.

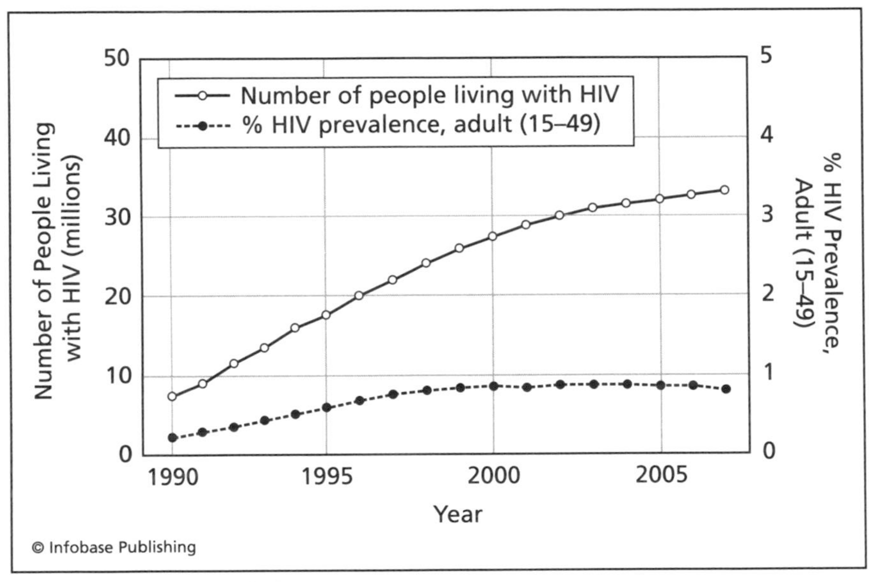

Source: UNAIDS 2007 Global Report, pp. 4–6.

3. MAJOR EPIDEMICS IN U.S. HISTORY

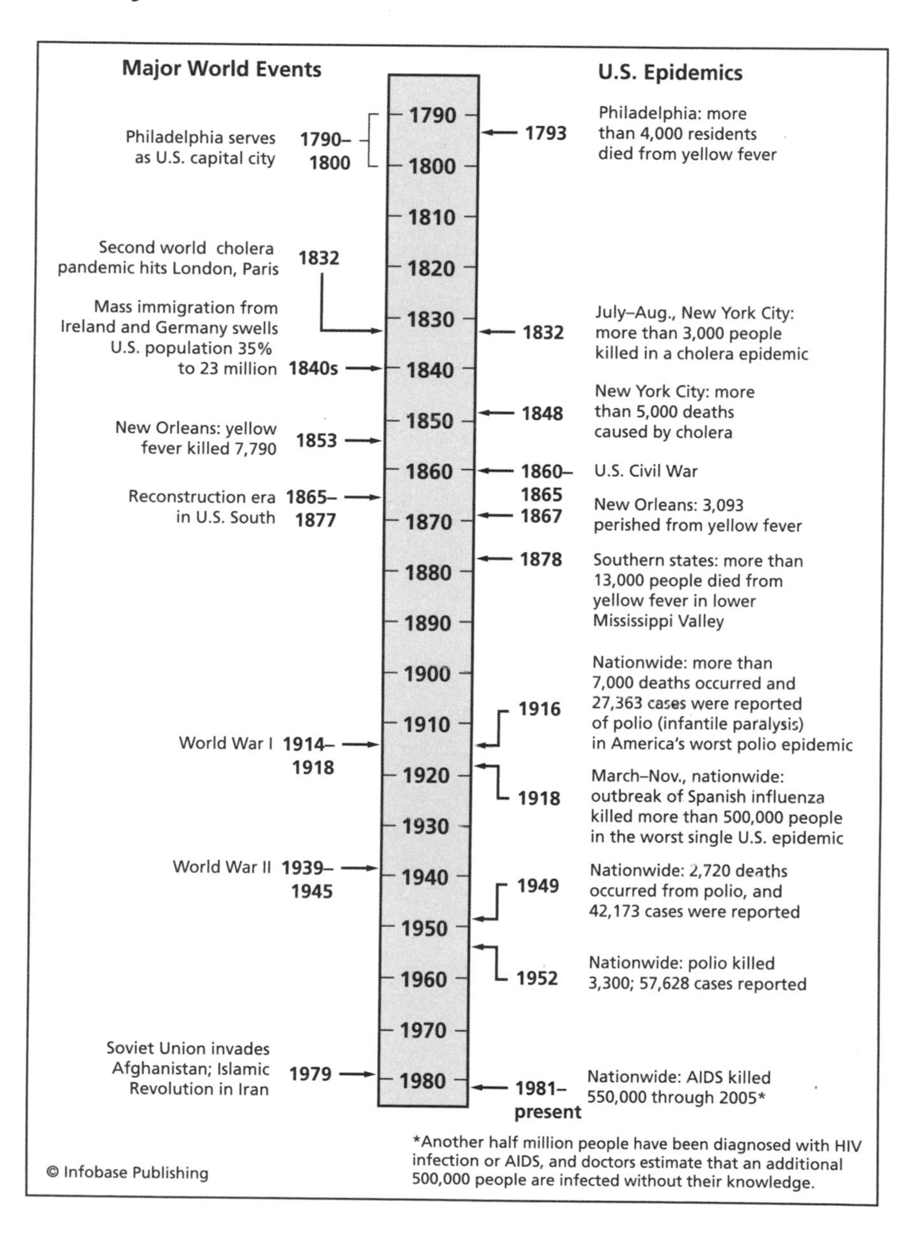

4. CASES OF NOTIFIABLE (CONTAGIOUS) DISEASE IN THE UNITED STATES

In order to monitor and control epidemic disease, U.S. law requires doctors and local health authorities to report all cases of most contagious diseases. The reported figures allow us to see the trends across time. Thankfully, many of the most serious diseases have been contained or even eliminated—but unfortunately not all of them. Sexually transmitted diseases, including chlamydia, are among the toughest problems.

Number of Cases Reported by Year

DISEASE	1950	1970	1990	2000	2002	2003	2004	2005
Diphtheria	5,796	435	4	1	1	1	—	—
Hepatitis A	—	56,797	31,441	13,397	8,795	7,653	5,683	4,488
Hepatitis B	—	8,310	21,102	8,036	7,996	7,526	6,212	5,119
Lyme disease	—	—	—	17,730	23,763	21,273	19,804	23,305
Meningococcal disease	—	2,505	2,451	2,256	1,814	1,756	1,361	1,245
Mumps	—	104,953	5,292	338	270	231	258	314
Pertussis (whooping cough)	120,718	4,249	4,570	7,867	9,771	11,647	25,827	25,616
Poliomyelitis	33,300	33	6	—	—	—	—	—
Rocky Mountain spotted fever	—	380	651	495	1,104	1,091	1,713	1,936
Rubella (German measles)	—	56,552	1,125	176	18	7	10	11
Rubeola (measles)	319,124	47,351	27,786	86	44	56	37	66
Salmonellosis, excluding typhoid fever	—	22,096	48,603	39,574	44,264	43,657	42,197	45,322
Shigellosis	23,367	13,845	27,077	22,922	23,541	23,581	14,627	16,168
Tuberculosis	—	37,137	25,701	16,377	15,075	14,874	14,517	14,097
Syphilis	217,558	91,382	135,590	31,616	32,912	34,270	33,401	33,278
Chlamydia	—	—	323,663	709,452	834,555	877,478	929,462	976,445
Gonorrhea	286,746	600,072	690,042	363,136	351,852	335,104	330,132	339,593
Chancroid	4,977	1,416	4,212	78	48	54	30	17

Source: National Center for Health Statistics, *Health, United States, 2007*. Available online. URL: http//www.cdc.gov/nchs/data/hus/hus07.pdf#summary.

5. GLOBAL SARS EPIDEMIC, NOVEMBER 2000 TO JULY 2003

The SARS epidemic touched every continent, but most countries were able to limit its impact, thanks to vigorous international cooperation and rapid action to contain the spread of infection within national borders. Note the high toll the disease took among health care workers.

COUNTRY	CASES	DEATHS	DEATH RATE (%)	HEALTH WORKERS	HEALTH WORKERS AS % OF ALL CASES
Australia	6	—	—	—	—
Canada	251	43	17	109	43
China	5,327	349	7	1,002	19
Hong Kong	1,755	299	17	386	22
Macao	1	—	—	—	—
Taiwan	346	37	11	68	20
France	7	1	14	2	29
Germany	9	—	—	1	11
India	3	—	—	—	—
Indonesia	2	—	—	—	—
Italy	4	—	—	—	—
Kuwait	1	—	—	—	—
Malaysia	5	2	40	—	—
Mongolia	9	—	—	—	—
New Zealand	1	—	—	—	—
Philippines	14	2	14	4	29
Republic of Ireland	1	—	—	—	—
Republic of Korea	3	—	—	—	—
Romania	1	—	—	—	—
Russia	1	—	—	—	—
Singapore	238	33	14	97	41

continues

continued

COUNTRY	CASES	DEATHS	DEATH RATE (%)	HEALTH WORKERS	HEALTH WORKERS AS % OF ALL CASES
South Africa	1	1	100	-	-
Spain	1	-	-	-	-
Sweden	5	-	-	-	-
Switzerland	1	-	-	-	-
Thailand	9	2	22	1	11
United Kingdom	4	-	-	-	-
United States	27	-	-	-	-
Viet Nam	63	5	8	36	57
Total	**8,096**	**774**	**9.6**	**1,706**	**21**

Source: World Health Organization. Available online. URL: http://www.who.int/csr/sars/country/table2004_04_21/en/index.html.

6. AIDS IN SUB-SAHARAN AFRICA

6.1 African Countries with the Largest Number of People Living with HIV

AIDS has devastated all regions in Africa. These 10 countries account for three-quarters of the total African caseload of people infected with the HIV virus.

COUNTRY	PEOPLE LIVING WITH HIV	WOMEN	CHILDREN	2005 AIDS DEATHS	AIDS ORPHANS*
South Africa	5,500,000	3,100,000	240,000	320,000	1,200,000
Nigeria	2,900,000	1,600,000	240,000	220,000	930,000
Mozambique	1,800,000	960,000	140,000	140,000	510,000
Zimbabwe	1,700,000	890,000	160,000	180,000	1,100,000
Tanzania	1,400,000	710,000	110,000	140,000	1,100,000
Kenya	1,300,000	740,000	150,000	140,000	1,100,000
Ethiopia	420,000–1,300,000	190,000–730,000	30,000–20000	38,000–130,000	280,000–870,000
Zambia	1,100,000	570,000	130,000	98,000	710,000
Dem. Rep. of Congo	1,000,000	520,000	120,000	90,000	680,000
Uganda	1,000,000	520,000	110,000	91,000	1,000,000
Total Sub-Saharan Africa	24,500,000	13,200,000	2,000,000	2,000,000	12,000,000

*Those under 18 who have lost one or both parents to AIDS

Source: UNAIDS 2006 Global Report

6.2 African Countries with the Highest Percentage of People Living with HIV

These 10 countries face a staggering challenge. Between one in 10 and one in three of all adults between 15 and 49 years old is infected with HIV, and will probably develop AIDS.

COUNTRY	% ADULTS AGES 15-49 INFECTED WITH HIV	PEOPLE LIVING WITH HIV	2005 AIDS DEATHS
Swaziland	33.4	220,000	16,000
Botswana	24.1	270,000	18,000
Lesotho	23.2	270,000	23,000
Zimbabwe	20.1	1,700,000	180,000
Namibia	19.6	230,000	17,000
South Africa	18.8	5,500,000	320,000
Zambia	17.0	1,100,000	98,000
Mozambique	16.1	1,800,000	140,000
Malawi	14.1	940,000	78,000
Central African Republic	10.7	250,000	24,000
Total sub-Saharan Africa	6.1	24,500,000	2,000,000

Source: UNAIDS 2006 Global Report

7. BLINDNESS AND DEVELOPING COUNTRIES

7.1 The Burden of Blindness

Blindness is often caused by infectious disease. Thus, it is more common in developing countries, where the impacts can be greater. In a world of poverty and few resources, blind people have less chance of living productive lives.

- There are an estimated 45 million blind people and 135 million visually impaired people worldwide
- Around 90% of people who are blind live in developing countries
- Worldwide, up to 70% of childhood blindness may be preventable
- An estimated 1.4 million children are blind, 320,000 of whom live in sub-Saharan Africa
- The global financial cost of childhood blindness (based on the loss of future earning capacity) is thought to be between US$6 billion and $27 billion
- An estimated 3.1% of deaths worldwide are directly or indirectly due to cataract, glaucoma, trachoma, and onchocerciasis
- In developed countries, for each decade after the age of 40 there is a threefold increase in the prevalence of blindness and vision loss
- In developing countries, it is believed that 60 to 80% of children who become blind die within 1–2 years

Source: Unite for Sight Website. Available online. URL: http://www.uniteforsight.org/eye_stats.php.

7.2 Onchocerciasis: Percentage of Blindness

The data below summarizes results from 2,315 villages in 11 West African countries, 1971–2001. For all those infected with onchocerciasis in a typical year, this chart shows what percent will go blind that year. The more microfilaria (larva) found in a skin sample, the higher the likelihood of going blind.

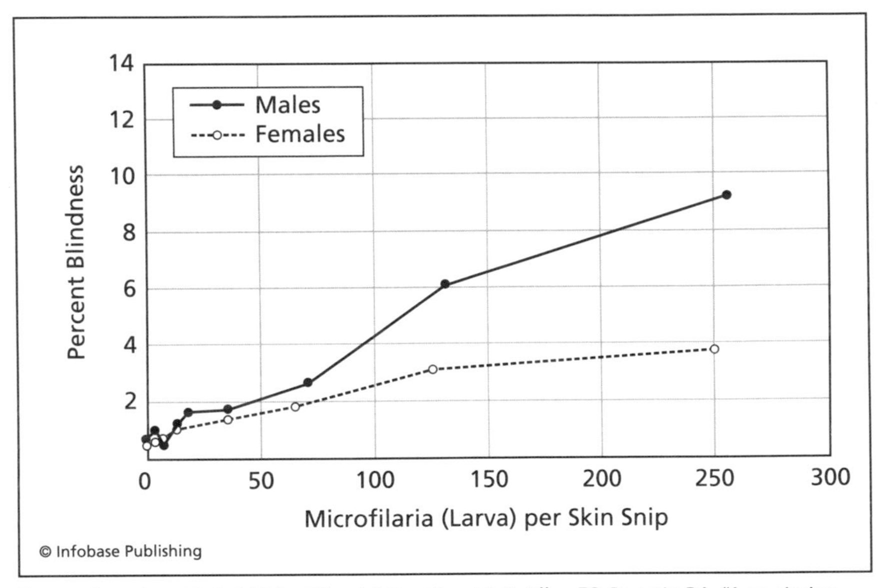

Source: Based on Little MP, Breitling LP, Basáñez M-G, Alley ES, Boortin BA. "Association between Microfilarial load and excess mortality in human onchocerciasis: An epidemiological study." *Lancet*. 2004; 363: 1514–1521.

7.3 Onchocerciasis: Mortality Rate

The data below summarizes results from 2,315 villages in 11 West African countries, 1971–2001. For all those infected with onchocerciasis, this chart shows what percent will die each year.

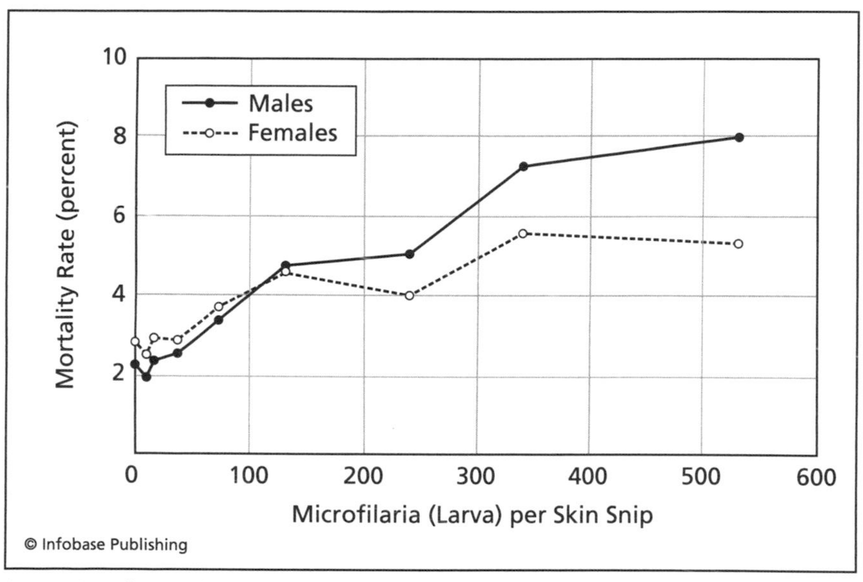

Source: Based on Little MP, Breitling LP, Basáñez M-G, Alley ES, Boortin BA. "Association between Microfilarial load and excess mortality in human onchocerciasis: An epidemiological study." *Lancet*. 2004; 363: 1514–1521.

8. MALARIA CASES AND DEATHS IN INDIA

8.1 Official Data

These figures were gathered and reported by the Indian government's National Anti-malaria Programme. They are probably accurate for the purposes of year-by-year comparison, but they do not include cases at private hospitals and clinics. Many experts believe the true numbers are a good deal higher.

YEAR	TOTAL MALARIA CASES (THOUSANDS)	*P. FALCIPARUM*† (THOUSANDS)	DEATHS (ACTUAL NUMBER)
1947	75,000	?	800,000
1961	49	?	—
1965	100	?	—
1976	6,470	750	59
1985	1,860	540	213
1990	2,020	750	353
1991	2,120	920	421
1992	2,130	880	422
1993	2,210	850	354
1994	2,510	990	1122
1995	2,930	1,140	1151
1996	3,040	1,180	1010
1997	2,570	990	874
1998	2,090	910	648
2002	1,840	870	973
2003	1,860	850	1,006
2004	1,910	890	949
2005	1,810	800	963
2006‡	1,040	460	890

†Cases involving the most deadly malaria parasite
‡Through November
Source: India National Anti-malaria Programme, as reported in Malaria Web site at URL: http://www.malariasite.com/malaria/malariainindia.htm.

8.2 Malaria Situation in Ahmedabad

The respected Malaria Research Centre of India (MRC) carefully studied the disease situation in Ahmedabad, a typical city. This chart compares the MRC's estimates (grey bars) to the reported results for the same city as published by the National Anti-malaria Programme (black bars).

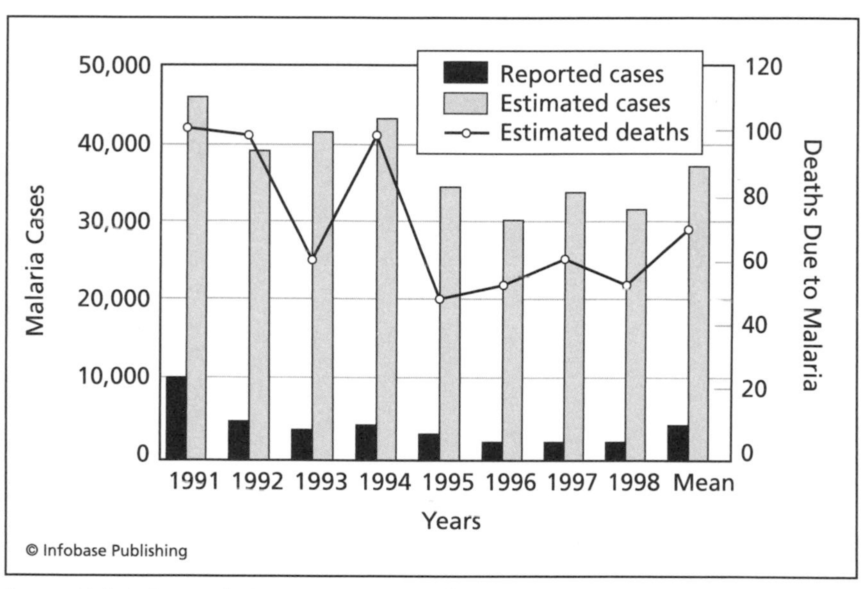

Source: Malaria Research Centre. "Estimation of True Incidence of Malaria." Available online. URL:http://www.mrcindia.org/MRC_profile/epidemiology/true_incidence.pdf.

9. CONFIRMED HUMAN CASES OF H5N1 AVIAN FLU

As of April 2, 2007, fewer than 300 human cases of avian flu had been reported since the epidemic began in 2003 among flocks of wild and domestic birds, although the death rate among these reported cases was nearly 60 percent. Many experts believe, however, that the virus could undergo mutations that would make it far more contagious between people. Avian flu could become the next great human pandemic.

	2003		2004		2005		2006		2007		TOTAL	
COUNTRY	CASES	DEATHS	CASES	DEATHS	CASES	DEATHS	CASES	DEATHS	CASES	DEATHS	CASES	DEATHS
Azerbaijan	—	—	—	—	—	—	8	5	—	—	8	5
Cambodia	—	—	—	—	4	4	2	2	1	1	7	7
China	1	1	—	—	8	5	13	8	5	3	27	17
Djibouti	—	—	—	—	—	—	1	—	—	—	1	—
Egypt	—	—	—	—	—	—	18	10	20	5	38	15
Indonesia	—	—	—	—	20	13	55	45	35	33	113	91
Iraq	—	—	—	—	—	—	3	2	—	—	3	2
Laos	—	—	—	—	—	—	—	—	2	2	2	2
Nigeria	—	—	—	—	—	—	—	—	1	1	1	1
Thailand	—	—	17	12	5	2	3	3	—	—	25	17
Turkey	—	—	—	—	—	—	12	4	—	—	12	4
VietNam	3	3	29	20	61	19	—	—	7	4	100	46
Total	4	4	46	32	98	43	115	79	74	49	337	207

Source: WHO. Available online. URL: http://www.who.int/csr/disease/avian_influenza/country/cases_table_2007_12_09/en/index.html.

8

Key Players A to Z

ABDURAZZAK (ZACKIE) ACHMAT (1962–) A South African health care activist, Zackie Achmat founded and led the Treatment Action Campaign (TAC), which leads the fight for improved social and medical treatment of people like himself infected with HIV/AIDS. Achmat was an activist and organizer against apartheid. He used South Africa's newfound freedom to win civil rights protection for gays and lesbians in the country's 1996 constitution. TAC was founded in Achmat's native Capetown in 1998, with the primary goal of assuring access to antiretroviral drugs for all those suffering from AIDS. Achmat drew attention to the issue by refusing to take the medicines himself unless they became available to the poor. Using the familiar tactics of grassroots organizing, noisy demonstrations, and even civil disobedience, TAC helped win dramatic changes in government policy, including a nationwide program to prevent mother-to-child transmission of HIV. TAC has drawn attention to the widespread problem of rape, especially as a factor in the spread of AIDS, and has protested the lack of treatment for HIV-positive inmates in the country's prisons.

ABHAY AND RANI BANG Abhay and Rani Bang are a married team of physician activists who developed protocols to dramatically reduce infant mortality in poor regions. After completing their education in public health at Johns Hopkins University, in 1986 they founded SEARCH (Society for Education, Action and Research in Community Health) in a poor rural region of Maharashtra State in India. At first focused on population control, the Bangs soon saw the need for a wider approach to women's (and men's) reproductive health; their research helped spread that understanding globally. SEARCH trains community health workers and traditional midwives to diagnose common infectious diseases of infants, and to counteract local customs that worked against maternal and infant health. They also showed that home neonatal care reduced mortality. By 1999 they reported a 75 percent decline in infant mortality, at a cost of less than $3 per life saved. SEARCH also runs programs to fight malaria and to reduce addiction to alcohol. Among many rewards they have received, the couple were named Global Heroes of Health for 2005 by *Time* magazine.

AGOSTINO MARIA BASSI (1773–1856) Agostino Bassi's discoveries in microbiology helped lay the groundwork for the germ theory of disease, developed in the following decades by his more famous colleagues, Louis Pasteur and Robert Koch. Bassi spent 25 years investigating the muscardine disease of silkworms, which was devastating the silk industry in his native Italy and France. He eventually proved that the disease was caused by a tiny parasitic fungus and that it was contagious; he published his findings in 1835. Bassi's recommendations for improved sanitation and disinfection, and for isolating and destroying infected caterpillars, revived the industry—and anticipated similar measures against human epidemics. Bassi's theory that other microscopic organisms were the cause of many plant, animal, and human diseases greatly influenced Pasteur.

BONO (PAUL DAVID HEWSON) (1960–) The Irish rock music star Bono has played a remarkable role in marshalling worldwide attention and support for the global effort to combat epidemic disease, among other humanitarian goals such as debt relief for poor countries. Lead singer and lyricist of the longtime hit band U2, Bono began using his celebrity in the service of global issues in 1979. Unlike some others who have followed a similar path, Bono has focused on coalition-building between activists, nongovernmental organizations, politicians of all political persuasions, government leaders, and business people. As a Christian, he has made explicit appeals to faith communities around the world to live up to the scriptural requirements of charity. In the 21st century he has drawn attention to the plight of sub-Saharan Africa, especially the HIV/AIDS pandemic. In 2005, he helped found Project Red in cooperation with major global corporations. The initiative aims to encourage exports from factories in poor countries that are committed to fair labor practices.

MARGARET CHAN (1947–) Margaret Chan's distinguished career in public health was capped when she was chosen to head the World Health Organization as director-general for a six-year term starting in 2006. Born in China and educated in Canada, Chan first joined the Hong Kong Department of Health in 1978, rising in 1994 to the position of director of health for the city, which became an autonomous region of China in 1997. She was the first woman to serve in that post. In her nine-year tenure she improved medical training, infectious disease surveillance, and international collaboration, all of which proved crucial during the avian flu epidemic of 1997 and the

SARS epidemic of 2003. At first criticized for complacency in the 1997 epidemic, she later pushed through the slaughter of 1.5 million chickens over political opposition. Joining WHO in 2003, Chan was later given responsibilities for Communicable Disease Surveillance and Response and for Pandemic Influenza. As WHO director-general Chan pledged to give priority to Africa and to women's health. She later called for a renewed fight against "neglected" infectious diseases, which affect about 1 billion people in developing countries, building on the progress already made against such ailments as leprosy, guinea-worm disease, and onchocerciasis.

NANCY COX (1948–) Nancy Cox is a leading researcher into human influenza viruses. As director of the U.S. Centers for Disease Control Influenza Division, she has played an important role in spurring international cooperation against seasonal flu viruses, and working toward national and international preparedness against the threat of a worldwide influenza pandemic. Since her family's brush with the deadly "Asian flu" epidemic of 1957, Cox has been a determined virologist, working since 1976 at the CDC in Atlanta. Her labs routinely select the strains of virus that are used in making the annual U.S. flu vaccine. She helped reconstruct the 1918 pandemic flu virus from preserved tissue samples. In recent years, Cox has worked on artificially developing viruses that combine avian flu and contagious human flu characteristics, in an effort to develop the vaccines that might stop a pandemic if such a combination emerged in nature.

GLADYS ROWENA HENRY AND GEORGE FRANCIS DICK (1881–1963) The husband-wife team George and Gladys Dick, physicians and researchers who married in 1914, conducted years of research that eventually conquered scarlet fever. The contagious childhood disease, caused by a bacteria called group A streptococcus, used to kill about one-quarter of those infected, and caused serious lifetime complications among many of the survivors. The Dicks isolated the bacteria that caused the disease and developed antitoxins to treat it. They also developed tests to determine susceptibility to the illness. Their decision to patent the toxin and antitoxin was controversial in its day.

RENÉ DUBOS (1901–1982) One of the key figures in the discovery and clinical use of antibiotics was the French-born American microbiologist René Jules Dubos. His early studies in agronomy in France gave him an appreciation for the natural environment that influenced all his later work.

After obtaining his doctorate in microbiology from Rutgers University in 1927, Dubos accepted a position at the Rockefeller Institute (now Rockefeller University) where he did almost all his scientific work. Asked to find a way to destroy the hard coating that protected certain toxic bacteria from all drugs, Dubos decided to search in soil, which contains organisms that can degrade any plant or animal. He found the first such chemical in 1930. In 1939 he was the first to systematically isolate a clinically useful antibiotic from the soil—gramicidin—which he tested on humans. Gramicidin proved of limited use, but Dubos's work stimulated renewed interest in penicillin, and encouraged other scientists who used his methods to developed more practical antibiotics. He also helped develop new therapeutic methods for treating tuberculosis. Dubos wrote several books on immunity and susceptibility to disease, and on tuberculosis and pneumonia.

Dubos's stress on the interplay of organisms in their natural environments led to his early warning that bacteria were likely to develop resistance to the new drugs. It also informed his later philosophical works on the balance of nature and human social evolution He became one of the most influential writers in the modern environmental movement, as an optimist who believed that nature, society, and science would be self-corrective. He coined the widely quoted phrase, "think globally, act locally."

PAUL EHRLICH (1854–1915) A brilliant pioneering organic chemist, Ehrlich helped explain how certain drugs acted within the cell to produce their therapeutic effects. For years he researched serum—a blood component that can contain antitoxins that are useful for fighting bacteria. He developed a successful antitoxin against diphtheria by infecting horses with the bacteria and refining horse serum. He also specialized in research into the immune system, for which he won a Nobel Prize in 1908. He was an early developer of chemotherapy—the use of various toxic chemicals to fight disease. After developing drugs against malaria and related parasites, he used one of them, Salvarsan, to fight syphilis, previously incurable.

GERTRUDE BELLE ELION (1918–1999) The American biochemist and pharmacologist Gertrude Elion built a remarkably prolific career as a theoretical and practical developer of drugs for a variety of human conditions, including infectious diseases. Denied a graduate research position due to her sex, Elion eventually joined the Burroughs-Wellcome company to work with George H. Hitchings. Alone and with Hitchings, Elion developed methods of drug discovery that relied on the biochemical differences between human cells and those of pathogens. The microbes could then be killed without harming the host cells. Among the discoveries she worked on were AZT, the first effective drug against HIV-AIDS, and successful medicines against malaria; bacterial infections that cause meningitis, septicemia, and urinary infections; herpes; and noninfectious diseases such as leukemia and gout. She won a Nobel Prize in Medicine in 1988.

PAUL FARMER (1959–) Paul Farmer, an American physician and medical anthropologist, has been a tireless campaigner for improved medical care in developing countries. Partners in Health, the nongovernmental global health organization that he founded in 1987 with Jim Yong Kim, has directly helped many hundreds of thousands of patients in Haiti, Peru, Rwanda, Russia and several other poor countries. PIH's programs have served as successful examples of how to deliver top-quality medical care in resource-poor countries. They have become the template for a spate of more recent NGO activities around the world. Indirectly, Farmer has helped spur the modern movement to make life-saving medicines available at reasonable prices in poor countries. Farmer has been inspired by concepts of social justice found in Catholic Liberation Theology. His practical success also derives from close ethnographic studies about health, disease, and medicine, in both developed and developing countries. Farmer opened a small clinic in rural Cange, Haiti, in 1983, and founded PIH largely to support this effort. It now serves 1,000 patients every day. In line with Farmer's model, local community health workers help assure that patients receive adequate food, clean water, housing, and education.

ANTHONY FAUCI (1940–) Dr. Anthony Fauci's name has been associated with the scientific and political struggle against HIV-AIDS since its recognition as an emerging disease in 1981. Director since 1984 of the National Institute of Allergies and Infectious Diseases (NIAID) of the National Institutes of Health, he is best known for helping to organize the U.S. government's response to the pandemic, and for keeping it in focus through years of controversy, disappointment, and then growing success. One of his strongest achievements was to bring together the often conflicting interest groups with a stake in the matter, including the research, business, political, and patient communities, and to win continued government funds for the effort.

Fauci's early research on the human immune system led naturally to his interest in AIDS. He turned his lab into a research center on AIDS just months after the syndrome was first reported; it has helped untangle HIV's effects on the immune system, which has aided in devising therapies. He has also focused on the long-term effort to develop AIDS vaccines.

RICHARD FEACHEM (1947–) Named as first head of the Global Fund to Fight AIDS, Tuberculosis, and Malaria in 2002, Sir Richard Feachem is a good example of the 21st-century global civil servant engaged in the fight against epidemic disease. Trained in both engineering and public health, Feachem began his career improving sanitation in Papua New Guinea and the Solomon Islands, and served for six years as dean of the celebrated London School of Hygiene and Tropical Medicine, followed by a four-year stint as director for Health, Nutrition, and Population at the World Bank. He has served as officer of many nongovernmental organizations including the International AIDS Vaccine Initiative, and he is founding director of the Institute for Global Health at the University of California at Berkeley. Feachem has written widely in the fields of water policy, sanitation, and public health.

ALEXANDER FLEMING (1881–1955) Fleming is considered the discoverer of penicillin, the first of the naturally occurring antibiotic drugs that revolutionized the treatment of infectious disease in the 20th century. He first made his mark as a microbiologist during World War I, by proving that the antiseptic then being used to clean wounds actually made things worse—they killed the white blood cells that were trying to fight the invading bacteria. In the 1920s he began studying natural substances that could work as nontoxic antibacteria agents, isolating the antibiotic lysozyme from human tears and mucus. In his famous accidental discovery of 1928, he found that a mold that had blown in an open window was killing staphylococcus bacteria. Later experiments showed that a common bread and fruit mold secreted a substance he called penicillin, which killed streptococci and pneumococci as well as staphylococci—all dangerous causes of human diseases. He gave the substance to animals and then to himself to prove it was nontoxic. Unfortunately, few doctors were interested in using the substance. It was hard to produce in pure form; besides the newly discovered sulfa drugs seemed to be more effective. In 1938 interest revived, and a team comprising the chemist Ernst Chain and the pathologist Howard W. Florey eventually purified the drug, which soon became a mass-produced "miracle drug," effective against a broad array of bacterial diseases. Chain and Florey, together with Fleming, were awarded a Nobel Prize in 1945.

ROBERT CHARLES GALLO (1937–) Biomedical researcher Robert Gallo discovered the first human retroviruses, and led the National Cancer Institute team that demonstrated that the HIV-1 retrovirus was the cause of AIDS. When AIDS first appeared in 1981, Gallo had been researching retroviruses for seven years, developing many of the tools later used by others in the field. In the race to find the pathogen behind AIDS, Gallo's team came in second behind Luc Montagnier's team at the Pasteur Institute in Paris. Montagnier charged that Gallo had isolated his virus from samples sent from Paris; an impartial group later confirmed that the French sample had contaminated Gallo's sample. Gallo did, however, succeed in proving the connection between the virus and the disease. He also developed the first tests to detect HIV in blood. Up to that point, thousands of people were infected during routine blood transfusions. In 1995 Gallo found that chemokines, a class of proteins produced by human cells, can interfere with HIV in the body, and slow down the progression to AIDS. His team has continued work toward developing an AIDS vaccine. Gallo now heads the Institute of Human Virology in Baltimore.

WILLIAM HENRY III (BILL) GATES (1955–) The richest man in the world, software entrepreneur Bill Gates has helped spark a substantial increase in charitable giving on behalf of global needs among wealthy people. Gates built Microsoft, Inc. into the world's largest software company, using tactics often condemned as predatory. The company was forced into an antitrust settlement with the U.S. Department of Justice in 2001, and with the European Union a few years later. Having amassed unprecedented wealth, Gates was reportedly inspired by the Rockefeller Foundation's global orientation when he founded the Bill and Melinda Gates Foundation in 2000. In turn, the foundation's widely publicized programs have inspired an increase in global charity, especially by others in technical industries. After transferring several billion dollars of their own money to the foundation (toward a pledged total of $30 billion), the Gateses in 2006 won a commitment from friend and fellow multibillionaire Warren Buffet to contribute $30 billion of his own Berkshire Hathaway stock over a period of years to the foundation. The foundation spends $800 million a year for health initiatives, about as much as the WHO and the U.S. Agency for International Development. It has financed child vaccination programs and malaria prevention programs around the world, and helps support HIV/AIDS research.

JULIE GERBERDING (1955–) Julie Gerberding's appointment as the first woman director of the prestigious and powerful U.S. Centers for Disease Control and Protection in 2002 capped a career as a doctor and public health administrator. Trained as an intern in San Francisco during the terrifying early days of the AIDS pandemic, Gerberding built a solid career in public health but achieved overnight celebrity with her forceful handling of the anthrax bioterrorism episode in 2001, when she was acting deputy director of the National Center for Infectious Diseases (NCID), a unit of the CDC. At NCID she had developed patient safety initiatives and programs to reduce medical errors and infections in the health care setting. As director, Gerberding has been an articulate and forceful public face for the CDC in an era when infectious disease threats have become a major public concern. However, her overhaul of the CDC's organizational structure has attracted criticism, and charges that nonscientific personnel have gained at the expense of lab scientists.

JOSEPH GOLDBERGER (1874–1929) A Hungarian immigrant to the United States, Goldberger's work at the U.S. Public Health Service (PHS) was instrumental in scientifically demonstrating and publicizing the connection between poor living conditions and epidemic disease. After several years working as an epidemiologist in the PHS fighting parasitic diseases in the U.S. South and the Caribbean, he was assigned to investigate pellagra, a disfiguring and fatal disease that was then endemic in several southern states. At that time pellagra was believed to be caused by either an infectious microbe or an undiscovered food toxin, but Goldberger suspected a connection with the corn-based, low-nutrition diet consumed by many poor residents of the South though low in nutrients. During a cotton depression in 1920, he warned that reduced income would lead to a huge increase in the case load. Despite criticism from parts of the medical establishment and from southerners who felt their culinary traditions were being insulted, Goldberger was eventually able to prove that a lack of Vitamin B was the culprit.

JOHN GRAUNT (1620–1674) Usually considered the founder of demography—the scientific, statistical study of human populations—the dry-goods merchant John Graunt also made important contributions to the study of epidemics. A resident of London, Graunt published a book in 1662 entitled *Observations on the Bills of Mortality*, a careful study of the lists of births and deaths published in the city over the previous century. He was able to draw important conclusions about life expectancy, about differences in death rates and causes as between the sexes and between urban and rural environments, and about the rise and decline of epidemics. Graunt's widely read book influenced later generations of epidemiologists.

BERNARDINE HEALY (1944–) One of the few women in her medical school class, Healy went on to carve out a career in public health and educational leadership, all the while continuing her practice as a clinical cardiologist. Her government service included a stint as deputy director of the White House Office of Science and Technology in the Reagan administration, and a two-year term as head of the National Institutes of Health (1992–93), the first woman to hold the position. She has been the bioterrorism adviser on the President's Council of Advisors on Science and Technology since 2001. In between she has been dean of the Ohio State College of Medicine and Public Health and president of the American Red Cross (1999–2001). She is known as innovative if sometimes controversial, and she has acquired a specialization in medical policy relating to women.

DONALD A. HENDERSON (1928–) Some successful doctors can boast of saving hundreds or even thousands of lives, but few can dream of matching the achievements of Dr. Donald A. Henderson, who headed the successful World Health Organization (WHO) campaign that eradicated smallpox in 1977.

Born in Ohio, Henderson received his medical degree in 1954. After his residency he served a stint in the Epidemiology Intelligence Service of the CDC, creating a Smallpox Surveillance Unit to guard against any imported epidemic. In 1966 he took charge of the WHO's Global Smallpox Eradication Campaign. After the disease was eliminated in Europe by 1972, Henderson energized a staff that overcame numerous technical and cultural challenges and pursued the virus to the far corners of the earth. In 1977 WHO was able to declare victory, when the last victim recovered in Somalia. No naturally occurring cases have emerged in the decades since then. In 1974 Henderson was instrumental in founding the WHO global immunization program, which yearly vaccinates 80 percent of the world's children against six serious diseases. After a 13-year term as dean of the Johns Hopkins School of Public Health, Henderson served in several key federal science advisory roles. In 1998 he set up a Center for Civilian Biodefense Strategies at Johns Hopkins, and he became its founding director. His work has won him many prestigious prizes, including the Presidential Medal of Freedom in 2002.

AUSTIN BRADFORD HILL (1897–1991) Austin Bradford Hill was a pioneering British epidemiologist with two famous achievements to his credit. First, he pioneered in developing the randomized clinical trial in medical research, while working as statistician for a major study on the use of the antibiotic streptomycin in tuberculosis. Second, together with Richard Doll he performed a series of studies in the late 1940s and early 1950s that demonstrated the close connection between cigarette smoking and lung cancer. One study compared lung cancer patients with healthy controls; another study followed some 30,000 doctors for a period of years, comparing smokers with nonsmokers. The evidence convinced most medical professionals that smoking causes cancer. Hill also had a long, distinguished career as a professor and writer on medical statistics, industrial diseases, and related topics. His nine "Bradford Hill criteria" are often used to determine the likelihood that a particular agent is the cause of a particular disease.

DAVID HO (1952–) An immigrant from Taiwan to the United States at the age of 12, David Ho has been a leader in AIDS research since the early 1980s, having published more than 250 scientific papers in the field. He is the founding head of the respected Aaron Diamond AIDS Research Center, which has been involved in much of the basic research in HIV and AIDS, including the initial speculation that the disease was caused by a virus. Ho is known for his studies into the complicated behaviors of HIV in those infected. To combat this versatile pathogen he has advocated the use of "combination therapy," using drugs that affect different stages in the reproduction of HIV within the body, including protease inhibitors, which Ho's lab helped develop. This tactic has proven to be the most successful in combating the virus; it has restored functional life to several million HIV-positive individuals, and it is being distributed to an even wider HIV/AIDS population in Africa and other poorer regions. Ho's teams have also worked to develop vaccines that might be able to dramatically slow the spread of the epidemic.

EDWARD JENNER (1749–1823) Eighteenth-century British physician Edward Jenner proved that people could be protected from smallpox by giving them a mild case of cowpox. Thanks to his careful work and his efforts to publicize his experiments, he can be considered the founder of vaccination. Vaccination against an ever-greater variety of microbes has spared untold millions from disease all over the world. After two centuries of slow progress, smallpox itself was wiped out in 1977.

Jenner was an irrepressibly curious naturalist who investigated a variety of topics while working as a doctor in his native Gloucestershire. His insight that angina pectoris (the chest pains that can precede heart attacks) was caused by blockage of the coronary arteries was borne out by later autopsies. He was the first to demonstrate that seasonal birds migrate (they were previously thought to hibernate), and he elucidated the fossil *plesiosaur* (a huge sea reptile). His work on the parasitic habits of cuckoo chicks remains a model of the scientific observation of nature.

As a child Jenner had a terrifying brush with a smallpox epidemic at his boarding school, where he was "variolated"—inoculated with fluid from a smallpox (*variola*) blister. The practice had been imported into England earlier in the century; it was widely practiced in Asia, the Middle East, and Africa. However, it did not always produce immunity, and a minority of subjects developed serious symptoms and died. Furthermore, the smallpox that variolation induced could itself be contagious.

Some years later Jenner heard that milkmaids who caught cowpox, a related but mild disease in both cattle and humans, never came down with smallpox. In the meantime, he was learning the rudiments of careful experimentation from the great surgeon John Hunter, and sharpening his observational skills by classifying thousands of specimens brought back by Captain James Cook's botanist, Sir Joseph Banks, in 1771.

After his son's nurse came down with cowpox in 1789, Jenner injected fluid from her blisters into his son and two other people who had also been exposed. As the disease was known in Latin as *vaccinia*, the practice became known as vaccination (the word is now used for all diseases). After they developed cowpox blisters, he injected them with liquid from smallpox blisters, but this variolation produced no rashes or other symptoms. In other words, vaccination made them immune to smallpox. Jenner repeated the experiment with a larger number of subjects, using different permutations of vaccination and variolation. A sociable and popular man, Jenner published his findings and educated wide circles of scientists and lay people. His work was soon translated, making him world famous.

ELIZABETH KENNY (1880–1952) Australian-born nurse and physical therapist Elizabeth Kenny developed a treatment for polio survivors that saved thousands of children from a lifetime of paralysis, in the years before the Salk vaccine was introduced. Sister Kenny (*sister* is British English for nurse) developed her techniques as a young woman, acting as a doctor for her many farm patients. She would keep the paralyzed limbs warm to relieve pain, and feel them for any signs of movement. By force of personality she convinced her patients that any remaining movement could be enhanced through conscious effort and training, and she thus returned many limbs to functional use. Rejected by the medical establishment in the United States, she finally found enough support in Minneapolis to set up an institute. Celebrated in the media and voted the most admired woman in the country, she was able to train many others to duplicate her successes.

JIM YONG KIM (1959–) A South Korea–born American physician and professor of social health, Jim Kim is a leading activist in the effort to assure access to medical care around the world, with a special focus on drug treatments for tuberculosis and HIV/AIDS. In 1996, while working in Peru under the auspices of Partners in Health (a global medical initiative he cofounded with health activist Paul Farmer in 1987) Kim developed practical treatment protocols for drug-resistant tuberculosis using the resources available in poor countries. He also led a campaign that won huge price cuts for TB drugs from pharmaceutical companies. In a three-year stint at the World Health Organization as head of its HIV/AIDS unit, Kim developed the "3 by 5 Initiative," an attempt to provide antiretroviral drug treatment to 3 million people living with HIV/AIDS in developing countries by the year 2005. The program missed its goal, but he did succeed in prodding governments and global agencies to triple the number of people enrolled in drug programs.

KITASATO SHIBASABURO (1853–1931) As a young man Kitasato studied at Robert Koch's famous laboratories in Berlin, becoming in 1889 the first person to develop a pure culture of tetanus bacteria. Together with Emil von Behring, the following year he helped prove that diphtheria antitoxin derived from the blood of diseased animals could give immunity against that disease to healthy animals. The discovery was an important foundation for the study of immunology, and won van Behring the first Nobel Prize in medicine and physiology in 1901. Kitasato founded a laboratory within the Tokyo Institute of Infectious Diseases, where he studied the use of dead virus in vaccinations. He also studied how tuberculosis is transmitted. In 1894 the Hong Kong government invited him and Alexandre Yersin from the Pasteur Institute to assist during a bubonic plague epidemic. Working separately, he and Yersin each was able to isolate the bacteria that causes plague, now called *Yersinia pectis.*

ROBERT KOCH (1843–1910) The germ theory of disease was already being taught by professor Joseph Henle when Koch studied medicine at the University of Göttingen. The student's own meticulous research was to put the theory on practical foundations, eventually earning Koch one of the first Nobel Prizes in physiology and medicine, in 1905. Working as a district medical officer, he first studied anthrax, then a common disease of cattle. Koch discovered that bacteria could lie dormant inside hard spherical spheres, and still retain their capacity to infect and sicken animals. His techniques for isolating, cultivating, and viewing bacteria became the foundation for all future microbiology. He even developed some of the standard equipment used since then in microbiology, including agar plates and Petri dishes. He also developed "Koch's postulates" for proving that a particular microbe caused a particular disease. Koch later discovered the bacteria that cause tuberculosis and cholera. He also developed the basic techniques for fighting cholera epidemics, but he was less successful in using serum from diseased individuals to enhance immunity in others. His discoveries, and his travels to epidemic zones around the world, made him world famous, and greatly enhanced the prestige of science and medicine in the modern era.

ARATA KOCHI (1949–) Japanese-born physician Arata Kochi is a combative and provocative leader in the global struggle against tuberculosis and malaria, two preventable and curable diseases that still claim millions of victims in poor countries. He has fought to institute cheap, easily duplicated programs around the world. As director of the UN's Stop Tuberculosis Initiative for several years after 1989, he forced through important changes in diagnostic and treatment practices and reinvigorated the fight against the disease; the percentage of TB patients around the world receiving adequate treatment increased dramatically during his tenure at Stop TB. Shortly after becoming director of the WHO's Global Malaria Program in late 2005, Kochi threatened to boycott 18 pharmaceutical companies that continued to sell artemisinin as a separate drug. Artemisin cures 90 percent of all cases of malaria, but drug-resistant strains of the malaria parasite have begun to emerge. Kochi (and most experts) argued that artemisinin should be used only as part of a "cocktail" of drugs; the companies and other international agencies using monotherapy quickly capitulated. He also antagonized many environmentalists by demanding an increase in the use of the pesticide DDT. DDT, when sprayed in homes in small doses, is safe and effective at killing and repelling mosquitoes. Unfortunately, for 40 years it has been a symbol of toxic chemicals for environmentalists in the West, and African countries are afraid that if they use the pesticide, the European Union might ban imports of their agricultural goods.

BERNARD KOUCHNER (1939–) To advance his humanitarian and human rights goals, Bernard Kouchner has served in leadership positions in the government of France (as health minister and, from May 2007, foreign minister) and in international organizations (including UN representative in Kosovo). However, his greatest impact is as cofounder of Médecins Sans Frontières (MSF, or Doctors Without Borders) and Médecins du Monde (Doctors of the World), which have sent thousands of volunteer doctors to work in poor countries, often to fight active or threatened epidemics. He founded MSF in 1971 after working as a Red Cross doctor in Biafra, Nigeria. The celebrated and media-savvy organization, which received a Nobel Peace Prize in 1999, has been instrumental in stimulating a renewed sense of global humanitarian concern in wealthy countries. Kouchner's support for international intervention in humanitarian and human rights crises, including at times military intervention, has earned him some criticism, but is in line with his activist creed as defined in his 1987 book *The Duty to Intervene.* MSF's $400 million budget comes mostly from private donations. The group deploys about 3,000 doctors and other health professionals to run programs in over 70 countries.

CHARLES-LOUIS-ALPHONSE LAVERAN (1845–1922) French physician Charles Laveran was the first scientist to discover that a protozoan (single-celled animal) could cause a disease in humans. Working for the French army health service, Laveran was posted in 1878 to Algeria, where he concentrated his studies on malaria, then a major problem for the army. Through his microscope he peered at numberless blood samples from patients, and he found one common element in all—bunches of tiny black spots. They were often concentrated in odd foreign bodies, which he concluded in 1880 were different life phases of a parasite, the cause of malaria. In Italy, in 1882, he tried to find the parasite in the soil, water, or air near swamps in malaria zones. When he was unable to find a single specimen, he guessed that mosquitoes were the transmitting agent. The medical establishment, which believed a bacteria caused malaria, rejected his findings, until they were endorsed by the celebrated Louis Pasteur in 1884. Laveran went on to study other human and animal diseases caused by parasites, including trypanosomiasis or African sleeping sickness, eventually publishing six influential books and hundreds of scientific articles. He was awarded the Nobel Prize in Medicine in 1907.

JOSEPH LISTER (1827–1912) Joseph Lister's advances in antiseptic surgery (in which all sources of infection are eliminated) were another important proof of the emerging germ theory of infectious disease. In his day, about one-half of all surgery patients died of infections, although most surgeons did not understand the bacterial origin of the problem. Lister himself believed the source was a "pollen-like" dust, until learning of Pasteur's theory that living organisms caused tissue decay. He began to use carbolic acid, which was then being used to disinfect sewage, and rates of postoperative sepsis plunged. His methods were quickly adopted in Germany, and eventually in all hospitals worldwide.

JONATHAN MANN (1947–1998) A native of Boston, Jonathan Mann began his medical career as an epidemiologist for the U.S. Public Health Service in New Mexico. He acquired his public health degree in 1980 just as the AIDS epidemic began to emerge, and his first major initiative (in 1984) was an AIDS program in Kinshasa, Zaire, called Projet SIDA (Project AIDS), which combined clinical and research work. The research demonstrated that AIDS could be spread by heterosexual sex, but that it could not be spread through mosquito bites. Mann was among the first international AIDS activists while teaching at the Harvard School of Public Health. As founding director of the World Health Organization's Global Programme on AIDS in 1986, he gave the group a "human rights" orientation—to prevent discrimination against those with AIDS or perceived as being at risk for AIDS. He opposed compulsory testing, a policy that was later questioned as contributing to the spread of the epidemic. He managed to secure increased funding for AIDS research, and helped build a world bureaucracy that later played an important role in fighting the epidemic.

In 1991 Mann founded Doctors of the World with the goal of building sustainable programs to protect health and human rights in the United States and around the world. He died along with his wife in a plane crash in 1998.

LUC MONTAGNIER (1932–) Luc Montagnier led one of the two teams that are credited for discovering the HIV virus, the cause of AIDS. In 1983 Montagnier's team at the Pasteur Institute in Paris isolated a retrovirus from lymph node tissue taken from an AIDS patient. He named it the lymphadenopathy-associated virus, or LAV. Shortly after, another team at the U.S. National Cancer Institute, led by Robert Gallo, announced its own discovery of a new retrovirus in tissue samples from AIDS patients. They named the virus T lymphotropic virus type III (HTLV-III). The two announcements precipitated a controversy: The two samples proved to be almost identical, despite the huge variety of HIV strains that have been identified. Montagnier charged that Gallo's team had used a sample he had sent them at their request. In 1986 the two names were dropped in favor of HIV. In 1990 a study at the U.S. National Institutes of Health confirmed that the two samples came from the same origin. Montagnier was involved in an additional controversy in the 1990s when he claimed that an elusive "cofactor" controlled how quickly HIV-infection could progress to AIDS.

FLORENCE NIGHTINGALE (1820–1910) Today's hospitals and clinics are key assets in the fight against infectious diseases, but before the career of Florence Nightingale they often served as unwitting agents in the spread of epidemics. Born to wealthy English parents in Italy, she devoted her life to a religious mission in the service of mankind, and became a powerful advocate for medical and social reform at an early age. Her famous efforts to improve sanitation at field hospitals during the Crimean War in 1854–56 cut the death rate among patients by two-thirds, and won her public support for efforts to reform the entire military medical system. Her disciplined campaigns were instrumental in improving sanitation and public health in both England and India. Her *Notes on Hospitals* of 1859 and *Notes on Nursing* of 1860 remained standard texts for many years. Nightingale founded an influential modern school of nursing in 1860, and the Women's Medical College in 1869. She was also a pioneer in the use of medical statistics and epidemiology.

LOUIS PASTEUR (1822–1895) One of the most famous scientists in history, Pasteur was a gifted chemist and microbiologist who, along with Robert Koch of Germany, established the germ theory of infectious disease on solid experimental grounds. Pasteur developed vaccines to protect farm animals from anthrax and cholera, using weakened forms of the bacteria. A century before, Edward Jenner had used natural cowpox virus to vaccinate against smallpox, but Pasteur's vaccines were the first to be artificially produced, a huge advance that prefigured most of the successful vaccines of the 20th century. He then developed a successful vaccine against rabies, which greatly reduced the scope of this previously fatal disease of animals and humans. This made him famous and led to the founding of the Pasteur Institute, one of the leading medical research laboratories in the world.

PETER PIOT (1949–) Born in Belgium and educated in medicine and public health, Piot became one of the most visible and influential figures in the anti-AIDS community after taking over as first executive director of UNAIDS, the Joint UN Programme on HIV/AIDS in 1994 (after four years as president of the International AIDS Society). He was also codiscoverer of the Ebola virus, which caused several outbreaks of fatal hemorrhagic fevers in African countries. His many activities against AIDS and other infectious diseases in Africa date back to the 1980s, and have earned him acclaim and awards throughout the continent.

STANLEY B. PRUSINER (1942–) A series of devastating brain diseases, in humans and animals, had long puzzled scientists. These diseases, including scrapie (among animals), Creutzfeldt-Jacob Disease (CJD, found among Europeans) and kuru (found among certain peoples on New Guinea), all caused progressive loss of mental function (dementia) and eventual death. Autopsies showed that brain tissue was pocked with holes and lesions. Based on epidemiological studies, some of the diseases appeared to be contagious, but no one could locate the cause, although scientists suspected a virus. Stanley B. Prusiner, a neurologist with extensive research experience, began research into CJD in 1974. By 1972 he concluded that the cause was a type of protein he called a prion, an entirely new type of infectious agent. When this protein folded incorrectly, it transferred this incorrect folding to other protein molecules, eventually causing the disease symptoms. After a number of years of controversy, Prusiner's conclusions were generally accepted, earning him a Nobel Prize in 1997. The field of prions became far more relevant with the rise in the 1990s of bovine spongiform encephalopathy (BSE), called "mad cow disease" or "variant CDJ," which is caused by a prion.

WALTER REED (1851–1902) A physician with thc U.S. Army, Walter Reed proved that yellow fever is transmitted by mosquitoes, rather than directly from person to person as had generally been believed. In 1893 he was appointed professor of bacteriology and clinical microscopy at the Army Medical College in Washington, D.C., where he conducted his important research. In 1899 and 1900 Major Reed visited Cuba, where yellow fever and other deadly tropical diseases were taking a heavy toll among the American troops who had defeated Spain in the Spanish-American War. He led experiments, using human volunteers, which conclusively identified the mosquito as the yellow fever vector. The discovery, followed by effective antimosquito measures, led to the near elimination of the disease in the United States, where it had claimed hundreds of thousands of lives. It also enabled the United States to build the canal through Panama, whose mosquito-infested swamps had defeated earlier attempts.

RONALD ROSS (1857–1932) Ronald Ross proved conclusively that malaria was transmitted to humans via mosquitoes, which had long been suspected. Born in India to a British general, he entered the Indian Medical

Service in 1881. He met scientist Patrick Manson in 1894 during a stay in England. He became convinced that Manson's theories about malaria (based on the earlier work of Alphonse Laveran) were correct, and he determined to prove them in India, where malaria had been a focus of his medical work. Struggling against bureaucratic and scientific resistance, Ross collaborated via the mail with Manson to devise the necessary experiments till he accumulated enough evidence to convince skeptics. By 1899 he had elucidated the entire life cycle of the *Plasmodium* parasite, both within the mosquito and in the human host, and he nailed down which mosquito species were involved. This and other achievements in the struggle against parasitic diseases won Ross the second Nobel Prize in medicine, in 1902. He devoted most of the rest of his life to the fight against malaria, focusing on mosquito control in Sierra Leone, Egypt, Greece, Mauritius, Spain, and Panama. He was also very active in founding antimalaria work across India, where his memory is honored. Ross was also a respected poet, playwright, writer, and painter.

JONAS SALK (1914–1995) After working on a flu vaccine for the U.S. Army during World War II, virologist Jonas Salk set up a laboratory at the University of Pittsburgh to investigate poliomyelitis (also known as infantile paralysis). Attracting the support of the National Foundation for Infantile Paralysis, Salk was able to take advantage of earlier research, including the work of John Enders in isolating and growing the polis virus. Salk beat out many other researchers in preparing an effective vaccine against the disease, which had taken an ever-increasing toll of death and paralysis among American children and children worldwide. Salk used killed polio virus in his vaccine, rather than attenuated live virus particles, as many of the competing research teams preferred to do. His skills at publicity, while criticized by many other scientists, helped make possible a groundbreaking nationwide test of the vaccine (which is still used today) among more than 1 million American schoolchildren. He went on to found and lead the important Salk Institute for Biological Studies in San Diego, California.

IGNAZ SEMMELWEIS (1818–1865) The careful observations and practical experiments of Hungarian physician Ignaz Semmelweis in the mid 19th century helped confirm the germ theory of disease. His campaign for improved hospital sanitary practices saved thousands of women from preventable deaths during childbirth. As a young surgical assistant at the Vienna General Hospital, Semmelweis noted that some 13 percent of all women giving birth in one ward died of puerperal or childbed fever, while only 2 percent died in childbirth at another ward in the same hospital. Doctors in the first ward, he discovered, moved from the autopsy room to the patient ward without washing their hands. He also noted that a doctor who cut his finger after an autopsy died of the same illness. Once doctors followed his instructions to wash their hands, deaths plunged to 2 percent in the first ward as well. Semmelweis was soon fired from the hospital for challenging authority. He was more successful in his native Hungary, and his views gained almost universal acceptance soon after his early death.

JOHN SNOW (1813–1858) John Snow is considered one of the main founders of the science of epidemiology. His achievements in research and public education helped stop the cholera pandemic that had spread through much of the world in the early and mid 19th century. A physician, Snow rejected the prevailing "miasma" theory of infectious disease. The miasmists believed that diseases such as cholera were breathed into the body through bad air, which supposedly contained minute particles of infectious matter. Snow's essay, "On the Mode of Communication of Cholera," claimed that the disease was ingested through the mouth in food or water. During a cholera epidemic in the London neighborhood of Soho in 1854, Snow carefully plotted all the cases, and traced the disease to a polluted water pump. Only those who drank water from that well got sick, while those who lived right by the source but did not drink the water remained healthy. This finding made Snow world famous, and helped win popular support for the germ theory of disease. Snow was also a pioneer in the scientific use of the anesthetics ether and chloroform.

CARLO URBANI (1956–2003) Carlo Urbani was a 21st-century hero in the fight against pandemics, who took great risks and ultimately sacrificed his life in this struggle. As an infectious disease doctor and researcher Urbani began working in the late 1980s to fight parasitic diseases in Mauritania. Hired by the WHO in 1993, and then working with Doctors Without Borders after 1997, he became respected and much in demand in poor tropical countries around the world. In 2003, as WHO's Western Pacific director of infectious diseases based in the Philippines, he raced to Hanoi to investigate one of the early cases of SARS, which he helped diagnose. His quick understanding and vigilant measures helped curb the epidemic in Vietnam; he also pushed the WHO into a more aggressive stance toward the Chinese government, which had tried to suppress news of the epidemic. Urbani himself caught the virus from treating patients in Hanoi and died in Bangkok soon after. His death was a further alarm bell, and the world health community raced into action, quickly suppressing a deadly and highly contagious new viral pandemic.

ANTONI VAN LEEUWENHOEK (1632–1723) A Dutch tradesman without any scientific education, Antoni van Leeuwenhoek was the discoverer of the world of microscopic organisms, including the tiny bacteria, protozoa, worms, and others creatures that cause the majority of infectious diseases. Leeuwenhoek refined the recently invented microscope, making some 500 of them during his long life. He was able to achieve a clear magnification of 200 times—objects appeared 200 times as large as they really were. Over decades, he tirelessly viewed countless samples, carefully recorded all he saw, and published innumerable papers at the Royal Society of London and other prestigious locales. The drawings and descriptions accurately depict many of the microorganisms familiar to scientists today. He chose to examine samples from a great variety of environments, including his own body, studying minerals as well as plant and animal matter. His 1676 discovery of single-celled organisms was met with disbelief, until a special team sent by the Royal Society confirmed his finding. Leeuwenhoek's exciting discoveries became widely known in his own lifetime and helped stimulate the growing field of microbiology.

SELMAN ABRAHAM WAXMAN (1888–1973) Selman A. Waxman was one of the pioneers in the discovery and development of modern antibiotic drugs. Winner of the 1952 Nobel Prize in Medicine, Waxman was a prolific experimenter and educator in the fields of soil and ocean bacteria, writing hundreds of articles and 18 books. He emigrated to the United States in 1911 after being denied admission to university in his native Russia because he was Jewish. In the 1930s, at Rutgers University in New Jersey, he became the world's expert on actinomycetes, a class of soil organisms that produce chemicals that destroy competing bacteria. In the late 1930s and early 1940s, he and his colleagues, including the French-born microbiologist René Dubos, exploited their carefully won knowledge of soil microorganisms to develop a series of antibiotic drugs, and to test them against bacteria that caused human diseases. Two of their drugs, streptomycin and neomycin, proved extremely effective against a wide range of ailments, and ushered in the era of the "wonder drugs." Waxman's success encouraged renewed research into penicillin.

WILLIAM HENRY WELCH (1850–1934) William Henry Welch was one of the founders of scientific medicine in the United States, through his own research as a pathologist and pathological anatomist, his tireless campaigns to improve and educate the medical profession, and as a founder and first dean of the Johns Hopkins University School of Medicine. He also helped found the Rockefeller Institute (now University) in New York, and he directed its extensive work in medicine and medical education in China. As a teacher at the Bellevue Hospital Medical College in New York, he developed the first laboratory courses in pathology in the United States and set up the country's first pathology lab, an important milestone in public health in New York and the nation. At the outbreak of World War I, the already world famous Dr. Welch played an important role (assisted by notable students) in directing the U.S. response to the terrible influenza epidemic of 1918–19.

ANNA WESSEL WILLIAMS (1863–1954) Anna Wessel Williams was a pioneering bacteriologist, one of the first prominent women in the field. In 1896 she brought rabies virus cultures from the Pasteur Institute back to America, to allow for large-scale vaccine production in the United States. Working for the New York City Health Department with William Park, she developed a practical, inexpensive antitoxin for diphtheria, thus helping to curb the disease in the developed world. Williams was aided by her curiosity and initiative in lab research. In 1919, she and Park demonstrated that the 1918 Spanish flu epidemic that killed tens of millions of people around the world had been caused by a virus, and not by pneumonia bacteria, as nearly all other scientists had believed.

LEE JONG WOOK (1945–2006) The first Korean to head a major international agency, physician Lee Jong Wook served as director-general of the World Health Organization from 2003 until his untimely death following brain surgery three years later. Lee joined the WHO in 1983, where he later headed up the Global Programme for Vaccines and Immunizations. Working with private industry, he helped develop better childhood vaccines. Later, as head of the Stop TB initiative, Lee built a coalition of 250 public and private entities and won consensus around aggressive new policies. His Global Drug Facility to fight tuberculosis served as a model for similar programs for drugs used in treating HIV/AIDS. From 1998 he helped direct the reform process within WHO.

ALEXANDRE YERSIN (1863–1943) Swiss-born physician and bacteriologist Alexandre Yersin was codiscoverer of the bacteria that causes bubonic and pneumonic plague, which was named *Yersinia pestis* in his honor. As a young researcher at the Pasteur Institute in Paris, he helped discover the toxin produced by the diphtheria bacteria. After gaining familiarity with Southeast Asian ports as a ship's doctor, Yersin was chosen by the French government and the Institute to investigate the pneumonic plague epidemic that was then devastating Hong Kong and South China in 1894. Together with Japanese researcher Kitasato Shibasaburo, he discovered the bacteria that caused the disease, which had terrified the civilized world in various epidemics over the centuries. He also isolated the bacteria from rats, confirming the source of transmission to humans. Back in Paris the following year, he produced the first antiplague serum. He then settled in Vietnam, where he was active for decades in medical and agricultural research.

ZHONG NANSHAN (1936–) Zhong Nanshan's efforts to combat the SARS virus in 2003, as director of the Guangzhou Institute of Respiratory Diseases, turned him into the most celebrated doctor in China. In 2005 he also emerged as a leader in China's surveillance and information efforts against the threat of avian influenza.

A strikingly fit athlete and graduate of prestigious Beijing Medical University, Zhong had treated many of China's top leaders in his long career, including Deng Xiaoping. Zhong had treated one of the earliest cases of SARS at the end of 2002, before the disease was named, and led the first major investigation for the provincial Health Department early the following year. He recognized that the disease was neither influenza nor bacterial pneumonia, and he fought to establish proper treatment protocols and isolation practices as quickly as possible. In the face of secrecy and mismanagement by the national government, Zhong helped Hong Kong researchers smuggle samples to their labs, where the SARS virus was eventually identified. He later aided efforts to identify and eliminate the animal reservoir of the disease. Once Beijing decided to attack the epidemic with a national campaign, Zhong was made the media symbol of the medical profession's heroic efforts.

9

Organizations and Agencies

There are thousands of organizations of all kinds that play a role in fighting epidemic disease and promoting public health around the world. In every developed and many less developed countries, health professionals, religious groups, businesses, private individuals, and governments have created and supported such organizations, working in their own and other countries. They vary from well-funded international alliances that can influence world strategies in dealing with specific diseases down to local groups of charitable volunteers who carry out small but vital projects in their own or more needy communities.

Any organization list must be a very limited sampling. The following selection includes some of the major agencies that are often mentioned in the media, as well as several smaller groups that may give an idea of the range of not-for-profit activity in the global public health field.

A Leg to Stand On
URL: http://www.altso.org
267 Fifth Avenue, Suite 301
New York, NY 10016
Phone: (212) 683-8805
Fax: (212) 683-8813

This modest organization provides orthopedic surgery and prosthetic devices for children in two locations in India and one in Colombia. More than 500 needy children have been provided with braces or artificial limbs and several dozen have undergone leg or foot surgery. Typical of many aid organizations organized around specific medical specialties, the group works with local medical professionals to open and maintain clinics that are intended to become self-sufficient.

Africa Fighting Malaria (AFM)
URL: http://www.fightingmalaria.org
1050 Seventeenth Street NW, Suite 520
Washington, DC 20036
Phone: (202) 223-3298

AFM calls itself a "health advocacy group," whose goal is to raise international awareness about malaria and promote government policy changes that could help the fight against the disease, which continues to infect hundreds of millions of citizens of poorer countries. Based in the United States and South Africa, the group, founded in 2000, conducts social and economic research, and disseminates the results through media and government channels. It pressures government to finance and implement effective malaria control policies, and promotes initiatives in the private sector. For example, it has tried to facilitate the distribution of antimalaria materials in poor countries by reducing tariffs and other bureaucratic barriers, and it has encouraged the wider use of DDT in control programs.

American International Health Alliance (AIHA)
URL: http://www.aiha.com
1225 Eye Street NW
Washington, DC 2005
Phone: (202) 789-1136
Fax: (202) 789-1277

For over a decade AIHA has run dozens of "twinning" programs in which communities in Africa, the Caribbean, and Vietnam are partnered with health care institutions and volunteer professionals in the United States in the struggle against the HIV/AIDS pandemic. It also has a network of similar programs in Eurasia (the former Soviet Union) that deal with other health issues in addition to HIV/AIDS. The organization supports a staff of 120 people in 18 different countries. It leverages its assistance by offering peer-to-peer training, exchange of information, technical assistance, and program management.

Access To Treatment
URL: http://accesstotreatment.org
7 Boulevard de la Madeleine
75001 Paris, France
Phone: (+33 1) 44-860-760
Fax: (+33 1) 44-860-122

Access To Treatment is a not-for-profit alliance between four major pharmaceutical companies that administers several programs providing free or no-profit medical products to people and institutions in poorer countries. These include drugs to treat HIV/AIDS, fungal infections, and cancer, as well as a 15-minute HIV diagnostic kit. Several hundred government and private agencies in 93 countries participate. The group, headquartered in Paris and Kampala, Uganda, claims to have treated over 3 million patients since its start in 2000. It aims to bring additional companies and products into the program.

Bill and Melinda Gates Foundation
URL: http://www.gatesfoundation.org
P.O. Box 23350
Seattle, WA 98102
Phone: (206) 709-3100

The Gates Foundation has quickly become the largest philanthropy in the world, with an endowment of $33 billion and pledges of billions more. Global health, especially in the developing world, has been a key focus. Its programs aim to increase access to vaccines and drugs that already exist and to develop practical, inexpensive solutions to diseases and other health problems. It also finances basic research in diagnosis, genetics, and other disease-related sciences. Apart from major grants to fight HIV/AIDS, malaria, and tuberculosis, the foundation has also taken aim at childhood diarrheal illness and pneumonia, which both take a heavy annual toll in poor countries. Another focus is reproductive, maternal, and newborn health, where small investments can often bring major results.

Catholic Medical Mission Board (CMMB)
URL: http://www.cmmb.org
10 W. 17th Street
New York, NY 10011
Phone: (212) 242-7757
Fax: (212) 807-9161

For 75 years the CMMB has supervised a variety of health care programs around the world, with a 2005 budget of around $300 million. It helps develop and train professional staff in local facilities in cooperation with governments, universities, NGOs, and the private sector, and it sends medical supplies and volunteers. It has offices in Zambia, Kenya, South Africa, and Haiti.

Dentaid
URL: http://www.dentaid.org
Giles Lane
Lanford, Salisbury
Wilts SP5 2BG
United Kingdom
Phone: (+44 1794) 324-249
Fax: (+44 1794) 323-871

Founded and run by British dentists, Dentaid specializes in refurbishing used equipment and instruments and shipping complete dentist offices to nonprofit groups in poorer countries. Since 1996 over 120 offices have been delivered to 43 countries, where they are used to treat half a million people a year. The group also provides educational materials and sends volunteers to help train dental professionals.

Direct Relief International
URL: http://www.directrelief.org
27 S. La Patera Lane
Santa Barbara, CA 93117
Phone: (805) 964-4767
Fax: (805) 681-4838

Direct Relief provides medical equipment, supplies, medicines, nutritional supplements, diagnostic material, and cash grants to local facilities in 56 countries around the world, based on requests from in-country professionals. Most of the material aid is donated by the private sector. The organization boasts of helping to serve more than 20 million clients a year. Most of the clients live in rural areas, and many are victims of natural disasters or war. The group has developed particular focuses on HIV/AIDS and maternal and child health.

Doctors Without Borders (Médecins sans frontières or MSF)
URL: http://www.doctorswithoutborders.org
333 Seventh Ave., 2nd floor
New York, NY 10001
Phone: (212) 679-6800
Fax: (212) 679-7016

The dramatic and widely reported work of Doctors Without Borders has helped inspire a new era of international volunteering, philanthropy, and advocacy for victims of disasters, wars, and endemic poverty around the world. Founded by French doctors in 1971, the organization now operates in more than 70 countries. Every year, the 19 national affiliates send a total of 4,700 doctors, nurses, and experts in logistics, water, and sanitation to work on emergency and ongoing projects; they work alongside more than 25,000 locally hired staff to supply basic and advanced health care and nutrition services. Since 1999, the group has pursued a Campaign for Access to Essential Medicines to ensure that residents of less developed countries can benefit from existing, abandoned, and new medicines against diseases that primarily strike the poor. MSF won the 1999 Nobel Peace Prize for its humanitarian work.

Family Care International (FCI)
URL: http://www.familycare.org
588 Broadway, Suite 503
New York, NY 10012
Phone: (212) 941-5300
Fax: (212) 941-5563

FCI works to improve the health of underserved women and adolescents in various countries in Africa, South America, and the Caribbean. Since its founding in 1987 it has focused on strengthening reproductive health and rights and opposing violence. It sponsors and publicizes research on improved pregnancy and childbirth care, and on preventing unwanted pregnancies. HIV/AIDS prevention education is another priority, as well as informational books and pamphlets for health care professionals. Between 2003 and 2005 the organization managed to upgrade some 100 health facilities in its target countries.

Foundation for International Medical Relief of Children (FIMRC)
URL: http://www.fimrc.org
P.O. Box 1132
Philadelphia, PA 19105
Phone: (888) 211-8575
Fax: (888) 735-6530

By sponsoring basic health care clinics in otherwise unserved rural regions in seven countries, FIMRC serves as an example of how modest aid efforts can help thousands of people. The group sends volunteers, both medical professionals and others, helps fund clinic upgrades, and advises recipients on developing further global volunteer resources. For example, FIMRC helps support a small hospital in Pignon on the Central Plateau in Haiti that serves 45,000 patients every year.

Global Alliance for TB Drug Development (TB Alliance)
URL: http://new.tballiance.org
80 Broad Street, 31st floor
New York, NY 10004
Phone: (212) 227-7540
Fax: (212) 227-7541

The TB Alliance is a good example of a major new trend in global health: a cooperative, well-funded project that brings together government, international agencies, NGOs and the private sector to coordinate the struggle against particular diseases or health care issues. The goal of the Global Alliance is to encourage the development and deployment of a new fast-acting tuberculosis drug within 10 years, to meet the threat of drug-resistant TB and the growing incidence of TB among HIV/AIDS patients. It also promotes development of new TB vaccines and diagnostic tools. Since its founding in 2000 it has built a large "pipeline" of potential drugs at participating companies and agencies, and has helped develop streamlined strategies to handle regulatory, testing, and patent issues. It has headquarters in New York, Brussels, and South Africa.

Global Forum for Health Research
URL: http://www.globalforumhealth.org
1–5 route des Morillons
P.O. Box 2100
1211 Geneva 2
Switzerland
Phone: (+41 22) 791-4260
Fax: (+41 22) 791-4394

The Global Forum is a research and advocacy group in the area of "neglected" diseases and conditions—those that primarily affect poor people in the developing world and have not benefited from adequate attention from the developed world. It conducts research in medicine, health care systems, and health-related behaviors. It holds conferences, supports a publishing program, and organizes coordinating committees.

The Global Fund to Fight AIDS, Tuberculosis, and Malaria
URL: http://www.theglobalfund.org
Chemin de Blandonnet 8
1214 Vernier
Geneva, Switzerland
Phone: (+41 22) 791-1700
Fax: (+41 22) 791-1701

Organized in 2002 within the framework of the World Health Organization (WHO), the Global Fund's mandate is to coordinate the effort to raise and distribute funding for programs to combat the three pandemics mentioned in its full name. To date, this alliance of the public, private, and NGO sectors has succeeded in raising commitments of $7.1 billion to the effort from governments and other sources, a major increase from past years. It has distributed large sums to coordinated country programs around the world. The group works to raise the profile of malaria and TB, which mostly strike the less developed world.

International AIDS Vaccine Initiate (IAVI)
URL: http://www.iavi.org
110 William Street, Floor 27
New York, NY 10038
Phone: (212) 847-1111
Fax: (212) 847-1112

IAVI is a leading nongovernmental organization promoting the development of HIV/AIDS vaccines. It works together with local scientists and clinicians in India and sub-Saharan Africa, where the pandemic is most intense. Six of its candidate vaccines have entered human trials in 11 different countries. Its goal is to speed the process of research, manufacturing, testing, and regulatory approval by using expert project management teams.

International Medical Corps (IMC)
URL: http://www.imcworldwide.org
1919 Santa Monica Boulevard, Suite 400
Santa Monica, CA 90904
Phone: (310) 826-7800
Fax: (310) 442-6622

IMC focuses on rapidly extending medical care to victims of war and natural disasters such as hurricanes, tsunamis, and earthquakes. Since 1984, when it was founded by volunteer doctors and nurses, IMC has helped teach over 35,000 doctors, nurses, community health care workers, midwives, and water and sanitation workers how to respond to emergencies and to rebuild health care systems. Health workers are trained to recognize and help treat trauma and acute mental illness. They are also alerted to issues of sexual exploitation and gender-based violence. IMC maintains a bank of medical volunteers who can respond immediately to emergencies.

Malariacontrol.net Project
URL: http://malariacontrol.net
c/o Swiss Tropical Institute
Socinstrasse 57
P.O. Box
CH-4002 Basel, Switzerland
Phone: (41) 61-284-81-11
Fax: (41) 61-284-81-01

The Malariacontrol.net Project uses the spare computer processing power of thousands of Internet-connected volunteers to run a malaria research program. The mathematics-based program, developed by the Swiss Tropical Institute (STI), tries to calculate the effect of various malaria control strategies (bed nets, vaccines, drugs) on the growth or decline of endemic and epidemic malaria. The project is sponsored by STI and CERN (European Organization for Nuclear Research), as the first phase of a plan to use spare computer power to address humanitarian problems in Africa.

Nothing But Nets
URL: http://www.nothingbutnets.net
c/o United Nations Foundation
Department 93
Washington, DC 2005

Nothing But Nets is a fundraising campaign that aims to buy and distribute insecticide-treated bed nets in endemic malaria regions in Africa, while increasing public awareness of the impact of malaria on less developed countries. It has recruited various business and media partners, and encourages "retail" fundraising in schools and churches. Over half a million nets have been purchased and distributed in the year since the organization was founded. The United Nations Foundation administers the program, using the Measles Initiative for distribution.

Operation Smile
URL: http://www.operationsmile.org
6435 Tidewater Drive
Norfolk, VA 23509
Phone: (888) 677-6453
Fax: (757) 321-7645

Founded in 1982 by an American plastic surgeon and his wife, a nurse, Operation Smile volunteers and local partners have performed more than 100,000 free facial repair surgeries for needy children. They also help train physicians in 25 countries in Latin America, Africa, Asia, and eastern Europe, and in underserved U.S. communities. The group also works to encourage sustainable health care for children and their families in target countries.

PATH—Program for Appropriate Technology in Health
URL: http://www.path.org
1455 NW Leary Way
Seattle, WA 98107
Phone: (206) 285-3500
Fax: (206) 285-6619

The cost of health care in wealthy nations continues to increase in part because of ever-new and more sophisticated technology. PATH aims at identifying, developing, and delivering lower-cost equipment, medicine, and procedures that can have a big effect in poor countries. Examples include the modification of vaccination equipment to meet local cultural and resource needs; cooperative research with local governments to prepare new vaccination campaigns against rotavirus, meningitis, and pneumonia; HIV/AIDS education among boy scouts in Kenya and Uganda; and research on simple solutions against postpartum hemorrhaging in Vietnam.

Project Hope
URL: http://www.projecthope.org
255 Carter Hill Lane
Millwood, VA 22646
Phone: (800) 544-4673

Starting in 1958 with a highly publicized hospital ship, this charity has grown into a major presence in many countries. Its focus is to build up health care facilities by training professionals, community health workers, and volunteers; granting seed money and loans to new facilities; supplying medicine and equipment; and promoting education about HIV/AIDS, tuberculosis, and other illnesses.

Roll Back Malaria (RBM)
URL: http://www.rollbackmalaria.org
c/o World Health Organization
20 Avenue Appia
CH 1211 Geneva 27, Switzerland
Phone: (+41 22) 791-2891

Since 1998 the Roll Back Malaria partnership has played a coordinating role in the revived effort to control and defeat endemic malaria in less developed countries. Founded by the WHO, United Nations Children's Fund (UNICEF), and the World Bank, it now has affiliates in many countries, including governments, NGOs, and the private and academic sectors. The group's mandate is to prevent and treat malaria so that by 2015 the disease will be "no longer a major cause of mortality," and will no longer be a bar to economic development of individuals and communities.

Schistosomiasis Control Initiative (SCI)
URL: http://www.schisto.org
c/o Department of Infectious Disease Epidemiology
Imperial College St. Mary's Campus, Room 312
Norfolk Place
London W2 1PG

SCI works to reduce the prevalence of schistosomiasis and intestinal worms among at-risk populations in sub-Saharan Africa, such as children, women, and those in certain occupations. It has chosen several countries for model programs, working with governments and NGOs to distribute the appropriate medicines to at least 75 percent of the target population. The goal is to encourage sustainable ongoing programs in every country affected by the diseases.

Sight Savers International
URL: http://www.sightsavers.org
Grosvenor Hall, Bolnore Road
Haywards Heath, West Sussex
RH16 4BX
United Kingdom
Phone: (+44 1444) 446-600

For half a century Sight Savers has worked to prevent, treat, and reverse blindness, and to ensure that blind people receive adequate education and training. Together with local partners they support several hundred projects in 32 countries in Africa, Asia, and the Caribbean, treating millions of people and restoring sight to over 200,000 people every year.

Treatment Action Campaign (TAC)
URL: http://www.tac.org.za
34 Main Road
Muizenberg 7945
South Africa

Phone: (+27 21) 788-3507
Fax: (+27 21) 788-3726

TAC is a militant advocacy and educational group fighting HIV/AIDS in South Africa, which has suffered from the pandemic more than any other country. The group has been instrumental in changing government policy toward actively preventing and treating HIV infection. They have won support for a nationwide mother-to-child transmission prevention program and antiretroviral drug distribution. TAC uses litigation, lobbying, and protests to oppose discrimination against HIV/AIDS patients and to ensure wide and equal access to treatment programs.

10

Annotated Bibliography

This annotated bibliography offers an abundant choice of books, Web sites, and other resources for anyone looking for more information about infectious diseases and global health. For ease of use, it is divided into the following subject areas:

- History of epidemics and infectious disease
- Specific diseases, such as HIV/AIDS or influenza, in alphabetical order by disease
- General works

HISTORY

Aberth. John. *The Black Death: The Great Mortality of 1348–1350: A Brief History with Documents.* New York: Palgrave Macmillan, 2005. This book is focused on some 50 historical documents from the era of the Black Death, from a variety of countries in Europe and the Near East. They illuminate topics such as the origin and spread of the plague, medical procedures used to combat it, social, political, and economic impacts, and artistic responses.

Ayliffe, Graham A. J., and Mary P. English. *Hospital Infection: From Miasmas to MRSA.* New York: Cambridge University Press, 2003. This is a well-written history of hospitals as a source of contagious disease, from the Middle Ages to the present. It traces theories of infection and the medical practices used in response, in military, civilian, and "lying-in hospitals" (for childbirth). Chapters examine the impact of the germ theory, antisepsis and asepsis, sterilization, and antibiotics. Several chapters deal with current problems, such as drug-resistant bacteria, and solutions, such as surveillance and organized infection control.

Barry, John M. *The Great Influenza: The Epic Story of the Deadliest Plague in History.* New York: Viking, 2004. This best-selling popular history delivers more than the title suggests. It is a history of American medicine and public health in the decades leading up to the 1918 influenza pandemic known as Spanish flu. In particular, the author follows the careers of some of the larger-than-life figures who helped put American medicine on a more scientific foundation, based on earlier European advances. Barry traces the epidemic itself to the U.S. Midwest, and claims a worldwide toll of up to 100 million deaths. A rapid scientific response to the pandemic together with informed public health measures probably helped keep the pandemic from taking an even worse toll. In any case, the experience provided many valuable lessons for the health professions.

Bollet, Alfred J. *Plagues and Poxes: The Impact of Human History on Epidemic Disease.* New York: Demos Medical, 2004. This general interest book covers the history of noninfectious diseases as well as infectious epidemics. It includes many less-known sidelights, for example, the price of Scotch whiskey increased during the 1918 flu pandemic in the United States, thanks to a widespread belief that the beverage helped control the symptoms of the disease.

Bray, R. S. *Armies of Pestilence: The Impacts of Disease on History.* New York: James Clarke and Co., 2004. A special feature of this book, which covers much the same ground as other general epidemic histories, is its excellent annotated bibliography, meant for nonspecialist readers. The author's dry wit helps get across an important message: Ancient and medieval history offers many opportunities for speculation. There may never be final answers to such questions as the diseases involved in ancient epidemics or the political impact of medieval scourges, but the detective work can be challenging and fun.

Byerly, Carol R. *Fever of War: The Influenza Epidemic in the U.S. Army during World War I.* New York: New York University Press, 2005. The dislocations and battle conditions of World War I almost certainly exacerbated the terrible Spanish flu pandemic of 1918, if it did not actually cause it. The author, a historical researcher for the U.S. Army, examines the response of army doctors to the epidemic, from their initial overconfidence to their failed attempts to persuade higher-ups to reduce crowding in barracks and on troop ships. The book also explores how guilt and despair helped suppress memories of the episode (which killed some 600,000 Americans).

Cantor, Norman A. *In the Wake of the Plague: The Black Death and the World It Made.* New York: The Free Press, 2001. Cantor, a noted scholar of the Middle Ages and writer of popular history books, turns his attention here to the Black Death of the 14th century, which killed some 40 percent of the population of Europe. In his concise yet readable book, the author can be quite graphic in his description of the horrors of the disease—and of the hard life of even healthy medieval Europeans. Yet he also finds a sardonic humor in the epidemic and its consequences, showing how they reflected the economic and social arrangements of the times. Cantor reexamines the epidemic using the latest scientific and medical knowledge, challenging some long-held beliefs. His narrative focuses on the plague's impact on England, and on the profound changes that the pandemic brought to European cultural, intellectual, and economic life. For example, the loss of a huge portion of the labor force allowed the surviving peasants in western Europe to improve their legal and economic status, and hastened the transition from feudalism to capitalism. In addition, Cantor maintains that the emotional impact of the plague and the helplessness of the traditional powers (church, feudal lords) helped undermine religious and traditional ways of thinking in favor of a more skeptical, scientific point of view.

Cartwright, Frederick F., and Michael Biddiss. *Disease and History.* 2nd ed. Stroud, U.K.: Sutton Publishing, 2000. This updated version of a classic history text is accessible to the general reader. It places the epidemics and health issues of today in the context of earlier episodes, from the classical world of Greece and Rome through the recent past.

Christensen, Allan Conrad. *Nineteenth-century Narratives of Contagion: Our Feverish Contact.* London: Routledge, 2005. Science was finally getting a handle on epidemics in the 19th century, as improved sanitation reduced cholera and tuberculosis, and as the germ theory gained force. However, contagious diseases were still a major problem in Europe, as reflected in novels. This book examines attitudes toward disease as manifested in the literature of the era.

Cockburn, Thomas Aidan, Eve Cockburn, and Theodore A. Reyman, eds. *Mummies, Disease and Ancient Cultures.* Cambridge: Cambridge University Press, 1980. Although focusing primarily on ancient Egypt and South America (the two main sources of mummified remains), the book also covers some deliberately or accidentally preserved bodies from Europe, Africa, North America, and Australasia. These remains can teach a great deal about health, nutrition, and infectious disease in times gone by, including places with few or no written records. The material is technical, but a general reader can skim the details and easily grasp the main points.

Crosby, Alfred W. *America's Forgotten Pandemic: The Influenza of 1918.* New York: Cambridge University Press, 2003. Ever since the 2003 SARS pandemic and the avian influenza fears that arose soon after, the 1918 episode can no longer be called forgotten. But this volume is among the better and readable of the recent books on the topic. Following a detailed depiction of the terrible months when 600,000 Americans died, the author explores the impact of the epidemic on the country and tries to understand how its memory was so quickly repressed.

DePaolo, Charles. *Epidemic Disease and Human Understanding: A Historical Analysis of Scientific and Other Writings.* Jefferson, N.C.: McFarland, 2006. This is a college-level book that tries to understand how previous generations understood epidemics of infectious disease. It examines scientific, religious, fictional, and other writings of various civilizations and cultures to analyze their approach to disease. Good for those interested in intellectual or cultural history.

Dormandy, Thomas. *The White Death: A History of Tuberculosis.* London: Hambledon and London, 2001. This lengthy and heavily researched book combines medical history with cultural history. Though the author is himself a physician, the book is written for the general public, and the writer finds room for humor and human interest amid the generally depressing account of this mass killer. The evolution of better examination techniques, diagnosis, and treatment forms a major theme; another is the accumulation of lifestyle and public health changes that may have played as great a role in controlling the disease as the antibiotic drugs that emerged in the 1940s. The author brings the story up to date with the reemergence of the disease in recent decades.

Friedman, Meyer, and Gerald W. Friedland. *Medicine's Ten Greatest Discoveries*. New Haven, Conn.: Yale University Press, 2000. Three of the 10 stories in this volume concern microbes and epidemics—"Antony Leeuwenhoek and Bacteria," "Edward Jenner and Vaccination," and "Alexander Fleming and Antibiotics." Each is written as a biographical sketch, placing the protagonist and his discoveries in the context of their time, place, and culture. The authors uphold the heroic reputation of their subjects; nevertheless, their keen eye for human foibles gives the stories a realistic and almost contemporary feel.

Gehlbach, Stephen H. *American Plagues: Lessons from Our Battles with Disease*. New York: McGraw Hill, 2005. Each of the chapters in this lively history of infectious (and noninfectious) diseases in the United States is devoted to a particular episode—an epidemic, an advance in medicine or public health, or a new public perception about a disease (e.g., lung cancer or heart disease). Most of the chapters focus on the lives and careers of the people most associated with these episodes, from the minister Cotton Mather, who championed inoculation during the 1721 smallpox epidemic in Boston, to physician Jonas Salk, who perfected the first successful polio vaccine in the 1950s. The biographies add a great deal of interest; together they trace the development of medical theory and practice in America. There are chapters on the statistical method of epidemiology, controlled clinical testing of treatments, improved public health measures, and the germ theory of disease. Many readers will be surprised to learn that some of today's worst "tropical" diseases were once common scourges in various northern and midwestern states, notably, yellow fever and malaria.

Greenblatt, Charles, and Mark Spigelman, eds. *Emerging Pathogens: The Archaeology, Ecology, and Evolution of Infectious Disease*. New York: Oxford University Press, 2003. Only serious students interested in science or medicine will want to try this book. For them, it is worth the effort to at least skim through it to get a sense of the exciting new developments in the field. The articles show how modern genetics, paleopathology (the study of ancient diseases), anthropology, and epidemiology are allowing the study of the evolution of infectious disease—the developments of the bacteria, viruses, and other pathogens themselves as well as their effect on their animal and human hosts.

Grob, Gerald N. *The Deadly Truth: A History of Disease in America*. Cambridge, Mass.: Harvard University Press, 2003. This well-written, thoughtful book begins with the premise that disease is an inevitable, natural part of life, and thus will never be eliminated. It accepts the enormous progress made in the 20th century, but insists that our longer life span is in part the result of better food and sanitation. The author traces the changing interactions between medicine, the environment, and society. Some of the material assumes knowledge of genetics and immunology, but much of the subject matter is accessible to any intelligent reader.

Annotated Bibliography

Hayes, J. N. *Epidemics and Pandemics: Their Impact on Human History.* Santa Barbara, Calif.: ABC-CLIO, 2005. A college-level historical survey that knowledgeable high school students can also use, this hefty book covers all aspects of the topic. It treats 50 epidemics from ancient time to the present, in Europe, Asia, and the New World, showing the local impact and medical responses in each case. There are several chapters covering current issues as well, including AIDS, mad cow disease, tuberculosis, and malaria.

Hoff, Brent, and Carter Smith. *Mapping Epidemics: A Historical Atlas of Disease.* London: Franklin Watts, 2000. This high school text covers 30 major epidemic diseases in human history. Each disease has a map showing where the epidemics have struck as well as a two- to six-page summary of important facts about the disease and about its historical impact.

Honigsbaum, Mark. *The Fever Trail: In Search for the Cure for Malaria.* London: Pan-Macmillan, 2002. This book combines an account of scientific research with an adventure story: the search by several 19th-century explorers through the jungles and mountains of South America to find the cinchona tree. The tree was the source of quinine, which was for a century the most important drug in treating malaria, but it was fast disappearing in the wild.

Kirby, David A. *Evidence of Harm: Mercury in Vaccines and the Autism Epidemic: A Medical Controversy.* New York: St. Martin's Griffin, 2006. In recent years some parents of autistic children have come to believe that mercury present in infant vaccines caused their children's disability. The medical community and government agencies believe they have disproved this theory. The author, a journalist, clearly sympathizes with the parents, but he tries to cover the issues fairly and thoroughly.

Kohn, George Childs, ed. *Encyclopedia of Plague and Pestilence: From Ancient Times to the Present.* 2nd ed. New York: Facts On File, 2007. Clearly written and accessible to the general reader, this book presents basic information about most of the major plagues of the past. It includes many suggestions for further reading and an extensive bibliography.

Kolata, Gina. *Flu: The Story of the Great Influenza Pandemic of 1918 and the Search for the Virus That Caused It.* Sagebrush, 2001. The author, a *New York Times* health reporter, tells the story of the terrible pandemic and its effects on American life. At the same time, she tells of the search for the actual virus that caused the disease. Scientists have been able to isolate viral DNA from tissue samples of flu victims buried in permafrost in Alaska or kept under seal at an army research facility. The book examines the prospects of similar pandemics in the future.

Little, Lester, ed. *Plague and the End of Antiquity: The Pandemic of 541–750.* New York: Cambridge University Press, 2006. This volume of essays brings together the latest research in a variety of fields that can shed light on this devastating ancient pandemic. It has often been claimed that the fall of the Roman Empire was caused by pandemic disease. Anyone wanting to reach their own decision on the issue should consult this dense, scholarly, but still readable work.

Mann, Charles C. *1491: Pandemics in Post-Columbian America*. New York: Knopf, 2005. In this fascinating history of the different peoples and civilizations of North and South America, the author focuses on the dreadful effects of the pandemics brought to the New World unintentionally by European explorers, conquerors, and settlers. He says that the native population dropped by as much as 95 percent in the first century and a half after European contact, since they lacked any immunity to smallpox, influenza, or the many other diseases brought by Europeans. Using new archaeological findings, he paints a picture of thriving, creative cultures covering most regions in North and South America, quite apart from the well-known Aztec and Inca civilizations of Mexico and Peru, respectively. The earliest European explorers in the Amazon forests, the Great Plains of today's United States, and the grasslands of South America all reported visiting heavily populated villages and towns, linked together in chains of commerce. These all disappeared, he argues, due to epidemics, leaving behind small, dispirited bands that could not keep their cultures intact.

Markel, Howard. *When Germs Travel: Six Major Epidemics That Have Invaded America and the Fears They Have Unleashed*. New York: Vintage, 2005. Written by a medical historian, this book treats six major infectious disease epidemics or scares: tuberculosis, bubonic plague, trachoma, typhus, cholera, and HIV/AIDS. The author's focus is on the emotional and social/political reactions of Americans, highlighting cases of anti-immigrant sentiment and even deportations. His main point that Americans cannot erect barriers against microbes from abroad is probably no longer controversial. He warns that the American public health system is flawed, and he calls for a global approach to fighting epidemics.

McBride, David. *From TB to AIDS: Epidemics among Urban Blacks since 1900*. Albany, N.Y.: State University of New York Press, 1991. This academic history book focuses on the African-American population, which became increasingly urbanized during the 20th century. It explores the social and economic context of black Americans in the South and in northern cities, the differences in health care resulting from racism, and the growth of the public health sector. It focuses on several diseases that impacted the African-American experience: TB in the 1920s, sexually transmitted diseases in the 1930s, the successful control of both problems after World War II, and the HIV/AIDS pandemic starting in the 1980s.

McNeill, William H. *Plagues and Peoples*. Garden City, N.Y.: Anchor, 1977. Although this book, by one of the most prominent historians of his era, has become outdated, it is still considered a classic. It is well worth the read, with its broad panorama sweeping across whole continents and centuries. Subsequent research has undermined some of the book's conclusions, but it remains a fine example of informed and reasoned history writing.

Oldstone, Michael B. A. *Viruses, Plagues, and History*. New York: Oxford University Press, 1998. Written by a virology researcher for a general audience, the book begins with clear, basic information about viruses and the immune system. It then tells the inspiring story of the conquest, or near conquest, of four viral diseases: smallpox, yellow fever, polio, and measles, and discusses the many new or familiar viral diseases that still plague the world.

Phillips, Howard, and David Killingray, eds. *The Spanish Flu Pandemic of 1918–1919: New Perspectives.* London: Routledge, 2001. This scholarly work brings together several different academic disciplines to example the 1918 pandemic. It includes articles on the virology, historiography, demography, and public health aspects of the disease, including its long-term medical, social, and demographic impact. Every continent and several countries are represented among the essays; the social reactions and government response sometimes varied dramatically, with dramatic results.

Porter, Dorothy. *Health, Civilization, and the State: A history of Public Health from Ancient to Modern Times.* London: Routledge, 1999. This book is considered valuable for its excellent exposition of the growth of the British public health system in the past 250 years.

Powell, Mary Lucas, Della Collins Cook, and Jerald T. Milanich, eds. *The Myth of Syphilis: The Natural History of Treponematosis in North America.* Gainesville: University Press of Florida, 2005. The syphilis pandemic that spread through the Old World immediately after Christopher Columbus's first journey to the Americas has long been "blamed" on the native peoples of North America, and much scientific evidence has been gathered to support that view. This book takes a dissenting view, bringing contrary evidence to suggest that venereal (sexually transmitted) syphilis may not have been present on the North American continent before the European conquest. Archaeology, history, and pathology are used to argue that the native disease that Europeans thought was syphilis may have instead been varieties of treponematosis, a bacterial disease.

Rice, Geoffrey. *Black November: The 1918 Influenza Pandemic in New Zealand.* Christchurch, N. Z.: Canterbury University Press, 2005. This is a grim account of the worst disaster in the country's history, which took 8,500 lives. It explores why the death rate was dramatically higher among Maoris, among young people, and among males. The author tries to draw lessons from the response at the time that may be relevant in meeting the threat of future influenza pandemics.

Rosen, George. *A History of Public Health.* Baltimore: Johns Hopkins University Press, 1993. While originally published in 1958, this book is still considered a classic in the field. It covers the ancient world up through the 1950s.

Rosenberg, Charles E. *The Cholera Years: The United States in 1832, 1849, and 1866.* Chicago: University of Chicago Press, 1987. This work, originally written in the 1960s, remains an excellent example of medical and public health history. The cholera pandemic of the 19th century was perhaps the "classic" epidemic of its era. The research techniques and public works projects (sewers and water supplies) that defeated the disease were among the triumphs of the early industrial era. The author conveys the human drama of the epidemics, the search for knowledge, and the eventual resolution of the problem.

Rosner, David, ed. *Hives of Sickness: Public Health and Epidemics in New York City.* Piscataway, N.J.: Rutgers University Press, 1995. The articles in this volume, sponsored by the Museum of the City of New York, take the story from colonial times to the present. They cover environment, housing, demography, and social conditions, as well as scientific progress.

Sallares, Robert. *Malaria and Rome: A History of Malaria in Ancient Italy.* New York: Oxford University Press, 2002. The book brings together literary and archeological evidence and the latest scientific research. The author concludes that *Plasmodium falciparum*, perhaps the most deadly of the malaria parasites, was already present in ancient Greece and Rome. He also demonstrates that malaria disease had major effects on population.

Slack, Paul. *The Impact of Plague in Tudor and Stuart England.* New York: Oxford University Press, 1984. The author explores the impact of the periodic epidemics of plague in England from the 15th through the 17th centuries. He discusses the effects on individuals, families, and communities, in rural areas, provincial towns, and London. The chief emphasis is on the ways in which various groups tried to explain, control, and come to terms with the epidemics, including the various public health measures that may have contributed to the disappearance of the disease.

Small, Hugh. *Florence Nightingale: Avenging Angel.* New York: Palgrave Macmillan, 1999. An excellent, concise biography of the famous nurse and health care reformer, this book helps burnish the already shining image of one of the giant figures of Victorian England. Using previously unknown letters, the author attributes Nightingale's long-time withdrawal from society to her guilt over her role in the Crimean War. He believes she felt responsible for thousands of unnecessary deaths by failure to improve the wretched sanitary conditions and sloppy methods in field hospitals. Eventually, these feelings spurred her to fight harder, and successfully, for major reforms.

Smallman-Raynor, Matthew R., and Andrew Cliff. *War Epidemics: An Historical Geography of Infectious Diseases in Military Conflict and Civil Strife, 1850–2000.* New York: Oxford University Press, 2004. This is a comprehensive scholarly look at the effects of war on epidemic disease among both military personnel and civilians. It includes material from the earliest times, but devotes the most attention to the wars of the past 150 years. The plentiful official documents of this era are carefully analyzed to tease out patterns. Most of the rich statistical and epidemiological material is put in appendixes, leaving the narrative accessible to general readers.

Snowden, Frank. *The Conquest of Malaria: Italy 1900–1962.* New Haven, Conn.: Yale University Press, 2006. From at least the time of the Roman Empire, malaria has been endemic in Italy, especially near marshlands. In the 19th and 20th centuries, it became a major social/political issue as well. The author describes the interplay between the medical and public health measures that eventually eradicated the disease and the various political movements and governments that contended for power.

Watts, Sheldon. *Epidemics and History: Disease, Power, and Imperialism.* New Haven, Conn.: Yale University Press, 1999. A very thorough, scholarly survey that focuses on seven major epidemic diseases that plagued humans from the Middle Ages to the present—bubonic plague, leprosy, smallpox, syphilis, cholera, yellow fever, and malaria. The author examines these diseases in part as "social constructs" reflecting the biases of time and place, and he examines their political, social, cultural, and economic impact. His politically charged criticism of "western" and "scientific" medicine, according to a review in the *New England Journal of Medicine*, "can be overlooked in this otherwise engrossing book."

Wilson, Daniel J. *Living with Polio: The Epidemic and Its Survivors*. Chicago: University of Chicago Press, 2005. The author, a survivor of the U.S. polio epidemic of the 1940s and 1950s, writes a personal memoir that is also a scholarly history of the epidemic. It is a chronicle of paralysis, hospital isolation, tough physical therapy, and a lifetime of disability. It also reveals the story of "post-polio syndrome" that many survivors began to experience decades after infection.

DISEASES

For all major diseases, there are comprehensive summaries and many useful links on the Web sites of the U.S. Centers for Disease Control and Prevention (CDC) (e.g. URL: http://www.cdc.gov/ncidod/dbmd/diseaseinfo/cholera_g.htm) and the World Health Organization (WHO) (e.g. URL: http://www.who.int/topics/cholera/en).

Bubonic (and Pneumonic) Plague

Dennis, David T. "Plague as a Biological Weapon," pp. 37–71. In Ignatious W. Fong and Kenneth Alibek. *Bioterrorism and Infectious Agents: A New Dilemma for the 21st Century*. New York: Springer, 2005. This chapter covers the epidemic history and all medical aspects of the disease. It includes sections on microbiology, the different clinical forms of the disease, and its symptoms, treatments, and possible prevention and control. In keeping with the overall topic of the book, it points out ways of determining whether an outbreak is natural or intentional. The language is rather technical.

Marriott, Edward. *Plague: A Story of Science, Rivalry, and the Scourge That Won't Go Away*. New York: Metropolitan Books, 2002. This book is part history, part current events, and part a warning about the future. It recounts the Hong Kong plague epidemic of 1894 in an exciting journalistic style, including the race between a French and a Japanese scientist to find the cause—the bacteria *Yersinia pestis*. After exactly 100 years another epidemic, in Surat, India, was met with coverups and then panic. As for the future, the author warns New York City that its vast population of rats constitutes an ever-present danger.

Orent, Wendy. *Plague: The Mysterious Past and Terrifying Future of the World's Most Dangerous Disease*. New York: Simon and Shuster, 2004. For many people, the term bubonic plague conjures up images of total horror and inescapable death played out in a medieval setting. In fact, the plague is very much alive in today's world (especially among rodents in rural areas). It is typically cured by ordinary antibiotics. Nevertheless, the author of this highly readable book believes the disease, particularly its airborne pneumonic form, retains the potential to cause havoc. Her main concern is that stocks of weaponized plague bacteria developed in the old Soviet Union are apparently missing. If they fall into the wrong hands, we are all in trouble.

Ebola

"Ebola," pp. 130–136. In Michael B.A. Oldstone, *Viruses, Plagues, and History*. New York: Oxford University Press, 1998. This chapter deals with this frightening and puzzling new virus, which first appeared in 1976 in northern Zaire, and has made periodic reappearances at various dispersed African locations.

Smith, Tara C. *Ebola*. New York: Chelsea, 2005. Part of the publisher's Deadly Diseases and Epidemics series, this brief book is aimed at young adults. It presents all the important facts about this emerging viral disease, which can cause severe and often fatal hemorrhaging in its victims.

HIV/AIDS

AVERT. "Averting HIV and AIDS," Available online. URL: http://www.avert.org. Accessed February 26, 2007. This is the health education and information Web site maintained by the British HIV/AIDS charity AVERT, which conducts AIDS prevention programs in southern Africa, India, and other countries. It contains a wealth of clearly written information about the disease, its prevention, treatment, and impact, all organized for easy access and presented in an attractive graphic format. It presents the ongoing issues and controversies in the field reasonably and without rancor, though it clearly supports "comprehensive sex education" for teens rather than "abstinence only." The authors are informed on the science and the latest developments. There are technical pages of interest to those with a biology background, yet most sections are written for the widest possible audience. A few topics are translated into Spanish.

Barnett, Tony, and Alan Whiteside. *AIDS in the Twenty-first Century: Disease and Globalization*. 2nd ed. New York: Palgrave Macmillan, 2006. This is a comprehensive look by two economists at the horrific social and economic impact of the HIV/AIDS epidemic, especially in Africa, the home of most of its victims. It deplores inadequate or failed responses to the epidemic and calls for specific measures toward its control. The authors, one of whom is South African, claim that the antiblack apartheid regime that prevailed in that country until 1994 helped spread the epidemic through its brutal labor and other policies. They also cite corruption and war in several black-led countries as contributing factors to the worsening epidemic.

Bartlett, John G., and Ann K. Finkbeiner. *The Guide to Living with HIV Infection*. 6th ed. Baltimore: Johns Hopkins University Press, 2006. This book it aimed at people who are infected with HIV and their families, friends, and health care givers. As a product of the Johns Hopkins AIDS clinic, it keeps its focus on practical issues, including information on the latest drugs (as of 2006), but there is no aspect of the pandemic that is not dealt with in clear, straightforward language.

Campbell, Catherine. *Letting Them Die: Why HIV/AIDS Prevention Programs Fail.* Bloomington: Indiana University Press, 2003. The author, a respected social psychologist specializing in HIV/AIDS, presents a provocative criticism of most HIV prevention efforts. She argues that human behavior is shaped in part by cultural and social factors, so that individuals are often not capable of acting on their knowledge of how to avoid infection. These people need the support of a "health-enabling community," she argues in this somewhat pessimistic book.

Conner, Ross F., and Luis P. Villarreal. *AIDS: Science and Society,* 5th ed. Boston: Jones and Bartlett, 2007. Intended as a college textbook for nonspecialist students, this book covers the biological, social, and psychological aspects of HIV/AIDS in accessible language and illustrations. It also aims to help students understand their own risk, learn how to avoid infection, and, for those already infected, live with the condition.

Duesberg, Peter A. *Inventing the AIDS Virus.* Washington, D.C.: Regnery, 1997. The author is world famous as a skeptic about HIV, arguing that the virus is not the primary cause of AIDS. The arguments presented in this book, while once seen as plausible, have long ago lost support from almost all scientists, even radical opponents of the medical establishment. In the past decade, drugs developed specifically to fight the HIV virus have eliminated or reduced the symptoms of AIDS in most patients, adding further proof that the virus causes the disease.

Fournier, Arthur, M., and Daniel Herlihy. *Zombie's Curse: A Doctor's 25-Year Journey into the Heart of the AIDS Epidemic in Haiti.* Washington, D.C.: Joseph Henry Press, 2006. The author, a physician who treated the first cases of HIV/AIDS in Miami, soon moved to Haiti to deal with the epidemic that was beginning to devastate that country. This book focuses largely on the confusion and blame that has faced patients and those who care for them. It concludes as a reaffirmation of the strength and courage the author discovers among the impoverished people of Haiti.

Fordham, Graham. *A New Look at Thai Aids: Perspectives from the Margin.* New York: Berghahn Books, 2004. This scholarly book by an anthropologist with extensive experience in northern Thailand is not an easy read for nonexperts, given its extensive academic terminology. However, it is a good example of how knowledge of local cultures and behavior is important for those who want to understand epidemics, and to devise prevention and treatment programs. Thailand has won praise for its campaigns to counter its serious epidemic of HIV/AIDS, but the author calls for more effective local efforts.

Frasca, Tim. *AIDS in Latin America.* New York: Palgrave Macmillan, 2005. The author, a journalist, covers the scope and impact of the disease on various Latin American countries. He stresses the participation of citizen activists and people with AIDS in pressuring national governments to take action. As a result, several Latin American countries, such as Brazil, have managed to contain HIV/AIDS within manageable limits and reduce both individual suffering and the negative social and economic impacts.

Green, Edward C. *Rethinking AIDS Prevention: Learning from Successes in Developing Countries.* Westport, Conn.: Praeger, 2003. This controversial book comes down squarely on the side of "ABC" techniques of AIDS prevention (Abstinence, Be faithful, and Condoms) as the best hope of slowing the pandemic in Africa. It also argues for increased support for religion-based organizations as the key to reaching local people with education that relates to their culture and needs. The author criticizes what he sees as an overemphasis on medical technology and products. Though many supporters of such an approach are conservatives and or religious Christians, the author's factual and reasonable prose has attracted praise from many camps in the AIDS community.

Guest, Emma. *Children of AIDS: Africa's Orphan Crisis.* Pluto Press, 2003. The author of this concise book combines case studies with a human-interest style as she investigates one of the saddest outcomes of the African AIDS crisis: the millions of children who have lost one or both parents to AIDS. She focuses on South Africa, Zambia, and Uganda, and manages to find inspiration in many stories of courage and resourcefulness.

Howe, Glenford, and Alan Cobley, eds. *The Caribbean AIDS Epidemic.* Kingston, Jamaica: University of the West Indies Press, 2000. The articles collected in this volume treat many diverse aspects of the epidemic—medical, social, economic, legal, educational, psychological, and others. Some articles focus on specific nations within the Caribbean, providing information not easily available elsewhere.

Hunter, Susan. *Black Death: AIDS in Africa.* New York: Palgrave Macmillan, 2004. The author, who has worked as an AIDS consultant in Africa for 20 years, is able to enrich this story with intimate accounts of many Africans living with AIDS or working to control the epidemic. In her view, the primary cause for the HIV/AIDS epidemic was "exploitation of developing nations by the West." Solutions are emerging locally, in her account, but they need continued help from the outside.

Hunter, Susan. *AIDS in America.* New York: Palgrave Macmillan, 2006. Unlike other, more optimistic accounts, this book warns against a possible upsurge in the illness. The author accused the U.S. government of concealing or downplaying the scope of the problem, especially among women and among the prison population. These failings may prove to have devastating result if, as the book warns, the virus soon manages to outwit the current batch of medicines by developing drug resistance.

Iliffe, John. *The African AIDS Epidemic: A History.* Columbus: Ohio University Press, 2006. The book is a concise treatment of the history of the HIV/AIDS pandemic in Africa. The author attributes the staggering size of the pandemic on the continent to the fact that it was able to spread for years before it was recognized by the medical profession. He also discusses the role of urbanization, demographic growth, and social changes in worsening the epidemic.

Kalichman, Seth C. *The Inside Story on AIDS: Experts Answer Your Questions.* Washington, D.C.: American Psychological Association, 2003. This book is structured around 350 questions commonly called in by the public to AIDS hotlines. It covers most medical and psychological information on the disease, including testing, prevention, and treatment.

Karim, Salim S. Abdool, and Quarraisha Karim. *HIV/AIDS in South Africa.* New York: Cambridge University Press, 2005. This encyclopedic work brings together contributions from experts in many fields to give a complete picture of the HIV/AIDS crisis in the Republic of South Africa, which has become one of the chief epicenters of the pandemic. Much of the information, of course, would be just as relevant in any other country. It includes a wealth of detailed data and balanced discussion of history, virology, transmission and prevention, symptoms, treatment, risk groups, social and economic impact, and projections for the future. The editors and many of the writers convey the passion that derives from years of struggle, often frustrating but often productive, against this scourge.

Levenson, Jacob. *The Secret Epidemic: The Story of AIDS and Black America.* New York: Anchor, 2005. African Americans now constitute about half of all new cases of HIV/AIDS diagnosed in the United States, and possibly more than half of undiagnosed cases. The author investigates the social, economic, and medical reasons for this disproportionate impact, and explores what it means for the black community and for race relations. The book is framed around personal stories of many individual lives destroyed or damaged by the epidemic.

Marlink, Richard, Alison Kotin, and Mildred Vasan. *Global AIDS Crisis: A Reference Handbook.* Santa Barbara, Calif.: ABC-CLIO, 2004. This high school textbook includes a historical and scientific survey of the HIV/AIDS pandemic, and a discussion of the various controversies concerning the disease and its treatment. There are profiles of key figures in the struggle against the disease, maps, charts, and lists of organizations working in the field.

Mayer, Kenneth H., and H. F. Pizer, eds. *The AIDS Pandemic, Impact on Science and Society.* Burlington, Mass: Academic Press, 2004. Many of the articles in this volume are quite technical, but others that focus on the social impact of the disease and prevention strategies are more accessible to the general reader. The book was widely praised as a comprehensive survey of the scientific and medical progress that has occurred during this decades-long pandemic.

Mendel, Gideon. *A Broken Landscape: HIV and AIDS in Africa.* Barcelona: Blume, 2003. A photographic documentary of the AIDS epidemic in Africa, this book focuses on the actual patients, their families, the villages they live in, and the local people who are trying to help. While not shrinking from the suffering and the terrible need for outside assistance, it finds a positive message in the strength and mutual support that AIDS has evoked among many people in Africa. It includes a series of interviews with some of the photographed individuals, telling their stories in their own words.

Panda, Samiran, Anindya Chatterjee, and Abu S. Abdul-Quader, eds. *Living with the AIDS Virus: The Epidemic and the Response in India.* Thousand Oaks, Calif.: Sage,

2004. This is a comprehensive volume about all aspects of the massive HIV/AIDS pandemic in India, which vies with South Africa for the largest AIDS caseload. It focuses on the various government and nongovernmental programs designed to control the disease and prevent its further spread. Some of the programs have successfully brought behavior changes among risk groups; but the size, population density, and widespread poverty combine to make for one of the most challenging public health problems in the world.

Pogash, Carol. *As Real as It Gets: The Life of a Hospital at the Center of the AIDS Epidemic*. New York: Plume, 1994. The book is a first-hand, human-interest story of the early years of HIV/AIDS at San Francisco General Hospital, one of the epicenters of the epidemic in the United States. The dedicated doctors, nurses, and patients had to find their own way in diagnosing and treating the disease and its social and economic impacts, which devastated the city's large gay community.

Poku, Nana K. *AIDS in Africa: How the poor Are Dying*. New York: Polity Press, 2006. Written by the research director of the UN's African AIDS project, this book traces the devastating effects of the epidemic on Africans. It does not spare the developed countries from criticism for what it considers bad economic advice and policy. Africa's marginalization during an era of globalization, this work argues, gets in the way of addressing the problem.

Shilts, Randy. *And the Band Played On*. New York: Penguin, 1988. This controversial book, written early in the AIDS epidemic, criticized the inadequate response by Americans to the new, puzzling threat. The author, a gay journalist who himself later died of the disease, saved much of his criticism for many gay and AIDS activists of the time, who he thought were in a state of denial. He called for the institution of the time-honored methods of fighting epidemics, especially sexually transmitted diseases, namely, contact tracing, testing, education aimed at changing behavior, and curbs on the commercial sex industry that, he felt, was fueling the disease.

Stine, Gerald J. *AIDS Update 2005*. Boston: Benjamin Cummings, 2005. This lengthy volume summarizes all the research into HIV and AIDS ongoing at the time, and is written for the nonscientist. It includes such topics as the virus itself, its impact on the immune system, its transmission, progression from infection by HIV to AIDS, HIV/AIDS prevention and treatment, opportunistic infections and cancers, epidemiology, and the social context.

Valdiserri, Ronald O., ed. *Dawning Answers: How the HIV/AIDS Epidemic Has Helped to Strengthen Public Health*. New York: Oxford University Press, 2002. Although the AIDS epidemic in the United States has involved substantial loss of life—over 500,000 mostly young victims—it has had some positive impact as well, according to the authors of these essays. They explore the development of community support and advocacy groups; increased government funding for treatment, especially for those in financial need; the emergence of safer social and sexual behaviors as a result of the epidemic; and improvement in the training of public health workers.

Whiteside, Alan. *HIV/AIDS: A Very Short Introduction*. New York: Oxford University Press, 2007. This book delivers on the promise of the title. In less than 150 pages, it presents a fairly thorough, balanced discussion of the virus, the disease, and the pandemic on an adult level. For those without the time to pursue the subject in depth, it could be a useful shortcut to basic knowledge.

Hepatitis

Askari, Fred K., and Deniel S. Cutler. *Hepatitis C: The Silent Epidemic.* New York: HarperCollins, 2001. Written by a scientist but meant for nonscientists, this short book covers all the main ground about this dangerous group of illnesses, and it is a helpful guide to those infected with the virus and their loved ones.

Blumberg, Baruch S. *Hepatitis B: The Hunt for a Killer Virus.* Princeton, N.J.: Princeton University Press, 2003. The Nobel Prize–winning author intended this book for nonscientists as well as professional colleagues. There is a lot of technical material, but also a great deal of human interest in this scientific autobiography, which takes the reader all over the world. The "hunt" uncovered vital new information about cancer and other health issues.

Palmer, Melissa. *Dr. Melissa Palmer's Guide to Hepatitis & Liver Disease.* New York: Penguin, 2004. This book, by a hepatologist, is a layman's guide to liver diseases. After a general introduction, it devotes over 100 pages to the major strains of viral hepatitis, known as A, B, C, and D. It includes information about transmission, symptoms, treatment, and possible long-term effects of these viruses, which have infected hundreds of millions of people around the world.

Influenza

Davis, Mike. *The Monster at Our Door: The Global Threat of Avian Flu.* New York: The New Press, 2005. Davis's book is a somewhat sensational response to the early human cases of avian flu. No one can gainsay his warnings that up to 100 million people could die in a global pandemic within two years, *if* the virus were to mutate so as to pass more easily between people, and *if* a pandemic takes hold before any adequate vaccine or antiviral can be deployed. However, similar predictions of doom can be made about a host of other threats to humanity, some of them perhaps more likely than a pandemic of human H5N1 virus. The author's tone may help evoke faster action from those who can help—but it may also contribute to public cynicism and apathy. In any case, the book is a tightly written, exciting read, impassioned and angry about perceived conspiracies of silence, corruption, disregard for poor people, and ignorance. The targets include China and other Asian countries accused of coverups, global corporations (including pharmaceutical and agricultural companies) accused of putting profits above all else, racism, and the capitalist system in general.

Farndon, Tom. *Bird Flu: Everything You Need to Know.* London: Icon Books, 2005. This is a concise, readable book for the nontechnical reader. It begins with the essential information about infectious diseases and viruses, and presents a concise history of influenza epidemics in the 20th century. The author tries to gauge just how real the threat of a human bird flu epidemic is, and how serious it might become. It discusses possible treatments and vaccines, and gives advice to ordinary people about what to do in case an epidemic does suddenly appear. It is written from the point of view of residents of the United Kingdom, but is just as relevant to readers anywhere.

Greger, Michael. *Bird Flu: A Virus of Our Own Hatching*? New York: Lantern Books, 2006. Issued by a vegetarian and naturalist publisher, this book develops the theory that avian influenza has become a serious threat because of recent changes in the way chickens are fed and raised for the market. The author, a physician who is director of public health for the Humane Society of America, criticizes the practice of raising animals and fowl in confined quarters, such as in modern factory farming. He claims that this has made "zoonotic" microbes (those that transfer from animals to humans) far more dangerous than ever before. The argument is made clearly and without animosity toward opponents. While most of the book's points are accepted science, the emphasis on farming methods as the key factor in today's epidemics is not a mainstream point of view.

Greene, Jeffrey, and Karen Moline. *The Bird Flu Pandemic: Can It Happen? Will It Happen? What to Do to Protect You and Your Family.* New York: St. Martins Griffin, 2006. This straightforward work aimed at the general public takes the view that a serious pandemic of avian influenza is quite possible. In any case, the commonsense measures the author recommends can hardly hurt—and could help in other possible epidemics or other catastrophes.

Knobler, Stacey L., et al., eds. *The Threat of Pandemic Influenza: Are We Ready?* Washington, D.C.: National Academies Press, 2005. The articles in this volume are written by some of the top experts in the field, and they cover just about every aspect of the problem: the history of past flu epidemics, the nature of the avian flu virus, opportunities and obstacles to preparedness, controlling the disease in birds and other animals, new drug and vaccine strategies, and the possible social and economic impact.

Liung, Ping-chung, and Paul A. Tambyah, eds. *Bird Flu: A Rising Pandemic in Asia and Beyond?* Singapore: World Scientific Publishing, 2006. This up-to-the-minute collection of scientific and epidemiological articles covers every aspect of avian flu. It includes essays about the virus itself, the history of the bird and human epidemics to the present, and the potential social and economic impact. Two articles examine the threat in Indonesia, and other articles detail the prevention and control measures adopted in Hong Kong and Singapore.

Neustadt, Richard E., and Harvey Fineberg. *The Swine Flu Affair: Decision-Making on a Slippery Disease.* Stockton, Calif.: University of the Pacific, 2005. The "affair" was the national reaction, or overreaction, to the perceived threat to the United States of a dangerous new flu virus that had surfaced in Asia in the mid 1970s. The book reconstructs the events and explains how decisions were made, using many interviews as well as official documents. It is a balanced account of an episode that raised serious questions about public health and disease control. The authors explore the costs of the mobilization (some vaccine deaths, great expense, and public mistrust) as balanced by the always present risks of inaction.

Siegel, Marc. *Bird Flu: Everything You Need to Know about the Next Pandemic.* Hoboken, N.J.: Wiley, 2006. Published by one of the major scientific, medical, and technical publishers, this book by a medical doctor is written for a wider audience, in a conversational though factual tone. The author adopts a somewhat debunking approach about the possibility of a deadly bird flu pandemic. In his view, popular misconceptions and even media hype lead people to focus on distant, unlikely health threats while ignoring much more dangerous threats like cigarette smoking. To the extent that a genuine threat exists, there is much the world can and probably will do to reduce the danger, and much that individuals can do to protect themselves and their families. In any case, after sifting through all the evidence, the author concludes that a deadly human avian influenza epidemic is not likely to happen after all.

Mad Cow (and Other Prion Diseases)

Klitzman, Robert. *The Trembling Mountain: A Personal Account of Kuru, Cannibals, and Mad Cow Disease.* New York: Perseus, 2001. The author spent a year among the Fore people of New Guinea in 1981, while they were enduring a terrible epidemic called kuru. The disease, caused by a prion similar to the cause of mad cow disease, was spread through ritual cannibalism of the dead, a practice since abandoned. The book's interest lies in its observations of a culture so different from our modern world, and in its personal stories of the victims.

Ridgway, Tom. *Mad Cow Disease: Bovine Spongiform Encephalopathy.* New York: Rosen Publishing, 2002. A short, concise, summary of mad cow disease written for the high school level, this book answers the main questions about the new and frightening disease.

Rhodes, Richard. *Deadly Feasts: Tracking the Secrets of a Terrifying New Plague.* New York: Simon and Shuster, 1998. Although written during the widespread panic over mad cow disease, this book is mostly a sober account of how scientists eventually unraveled the cause of the disease, and of the related human prion diseases.

Yam, Philip. *The Pathological Protein: Mad Cow, Chronic Wasting, and Other Deadly Prion Diseases.* New York: Springer, 2006. Although written for the general reader in an entertaining style, this book tackles the complex science behind prions. These tiny protein particles have been discovered only in recent years, thanks to the epidemic of mad cow disease and the related human epidemics of Creutzfeldt-Jakob brain disease and kuru. He treats the early human cases as a forensic challenge and follows the story as scientists begin to understand what is going on. So far, the medical community has found no treatment for or protection against misformed prions, but the book discusses the various research projects now underway.

Malaria

Day, Nancy. *Malaria, West Nile, and Other Mosquito-Borne Diseases.* Berkeley Heights, N.J.: Enslow, 2001. Although written for tenth-grade level, this short book presents a good summary of all the diseases that can be passed by mosquitoes, including yellow fever and dengue fever. It covers the anatomy and life cycle of the troublesome insects. The book explores the various strategies used to combat these diseases, and the downsides of each.

Desowitz, Robert S. *The Malaria Capers: More Tales of Parasites and People, Research and Reality.* New York: W.W. Norton, 1993. Although this book has become a bit outdated, its portrait of deteriorating public health systems in many poor countries is unfortunately still accurate. The author blames ineptitude and greed in both the public and the private sectors for the many failures in the antimalaria struggle, and for the lack of a viable antimalaria vaccine. (Such vaccines have since been developed and are being widely tested.)

Kakkilaya, B. S. "Malaria Site." Available online. URL: http://www.malariasite.com/. Accessed February 1, 2007. This is a comprehensive and rich Web site, maintained by a physician, with a large number of pages about every aspect of the disease. It is accurate but written in a popular style. It covers history, epidemiology, diagnosis, treatment, control, and prevention. It includes FAQs for general readers and for physicians unfamiliar with the disease, definitions, useful links (check the Web ring as well), and frequent medical and epidemiological news updates—including controversies as well as discoveries. The Indian subcontinent receives particular attention, but all other endemic regions are covered as well. Serious questions are entertained from readers and responded to in detail.

Reuben, R. "Obstacles to Malaria Control in India—the Human Factor," pp. 143–154. In Michael W. Service, *Demography and Vector-Borne Diseases.* Washington, D. C.: CRC Press, 1989. This article explores the reasons that India's malaria eradication program fell short of its goal. It deals with changes in land use and agricultural practices, deforestation, irrigation, and population movement. On the human behavior side, it reports growing resistance to indoor spraying and criticizes the health care delivery system.

Roll Back Malaria Partnership, *World Malaria Report 2005.* Geneva, Switzerland: WHO, 2005. Available online. URL: http://www.rbm.who.int/wmr2005/index.html. This remarkably well-written status report contains a wealth of information about the effort to control and prevent malaria around the world. It summarizes several years of research and action under the umbrella of Roll Back Malaria, a partnership of UN agencies, the World Bank, and many other public and private sector organizations. Region and country surveys take up most of the work. It includes frank discussions of policy issues and ways of evaluating progress. A set of maps and tables makes this an excellent first stop in any research on malaria today. The report's can-do optimism is summarized on the first page: "the tide may be beginning to turn against malaria as control and prevention programmes start to take effect."

Singer, Burt, Awash Teklehaimanot, Andrew Spielman, and Allan Schapira. *Coming to Grips with Malaria in the New Millennium.* New York: Earthscan, 2005. This work is part of the United Nations "Millennium Project," aimed at eliminating world poverty. The premise is that malaria is a major impediment to economic growth and general health in many poor countries. The work presents a straightforward presentation of antimalaria strategies including early diagnosis, drug therapy, indoor spraying, treated bed nets, and improving housing, education, and the environment.

Tren, Richard, Roger Bate, and Harold M. Koenig. *Malaria and the DDT Story.* London: Institute of Economic Affairs, 2001. Passionately written by experts in the field, this book pursues the argument that anti-DDT environmentalists in prosperous countries caused serious harm to people in several developing countries who desperately needed the powerful antimosquito insecticide. When DDT became limited or unavailable, cases of malaria soared. Whether or not the effects of the anti-DDT campaign were as bad as the authors claim, they make a convincing case of how complex global issues can be. Even with the best of intentions, people solving one problem can sometimes create new problems in other areas.

Onchocerciasis and Other Worm-Borne Diseases

Beigbeder, Yves. "Controlling Onchocerciasis," pp. 87–94. In *International Public Health: Patients' Rights vs. the Protection of Patents.* This book, as the title indicates, deals with issues concerning the availability of life-saving drugs in those countries or sectors that lack the money to compensate drug companies for their intellectual property. The author uses the struggle against onchocerciasis as one example of "public-private partnerships for health."

Bynum, Helen. *Success in Africa: The Onchocerciasis Control Programme in West Africa, 1974–2002.* Geneva, Switzerland: WHO, 2002. This is an official version of the successful campaign to eliminate river blindness in West Africa. The program not only saved large numbers of people from disability and early death but also allowed resettlement of fertile riverside land.

Division of Parasitic Diseases. "Dracunculiasis: Guinea Worm Disease." Washington, D.C.: Centers for Disease Control and Prevention, 2004. Available online: URL: http://www.cdc.gov/ncidod/dpd/parasites/dracunculiasis/2004_PDF_Dracunculiasis.pdf. This fact sheet explains all the basic facts about guinea worm disease, which is endemic in parts of Africa. It includes the parasite's life cycle, method of transmission, symptoms of the disease, treatments, and the international campaign to control or eliminate the parasite.

Levine, Ruth, Molly Kinder et al. "Controlling Onchocerciasis in Sub-Saharan Africa," pp. 57–64. In *Millions Saved: Proven Successes in Global Health.* Washington, D.C.: Peterson Institute for International Economics, 2004. This book is premised on the belief that one of the best ways to win public support for expensive global public health programs is to show how successful many of these programs have been. The authors consider onchocerciasis to be one of the most inspiring success stories. A summary page provides all the basic information on this endemic disease. The remainder of the chapter details the global response to this disease, which began slowly in 1968 but has since had dramatic success, using both vector (insect) control and antiparasitic drugs.

McNeil, Jr., Donald G. "Dose of Tenacity Wears Down a Horrific Disease." In *New York Times,* March 26, 2006. Also available online at URL: http://www.nytimes.com/2006/03/26/international/africa/26worm.html?ex=1172725200&en=7e99d5 ab8104ac38&ei=5070. The online version of this report on the campaign to eliminate guinea worm disease includes several helpful multimedia features. Its tells of hard-won progress in prevention and eradication of this painful and debilitating affliction.

SARS

Abraham, Thomas. *Twenty-first Century Plague: The Story of SARS.* Baltimore: Johns Hopkins University Press, 2004. This is a concise, straightforward study of the 2002–03 SARS epidemic, written by a prominent Asian journalist with years of experience in Hong Kong. Using his intimate knowledge of the local cultures and prominent figures, he traces the epidemic from the earliest cases through its international breakout and its final suppression. While maintaining a dispassionate, objective tone, the author does not hesitate to deal with controversial issues concerning SARS and other pandemics. He ends with a strong warning against the dangers of viral pandemics, focusing on avian flu.

Brookes, Tim, and Omar A. Khan. *Behind the Mask: How the World Survived SARS, the First Epidemic of the Twenty-first Century.* Washington, D.C.: American Public Health Association, 2004. This is a clearly written nontechnical book, giving a complete timeline of the SARS epidemic from its inception in late 2002 to the final cases early in 2004. Interviews with some of those involved in the fight against the new virus add immediacy to the text.

Greenfeld, Karl Taro. *China Syndrome: The True Story of the 21st Century's First Great Epidemic.* New York: HarperCollins, 2006. A *Time* magazine editor and journalist with years of experience in Asia, Greenfeld offers a very readable account of the SARS epidemic. He presents all the basic medical and scientific information, explained clearly for the layman. The author builds the story of the terrifying epidemic day by day, almost as a diary, writing from the point of view of several actual patients and health workers. The book sets the stage with fascinating descriptions of life in today's urban China, including the rapid growth in production and prosperity, and the downside—overcrowded, unregulated, and unhealthy living and working conditions that could provide an ideal breeding ground for epidemics, especially given the growing popularity in China of wild animal food. The book sings the praises of many of the vigilant scientists and doctors of Hong Kong, who play a key ongoing role in protecting the world's population from a perennial threat of pandemic influenza, as well as their colleagues and counterparts in the United States, at the World Health Organization, and around the world. *China Syndrome* is one of the most accessible books in the field—although perhaps less cautious in its judgments and opinions than a strictly scientific work would be.

Kleinman, Arthur, and James L. Watson, eds. *SARS in China: Prelude to Pandemic?* Palo Alto, Calif.: Stanford University Press, 2005. Contributions by a journalist, doctors, scientists, and public health professionals help to make this a lively and informative collection that covers every aspect of the SARS pandemic of 2003. They deal with issues of national sovereignty versus global responsibility, and draw lessons from the response to SARS for possible future pandemics, such as avian flu.

Leung, P. C., and E. E. Ooi, eds. *SARS War: Combating the Disease.* Singapore: World Scientific, 2003. Although written in mid 2003 in Hong Kong and Singapore, which were then at the center of the frightening epidemic of SARS (severe acute respiratory syndrome), this book managed to retain a level-headed tone and approach. The authors, one a prominent doctor in Hong Kong, the other a virus researcher in Singapore, called for stronger public health measures, but warned against panic and overreaction. In plain, simple language, the book describes the disease, traces the course of the epidemic around the world to that point, discusses the treatment protocols then being used (including traditional Chinese herbs), and gives clear instructions as to personal and public hygiene measures that could control the outbreak. As a snapshot of an epidemic in progress, the book is well worth reading.

McLean, Angela R., et al. eds. *SARS: A Case Study in Emerging Infections.* New York: Oxford University Press, 2005. This is a collection of essays by experts concerning all aspects of the brief but deadly SARS pandemic of 2003. The aim is to learn lessons about what must be done if—or when—the next new or revived infectious disease epidemic arrives. Topics covered range from new mathematical modeling of how epidemics can spread via airline networks, to the ethical concerns raised by enforced quarantines, to the dynamics of the spread of microbes within nonhuman animal hosts.

Suok, Kai Chew. *SARS: How a Global Epidemic Was Stopped.* Manila, Philippines: WHO Regional Office for the Western Pacific. The office that published this inside account was closely involved with the SARS epidemic from before the disease was named. The result is an authoritative look at what happened, as this potential world disaster was controlled through unprecedented international cooperation.

Smallpox

Carrell, Jennifer. *The Speckled Monster: A Historical Tale of Battling the Smallpox Epidemic.* New York: Dutton, 2003. A detailed account of the early days of smallpox inoculation in Europe and America, the book reads like a novel (complete with imagined conversations). It focuses on two figures who were instrumental in promoting the practice during the epidemics of 1721 and 1722: Lady Mary Wortley Montagu in London and the Boston physician Zabdiel Boylston. Those interested in social history and in European attitudes about women and non-European cultures will find this rather long book well worth reading.

Fenn, Elizabeth Anne. *Pox Americana: The Great Smallpox Epidemic of 1775–82.* New York: Hill and Wang, 2002. This scholarly account of one epidemic includes many original documents from the era. Among other interesting incidents, it credits George Washington with saving the Continental Army by inoculating the troops.

Finer, Kim Renee. *Smallpox.* New York: Chelsea House, 2004. Like many of the volumes in this series, this book is a well-written and comprehensive account of the disease and its epidemic history designed for high school students.

Glynn, Ian, and, Jenifer Glynn. *The Life and Death of Smallpox.* New York: Cambridge University Press, 2004. Surprisingly, this very readable and well-illustrated survey of smallpox throughout history is a pleasure to read. The story illustrates the effects of the disease by showing how it touched the lives of prominent historical figures such as Queen Elizabeth I, Voltaire, Mozart, and Abraham Lincoln. The authors detail the frightening treatments used in the past, almost as harmful as the disease. They then trace two centuries of progress from the time Edward Jenner promoted inoculation to the final eradication of the disease in 1977.

Preston, Richard. *The Demon in the Freezer: A True Story.* New York: Random House, 2002. This best-seller reads like a crime thriller, but it is nevertheless a serious examination of the issue—what should the world do with the remaining samples of smallpox virus residing at secure labs? All remaining smallpox samples, as far as is known, are kept in just two high-security facilities, one in Russia and one in the United States, although some former Soviet samples may have gone missing. Should the official samples be destroyed to avoid the danger of accidental, terrorist, or criminal release? Should they be saved for research, especially to protect against future epidemics? Are such epidemics possible, if the virus still exists somewhere in nature or in hidden labs?

Tucker, Jonathan B. *Scourge: The Once and Future Threat of Smallpox.* New York: Grove Press, 2002. A scholarly book full of both scientific and historical detail, this is considered one of the best works on the topic for the serious reader. It also covers the possible use of "weaponized" smallpox in future bioterror events. Although technical, it is not dry, certainly not in its portraits of the heroic physicians and scientists who worked to control and then defeat this ancient scourge.

Syphilis and Other STDs

Barlow, David H., Ali Mears, and Dip Gum. *Sexually Transmitted Infections: The Facts.* New York: Oxford University Press, 2006. This mass market book offers clear information about all the major serious sexually transmitted diseases, mostly from the standpoint of individuals seeking advice about prevention, diagnosis, and treatment. The book is written with British readers in mind, but nearly all the information would be relevant to readers anywhere. Apart from the most well-known illnesses, it treats gonorrhea, herpes, genital warts, and a variety of tropical and other infections.

Eng, Thomas R., and William T. Butler. *The Hidden Epidemic: Confronting Sexually Transmitted Diseases.* Washington, D.C.: National Academies Press, 1997. This book deals with the wide variety of STDs that still damage the health and economic well-being of many Americans, and that may be overlooked in the attention given to HIV/AIDS, currently the most deadly of the STDs. The authors maintain that most epidemics of STDs are largely invisible to the public, because they are often asymptomatic (the patients do not experience any clear symptoms); the serious consequences, such as sterility and cancers, usually do not show up until years after the initial infection; and, of course, there is still a stigma or shame associated with STDs that lead many people to put up with symptoms they believe are not life-threatening. As befits a product of the National Institute of Medicine, the prose is dry and scholarly, but the book pulls together information that is crucial to this problem. The authors make recommendations toward establishing "an effective national system to prevent STDs."

Suiter, Elizabeth. "Waging War on STDs—and Drugmaker Apathy—with Microbicides." In Mary Worcester, and Marianne H. Whatley, *Women's Health: Readings on Social, Economic, and Political Issues,* pp. 602–604. Dubuque, Iowa: Kendall/Hunt, 2004. The article discusses the general threat to women's health from a variety of sexually transmitted diseases. The author's premise is that women are often unable to insist on safer sex practices, and therefore they need the protection that new microbe-killing substances might provide.

Tuberculosis

Daniel, Thomas M. *Captain of Death: The Story of Tuberculosis.* Rochester, N.Y.: University of Rochester Press, 1999. This book for general readers gives an authoritative overview of the disease, for many years one of the world's most deadly. As long as the disease remains prevalent in certain poorer countries such as Haiti, Daniel warns, antibiotic-resistant strains threaten people everywhere. Written by a doctor, this account celebrates the lives of the famous and anonymous doctors who helped contain tuberculosis. A good part of the book is devoted to a clear exposition of how the microbe does its damage to the body, and how the body fights back. This information unfolds as an entertaining historical detective story.

Draus, Paul Joseph. *Consumed in the City: Observing Tuberculosis at Century's End.* New York: Oxford University Press, 2004. The author was a fieldworker in New York and Chicago during the small but frightening tuberculosis epidemic that emerged during the 1990s. The revival of a once-dreaded disease that had all but disappeared in America was a side effect of the HIV/AIDS pandemic. People with weak immune systems were easy victims for the bacteria, which had mutated into strains more difficult to treat. The disease was just one more blow to a subpopulation of poor urban residents.

Gandy, Matthew, and Alimuddin Zumla, eds. *The Return of the White Plague: Global Poverty and the "New" Tuberculosis.* New York: Verso, 2003. In the 19th and early 20th centuries endemic tuberculosis was a major killer all over the world, until it was almost eliminated by public health measures, higher living standards, and antibiotics. In recent decades, however, it has reemerged in several countries, especially among AIDS patients, due largely to the bacteria's growing resistance to drugs. This collection of essays explores the scientific and medical aspects of the renewed epidemic, as well as the social and economic background—most of those who become infected are poor. Several of the authors call for a combined approach of antipoverty measures alongside new drugs and vaccines.

Reichman, Lee B., and Janice Hopkins Tanne. *Timebomb: The Global Epidemic of Multi-Drug-Resistant Tuberculosis.* New York: McGraw-Hill, 2004. This is a thorough treatment of a serious new threat. Tuberculosis was responsible for one in four deaths in the United States in the 19th century. It was controlled, at least in developed countries, by the new antibiotics of the 1950s, but strains of the bacillus have slowly become resistant to almost every drug thrown against them, in part because the drugs are not always carefully dispensed. Considering how easy it is to spread (a single cough will do it), epidemiologists are concerned. Complicating factors are the spread of HIV/AIDS, which lowers resistance, the rise in prison populations, and the simple fact that, the author claims, 2 billion people are already infected with latent TB; 2 million die of the disease each year.

Yellow Fever

Dickerson, James L. *Yellow Fever: A Deadly Disease Poised to Kill Again.* Amherst, N.Y.: Prometheus, 2006. This book details the history of yellow fever, its suppression in the developed world early in the 20th century, and its survival in certain parts of the developing world. The author warns that the parasite could make a deadly comeback, either in weaponized form during bioterror attacks or as a result of global warming. A rise in temperatures, he argues, might expand the natural range of the mosquitoes that transmit the yellow fever parasite.

Pierce, John R., and James V. Writer. *Yellow Jack: How Yellow Fever Ravaged America and Walter Reed Discovered Its Deadly Secrets.* Hoboken, N.J.: Wiley, 2005. Yellow fever was a serious endemic disease in the American South for generations. The author retells the oft-told story of how it was defeated, at the cost of the lives of several researchers. Army physician Walter Reed headed up a Yellow Fever Board that proved that mosquitoes were the transmitters of this disease. Almost overnight the plague was eliminated from Cuba, opening up many tropical areas to heavier settlement and economic development.

GENERAL

Akukwe, Chinua. *Don't Let Them Die: HIV/AIDS, TB, Malaria, and the Healthcare Crisis in Africa.* London: Adonis and Abbey, 2006. The author of this concise appeal to the world's conscience is an academic/activist on global health issues. All the diseases he explores are preventable and treatable, yet millions of Africans are still being infected, and millions are still dying every year.

Akukwe examines the issues of health care policy surrounding theses diseases, and he shows the feedback connection between them and poverty in Africa.

Alcamo, I. Edward. *Microbes and Society: An Introduction to Microbiology.* Boston: Jones and Bartlett, 2002. This college-level survey is designed to be used by nonscience students. The many graphics and illustrations help make it accessible to serious high school students as well. It covers the role of microbes in agriculture, industry, the environment, and in our bodies. About one-fourth of the volume deals with the role of viruses and bacteria in infectious disease.

Anand, Sudhir, Fabienne Peter, and Amartya Sen, eds. *Public Health, Ethics, and Equity.* New York: Oxford University Press, 2006. The essays in this collection are written by experts from several fields including medicine, economics, anthropology, and philosophy. They deal with differences in the health status between populations, globally and within individual countries. Apart from unequal access to modern medicine and inadequate public health infrastructure, these differences can be caused by varying behaviors and values. Should these differences be ironed out in the interests of better health? Can health outcomes be similar when there are social and economic differences between groups? How can society balance individual responsibility for health with desired goals for society as a whole? These and similar questions are treated from many different points of view.

Armus, Diego, ed. *Disease in the History of Modern Latin America: From Malaria to AIDS.* Durham, N.C.: Duke University Press. Following current academic practice, this book treats disease as a "social and cultural construction." To that end, the contributors study the way different countries understood and responded to the concepts of health and disease, and to various specific disease epidemics at different times, from the late 19th century through the contemporary era. Certain epidemics, they maintain, helped further the process of nation-building. Several articles stress the interaction between medical ideas and concepts of sexuality, nation, and modernity.

Beaglehole, Robert, and Ruth Bonita. *Public Health at the Crossroads: Achievements and Prospects.* New York: Cambridge University Press, 2004. Used as a textbook in public health, this book defines and explains most of the topics in the field. While it surveys public health systems and practices in several individual developed and poor countries, the focus is on the growing globalization of problems and solutions. It concludes on a note of "cautious optimism" about growing public awareness and improved techniques in combating epidemics and improving health.

Bourdelais, Patrice. *Epidemics Laid Low: A History of What Happened in Rich Countries.* Baltimore: Johns Hopkins University Press, 2006. The author recounts the history of epidemics in Europe and describes how infectious diseases have been contained there. He attributes success to economic growth, the public's demand, medical research, and the ideology of progress. In other words, Europeans believed that modern times would bring an end to the scourges that had plagued them for so long—and this very belief helped drive the struggle against epidemics. The book (translated from French) ends with concern for the future, due to the rise of resistance against antibiotics and the emergence of "the Thunderbolt: AIDS."

Cliff, Andrew, Peter Haggett, and Matthew Smallman-Raynor. *World Atlas of Epidemic Diseases*. London: Hodder Arnold, 2004. This books consists of a thorough presentation of over 50 major epidemic diseases, nearly all of which are still around at least to some degree in the 21st century. Maps, graphs, and many illustrations help make the material accessible, although the articles themselves are not particularly tailored to nonprofessional readers.

Cueto, Marcos. *Return of Epidemics: Health and Society in Peru during the Twentieth Century*. Aldershot, U.K.: Ashgate, 2001. The author examines the causes, impact, and social response to a series of epidemic diseases that have hit Peru in the 20th century, from bubonic plague, which broke out in 1903, to the cholera epidemic of 1991. He emphasizes the social, political, and cultural response to the disease, among different strata of society and in different regions of the country. The premise is that the history of medicine and public health can contribute to understanding the changing social history of a country.

DeSalle, ed. *Epidemic! The World of Infectious Disease*. New York: The New Press, 1999. Published in conjunction with the American Museum of Natural History, this book was inspired by a traveling exhibit of the same name organized by the museum. Attractively designed and clearly written, the book consists of more than 20 fairly brief essays, written by prominent experts in the field, covering such topics as: how and why new diseases arise; how doctors and scientists can diagnose diseases and track outbreaks; how diseases are transmitted and diagnosed; how they spread and how they can be resisted and treated; and the various historical and social dimensions of epidemics. Each section is introduced by the editor with a series of key questions that are answered in the essays. Also included are several historical and contemporary case studies on infectious and epidemic disease, and profiles of a number of leading figures in the struggle against them. Thanks to the wide range of approaches and styles in the essays, the arresting illustrations, and the clear organization of material, the book can be recommended as an excellent introduction to the field for serious students.

Drexler, Madeline. *Secret Agents: The Menace of Emerging Infections*. Washington, D.C.: Joseph Henry Press. As the title promises, this book is a testimonial to a small group of individuals and agencies on the front line in the world's battle with new or revived epidemic disease. The science is presented clearly and readably, and the episodes give the satisfaction of solved crimes. The author treats the historical and public policy issues fairly as well, including the threat of bioterror. She calls for dramatically increased spending to counter the altered microbes that criminals or terrorists might in the future release.

Dudley, William and Mary E. Williams, eds. *Epidemics: Opposing Viewpoints*. Santa Barbara, Calif.: Greenhaven Press, 2005. The book presents a series of more or less controversial issues in the field of epidemics and infectious disease. Each issue is explored in a series of articles selected from various journals. Questions include: do epidemics threaten the future of mankind? how can the HIV/AIDS pandemic be controlled? how can food-borne illnesses be prevented? and are vaccines harmful?

Eward, Paul W. *Evolution of Infectious Disease.* New York: Oxford University Press, 1994. Those with a strong interest in or knowledge of biology may find this book fascinating. It summarizes the results of decades of research and tries to explain the coevolution of pathogens like viruses, bacteria, and protozoa along with their hosts, including insects, humans, and other animals. Pathogens can evolve to become more or less dangerous as a result of natural selection, changes in their ecologies, or medical intervention (e.g., doctors pass pathogens between patients, pathogens evolve to fight off antibiotics). The author writes in a crisp tone leavened with humor. He focuses special attention on HIV/AIDS, and he recommends that any strategies to control future epidemics must take evolution into account. The material avoids technical words and jargon, but it still requires a careful read.

Garrett, Laurie. *Betrayal of Trust: The Collapse of Global Public Health.* New York: Hyperion, 2001. Those who want an antidote to the optimism one may find these days in the global health field will welcome this book. Long (768 pages), dense, and heavily researched, it explores what the author sees as the collapse of public health systems in many regions, including Africa and eastern Europe, and the weakening of health care for many in the United States and elsewhere. It is written with all the techniques of a skilled reporter writing a gripping exposé. The book criticizes what it calls too much reliance on expensive technology and medicines, and the author calls for more attention to prevention and hygiene.

Hays, J. N. *The Burden of Disease: Epidemics and Human Response in Western History.* Piscataway, N.J.: Rutgers University Press, 1998. This is a readable historical survey of how Western civilization responded to disease and epidemics, from ancient Greece to the present global culture. It follows the continuity of ideas between magic, religion, medicine, and scientific research. All the main areas are covered: the ancient and medieval experience, the great plague pandemic from the 15th to the 17th centuries, early modern science and rationalism, improvements in sanitation and living conditions, the expansion of the West and pandemics, the optimistic era of disease eradication in the mid 20th century, and the emergence of horrifying new pandemics and pandemic threats by century's end.

Janse, Allison, and Charles Gerba. *The Germ Freak's Guide to Outwitting Colds and Flu: Guerrilla Tactics to Keep Yourself Healthy at Home, at Work and in the World.* Deerfield Beach, Fla.: HCI, 2005. Despite the amusing title, this book actually does provide some good advice on avoiding flu and colds, some of which will probably be news to most readers.

Karlen, Arno. *Man and Microbes: Disease and Plagues in History and Modern Times.* New York: Simon and Shuster, 1996. This popular book has an alarming thesis: changes in human behavior and the environment make it likely that the "epidemic of epidemics" of recent decades (Legionnaires and Lyme diseases,

AIDS, etc.) will continue and may worsen. The author contrasts the current situation with the optimism of the very recent past, which may have been shortsighted; after all, epidemics have been with us since earliest civilization. The book is well written and entertaining. However, it must be said that the years that have passed since it appeared have not borne out its most alarming predictions.

Lee, Kelly, ed. *Health Impacts of Globalization: Towards Global Governance.* New York: Palgrave Macmillan, 2003. Infectious diseases went global centuries ago; any attempt to control them must be global in scope as well. However, the positive and negative effects of today's economic and cultural globalization on health can be very complicated. The essays in this collection discuss such issues as HIV/AIDS, mad cow disease, cholera, resistance to antibiotics and other drugs, tobacco, nutrition, international trade, and global governance—the attempt to organize responsibility for these matters apart from national governments and corporations.

———, Kent Buse, and Suzanne Fustukian, eds. *Health Policy in a Globalising World.* New York: Cambridge University Press, 2005. The essays in this book, aimed at professionals in the field, concern the impact of economic and cultural globalization on public health systems around the world. It covers emerging diseases, environmental degradation, and demographic change.

Levine, Ruth, and Molly Kinder. *Millions Saved: Proven Successes in Global Health.* Washington, D.C.: Institute for International Economics, 2004. This volume has an almost old-fashioned American tone of optimism. Its message is that hard work, good will, an internationalist perspective, and money, when invested in global public health, can save millions of lives and bring significant political and economic benefits as well. Seventeen cases are explored in detail, including polio in Latin America, measles in southern Africa, and HIV/AIDS in Thailand.

Levy, Elinor and Mark Fischetti. *The New Killer Diseases: How the Alarming Evolution of Mutant Germs Threatens Us All.* New York: Crown Publishers, 2003. Immunologist Levy and science journalist Fischetti devote a chapter to each of the infectious disease epidemics, episodes, and scares of recent years, using actual case histories. Subjects include SARS, "flesh-eating bacteria," bioterrorism, mad cow disease, E coli, flu, tuberculosis, and antibiotic resistance. Their picture of a world out of control may be alarmist or exaggerated, but their accounts are factual.

McKenna, Maryn. *Beating Back the Devil: On the Front Lines with the Disease Detectives of the Epidemic Intelligence Service.* New York: Free Press, 2004. The disease detectives of this agency of the CDC, all doctors and nurses, are routinely summoned to travel to locations anywhere in the world to investigate and treat possible outbreaks of epidemic disease. This book recounts 11 dramatic case studies covering epidemics, environmental disasters, and terrorism. EIS workers tell the author of their struggles against disease as well as corrupt, brutal, or incompetent authorities. The book also describes the recruitment and training process of these often heroic men and women.

McMichael, Anthony J., and Pim Martens, eds. *Environmental Change, Climate, and Health: Issues and Research Methods.* New York: Cambridge University Press, 2002. It has become a truism that changes to the environment and to climate will have impacts on epidemics and public health in general. The essays in this collection try to assess just what those impacts will be, and what can be done about them. The tone is scholarly and sober, unlike many popular books in this field.

Merson, Michael H., Robert E. Black, and Anne J. Mills, eds. *International Public Health: Diseases, Programs, Systems, and Policies.* Boston: Jones and Bartlett, 2005. This technical volume serves as a textbook for students of global public health, but it can also be a mine of useful information and ideas for anyone interested in the field. Apart from epidemic diseases, it covers nutrition, disasters, mental health, environmental health and other public issues. Articles about the design and management of national health systems impact all these fields. Two concluding chapters analyze the increasing globalization of health issues and growing international cooperation.

Morse, Stephen S., ed. *Emerging Viruses.* New York: Oxford University Press, 1996. Listed by *American Scientist* as one of the 100 best science books of the 20th century, this book brings together noted experts in virology, epidemiology, and public health to give an authoritative account (for its time) of the new and renewed viral diseases, their evolution and spread, and attempts to control them. It puts the emerging viruses in historical context, warns that others will also emerge, but avoids any doomsday predictions or despair. Instead it calls for renewed research and action, not only for the well-known viruses like HIV and Ebola but also for the field of viral evolution in general. It is well written but assumes some knowledge of the field.

Needham, Cynthia, and Richard Canning. *Global Disease Eradication: The Race for the Last Child.* Washington, D.C.: ASM Press, 2003. Published by the American Society for Microbiology, this book examines the issues and problems involved in the global attempt to eliminate major epidemic diseases. For evidence it analyzes three campaigns—the successful fight against smallpox that ended in 1977, the unsuccessful attempt to eradicate malaria, and the ongoing struggle to end polio. The costs of eradication are computed, especially against alternative needs, as well as the possible dangers that face humanity if a pathogen is eliminated from nature, leaving humanity without immunity in the face of bioterror attempts.

Preston, Richard. *The Hot Zone: A Terrifying True Story.* New York: Anchor, 1995. A best-seller later made into a motion picture, this book relates the story of an accidental outbreak of Ebola virus disease at a lab in Reston, Virginia. The author spares no gory details in describing the physical effects of Ebola and similar viruses. He attributes their emergence, and the emergence of AIDS, to human disruption of tropical rain forests.

Price-Smith, Andrew T., ed. *Plagues and Politics: Infectious Disease and International Policy.* New York: Palgrave, 2001. The authors of the articles in this anthology include some well-regarded professors of international relations, history, political science, laws, economics, public health, the environment, and epidemiology. Their focus is not the scientific and medical aspect of epidemic disease, but the economic and political aspect. The tone is sober, but nontechnical readers should be able to follow many of the arguments. Nearly half the chapters are reproduced from scholarly journals and books published in the late 1990s; therefore, the book is a bit less up-to-date than the publication date indicates. There is also a certain amount of duplication and overlap between the articles. Nevertheless, the volume is worth browsing for anyone interested in topics such as the impact of biodiversity on health; the effect of economic growth on infectious disease patterns; the impact of epidemics on economic activity and trade, especially in poor countries; the threat that diseases pose to world peace and security; the role that intelligence agencies can play in gathering adequate epidemic information around the world, especially when governments suppress that information; and the history of international public health law.

Riley, James C. *Rising Life Expectancy: A Global History.* New York: Cambridge University Press, 2001. Even in an age of pandemics (HIV/AIDS) and endemic infectious disease (malaria, etc.), it is perhaps worth stopping to acknowledge the overall gains that have been registered in public health. This book is a fascinating account of just how the human race increased its life expectancy from 30 years in 1800 to 67 years in 2000. It presents evidence from many countries, economies, and cultures. Advances against epidemic disease and improvements in public health were among the major factors in this change.

Siddiqi, Javed. *World Health and World Politics: The World Health Organization and the UN System.* Columbia: University of South Carolina Press, 1995. This scholarly book analyzes the history of the World Health Organization (WHO) in the first few decades of its existence. The author praises the WHO's universal, decentralized structure, although he spares no criticism about its early failures, such as the malaria eradication campaign.

Spielman, Andrew, and Michael D'Antonio. *Mosquito: A Natural History of Our Most Persistent and Deadly Foe.* New York: Hyperion, 2001. This mostly entertaining book of popular science is not for squeamish readers. It details everything a reader wanted or did not want to know about mosquitoes, their life cycle, the deadly illnesses they transmit, and their impact on history. Noting the resilience of these insects (which come in 2,500 kinds), the author warns that the story of mosquitoes and epidemics is far from over.

Staples, Jeffrey et al. "Preparing for a Pandemic." *Harvard Business Review* (May 1, 2006). A serious flu pandemic could disable many businesses and other organizations. The brief articles in this essay deal with issues that organizations should be planning for today. It discusses preventive health measures for employees, contingency plans to carry on during the pandemic, legal aspects, and anticipated responses by various governments around the world.

Walters, Mark Jerome. *Six Modern Plagues, and How We Are Causing Them.* Washington, D.C.: Shearwater Books, 2004. This book, published by an environmental press, covers a topic that is often sensationalized, but the author treats it calmly and helpfully. It examines the role of changing industrial, commercial, and ecological practices in causing or exacerbating epidemics. The six epidemics treated here are all either passed from animals to humans today or first infected people by jumping from an original animal host: mad cow disease, HIV/AIDS, salmonella DT 104, Lyme disease, hantavirus, and West Nile virus. The author, a veterinarian, calls for renewed attention to the impact of human actions on the natural world and on food animals.

Wills, Christopher. *Yellow Fever, Black Goddess: The Coevolution of People and Plagues*. Boston: Addison-Wesley, 1997. Pathogens, this book maintains, have helped develop and maintain human biological diversity while serving as agents of historical change. In fact, they are an important factor in the evolution of ecosystems. The book covers many of the most famous historic epidemics, and surveys the many pathogens that plague and threaten us today. It finds comfort in scientific progress, and in the idea that nature works to keep pathogens in balance with their hosts.

Zelicoff, Alan P., and Michael Bellomo. *Microbe: Are We Ready for the Next Plague?* AMACOM (American Management Association), 2005. This mass market but accurate book covers most of the diseases that have emerged in the past 30 years, as well as terrorism and weaknesses in the U.S. public health system.

Zubay, Geoffrey, ed. *Agents of Bioterrorism: Pathogens and Their Weaponization.* New York: Columbia University Press, 2005. The topic of bioterrorism rose to the fore after the anthrax mailings that killed several Americans in late 2001 and have still not been solved. The scientists who wrote the articles in this anthology examine 13 different disease-causing organisms, including anthrax, smallpox, and influenza. They present a summary of everything that is currently known about the organisms, how they harm people, and how easy or difficult it might be for terrorists or criminals to abuse them. The authors discuss possible approaches in developing drugs or vaccines against these microbes, and they explore others way to protect the public against them. The tone is calm and balanced, despite the sensational subject matter.

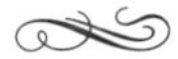

Chronology

3180 B.C.E.

- According to Manetho, a third-century B.C.E. Egyptian historian, a great pestilence occurs during the reign of the First Dynasty pharaoh Mempses.

2700 B.C.E.

- Traditional date for the *Nei Ching*, usually called the *Yellow Emperor's Classic of Internal Medicine.* This book, which many historians believe was written some 1,000 years later, lays the foundations for traditional Chinese medicine. It includes malarialike symptoms in its catalog of diseases.

2400 B.C.E.

- Several Old Kingdom mummies show evidence of tuberculosis.

2300 B.C.E.

- According to the Eshmuna Code in Mesopotamia, "If a dog is mad and the authorities have brought the fact to the knowledge of its owner, if he does not keep it in, and it bites a man and causes his death, then the owner shall pay two-thirds of a min of silver." This may be the first municipal rabies ordinance.

c. 1500 B.C.E.

- According to the book of Exodus in the Hebrew Bible (which took written form several hundred years later) several major disasters strike Egypt at around this time. They lay the ground for a plague of cattle, followed by a human plague manifested in skin boils, and then by a deadly plague that kills many Egyptians. The Israelites take advantage of this situation to flee the country. In the desert their leader Moses imposes laws, some of them health-related: quarantine for certain illnesses and prohibition of eating animals that died on their own or that show evidence of internal disease.

Chronology

14TH CENTURY B.C.E.

- A 20-year plague, apparently brought by Egyptian prisoners of war, devastates the Hittite nation in modern-day Turkey. This may be smallpox, which was first mentioned in Egyptian papyrus texts at this time. If so, this is the first time the disease appears outside of Africa, believed to be its place of origin.

1143 B.C.E.

- Egyptian pharoah Ramses V dies of smallpox at the age of about 35. His mummy shows ample evidence of the disease.

MID-11TH CENTURY B.C.E.

- According to I Samuel in the Hebrew Bible, the Philistines, who dwell along the southern coast of ancient Israel, suffer a debilitating epidemic characterized by swellings or tumors in the groin area. This might indicate bubonic plague, or possibly dysentery, according to medical historians.

1000 B.C.E.

- Smallpox is first mentioned in India.

C. 600 B.C.E.

- An early vedic poem in India refers to lepers, and warns that they should be driven away from villages with stones. This may indicate a rudimentary understanding of contagion. In later works leprosy is often considered a punishment or curse, although some great saints may have been lepers.

480 B.C.E.

- The Persian army is laid low during its invasion of Greece by an epidemic that appears to have been dysentery. According to the Greek historian Herodotus, who described the epidemic in detail, the incident contributed to the eventual Persian defeat.

C. 470 B.C.E.

- Birth of Hippocrates, perhaps the most famous physician of ancient times, and considered a founder of empirical medicine. He describes many infectious endemic and epidemic diseases in his work *Epidemics*, including the first mention of jaundice. He also explores the relationship between environment and health.

452 B.C.E.

- According to later Greek and Roman historians, the city of Rome and much of Italy are devastated by an extremely contagious epidemic. It kills most slaves in the city and one-half of the citizen population. Many patrician families are wiped out, and the commoners gain political strength at the expense of the historic aristocracy.

430–427 B.C.E.

- The "plague of Athens" breaks out, according to the celebrated Greek historian Thucydides. He reports that the epidemic began in Ethiopia, moved north through Egypt and Libya, and then arrived in Piraeus, the port of Athens. It kills a good part of the population and changes the course of the Peloponnesian War. For the first time in antiquity, an accurate empirical historian is present to observe and record the symptoms and progress of the disease. Even so, modern physicians have been unable to identify it as any known disease.

C. 400 B.C.E.

- Indian and Chinese medical texts describe leprosy.

323 B.C.E.

- Alexander the Great dies in Babylon of a fever that appears to be malaria. The army he had led into India a few years before had been decimated by a combination of climate and infectious disease.

300 B.C.E.

- Rabies is mentioned clearly in a medical text for the first time, in India.

SECOND CENTURY B.C.E.

- A medical treatise found in a Chinese tomb dated to this period mentions the Qinghao plant; in 340 C.E. the plant was cited in another work for its antifever properties. Qinghao is the source of artemisinin, which was isolated by Chinese scientists in 1971 and is today considered perhaps the most potent treatment for malaria.

48 C.E.

- Smallpox appears in China.

164–180

- A pandemic, often called the Antonine Plague, sweeps throughout the vast territories of the Roman Empire. It first appears among Roman troops fighting against Parthian Persia, and is apparently spread by them as they return to their posts throughout the empire, which was then at its territorial peak. It hits the city of Rome in 166. Many rural areas lose population, and conquered peoples from outside the empire's borders are drafted to replenish the ranks of the army. Many of these "barbarians" are even settled on newly vacant land.

Judging by the symptoms, the pandemic may have been a simultaneous attack of measles and smallpox.

251–270

- Another terrible epidemic, the Cyprian Plague, ravages the Roman Empire, possibly a resurgence of the diseases that caused the pandemic of the previous century. It is particularly devastating in Egypt, which loses a great deal of its population at this time; the city of Alexandria is reduced by two-thirds. Farmland throughout the empire is neglected and the economy shrinks drastically, ruining many of the urban middle classes. The army becomes perpetually short of recruits.

410

- Alaric, the Visigoth conqueror of Rome, dies of malaria, which has become endemic in central Italy.

541

- Outbreak of the "plague of Justinian," named for the Byzantine emperor who ruled from Constantinople, where up to 5,000 people died each day at the peak of the epidemic. It marks the entry of bubonic plague into history, and it kills millions of victims. The disease strikes almost everywhere in Europe, North Africa, the Middle East, and Central and South Asia; by 600 it reaches China, where the effects are similarly disastrous. Over the next two centuries bubonic plague returns every few decades, but now more localized and less deadly. By the mid eighth century, the European population is down by half. It may be coincidence, but this era is considered to mark the final decline of the Roman Empire in the West and the beginning of the "Dark Ages" of European history. It also marks the Arab conquest of the Middle East and North Africa.

552

- Severe epidemic breaks out in Japan, the first recorded in that country. It is believed to be either measles or plague. Believing that the disease was a punishment by native gods for the recent introduction of Buddhism, mobs destroyed temples and statues of Buddha, and they beat up priests and nuns.

585–87

- A severe epidemic hits Japan, now believed to have been smallpox, which was apparently brought to the country from Korea. As in the earlier epidemic of 552, the epidemic spurs a popular anti-Buddhist reaction by peasants, who believe the disease was a punishment meted out by Shinto spirits in protest against the new Buddhist temples and images.

994–95

- A virulent epidemic exterminates more than half the population of Japan. Since few records were kept during this catastrophe, medical historians have been unable to agree on a cause.

1179

- Pope Alexander III orders that lepers must wear the letter "L" on their clothing; they must neither touch nor look at nonlepers. In medieval Europe lepers were sometimes given land to form their own hospitals in isolation from the rest of society. At the height of the disease in the 13th century over 200 leper hospitals existed in England alone. The disease began to decline shortly thereafter, for unknown reasons.

1325

- Cholera appears clearly for the first time in India, although the great fifth-century physician Susruta had described a disease that may have been cholera. It is subsequently reported in different regions of the country in 1438, 1503, and 1612.

1347

- A pandemic of bubonic and pneumonic plague begins. Entering Europe from the Middle East, the plague kills about one-third of the continent's population. It causes profound economic, religious, social, and cultural changes. Subsiding in Europe by 1351, the plague continues its course to India and China. By the end of the century it has killed some 75 million people. The disease reemerges every few decades in one place or another in the Old World for some 300 years.

1489–90

- Epidemic of typhus kills 17,000 people in Spain.

1492

- Christopher Columbus lands in the New World, beginning the era of conquest and colonization by Europeans. Old World bacteria and viruses stow away on his and later European ships; they are soon transmitted to the New World peoples, who lack any previous exposure or immunity to these diseases. Smallpox epidemics decimate Mexico (1519) and Peru (1532), enabling the Spaniards to capture the great Aztec and Inca empires with tiny forces. By 1650, smallpox, typhus, influenza, diphtheria, hepatitis, and other diseases wipe out most of the indigenous population of South and North America.

Chronology

1493

- Genital syphilis first appears in Europe. Most scholars believe it is introduced by explorers and sailors returning from trips to the Americas. Within one or two years it can be found all over Europe and the Middle East, and it finds its way to China within a few years.

1662

- Spanish doctor Pedro Barba successfully treats a malaria patient with an extract of cinchona bark. Indians had shared the fever remedy with Jesuit missionaries.

1665–66

- Great Plague of London kills 75,000 to 100,000 people, about one-fifth of the city's population. It was probably the last major epidemic of the "second bubonic plague" that had decimated Europe 300 years before. Only a few other localities in England were effected.

1667

- The newly reorganized police force of Paris, France, establishes a commission of physicians to advise the government on matters of public health.

1668

- A yellow fever epidemic hits New York, then a small town. The disease returned in 1702 in greater force. It killed 500 people, some 10 percent of the population at that time.

1720

- An outbreak of plague in Marseilles in France kills one-third of the city's population.

1721–22

- A major smallpox epidemic hits Boston. More than half the population of 11,000 is infected, and 844 people die. For the first time in the Americas a handful of doctors, supported by the leading clergymen of the city, use inoculation. Only a handful of those who are inoculated with smallpox pus come down with the disease. These results eventually convinced skeptics to adopt the practice.

1741

- Typhus kills 30,000 Austrian soldiers defending the city of Prague, which then falls to the French and Bavarian armies. This disease, spread by lice, has long been the scourge of armies at war, who live and travel under very crowded conditions and lack adequate bathing facilities. For example, in 1643 the contending armies in the English Civil War are both struck with the disease, which forced the king to give up his attempt to recapture London.

1774

- King Louis XV of France dies of smallpox.

1781–82

- The first carefully recorded influenza pandemic spans the winter of 1781 through the summer of the following year. Although some experts consider the phenomenon to be a series of unconnected local epidemics, the majority of historians believe the pandemic began in either China or eastern Russia, and spread to India, Europe, and North America. The term influenza had only recently come into common use from its origin in 16th-century Italy; the presence of Western observers familiar with the term in East and South Asia at this time makes it likely that the various local epidemics all represented the same disease. Even in the absence of railroads and steamships, the disease could cover many miles a day.

1798

- British physician Edward Jenner announces his successful experiments to prevent smallpox by vaccinating people with cowpox. His vaccine is the basis for the vaccines that will finally eliminate smallpox from every country in the world by 1977.

1803

- A French army, trying to put down a slave rebellion in Haiti, suffers huge losses from yellow fever. In reaction the French emperor Napoléon I withdraws from Haiti and sells the Louisiana territory to the United States, which thus become a continental country. The slaves, some of whom at least are immune to the disease, set up the first African-ruled government outside the continent of Africa.

1812–13

- Weakened by hunger and cold, Napoléon's army in Russia is utterly devastated by typhus and dysentery. Some 95 percent of his 600,000 troops die.

1817–23

- The first recorded cholera pandemic begins in Bengal, India, in the fall of 1817. It was already endemic in that country, possibly using the Ganges River as its reservoir, but it was unknown outside. Most subsequent cholera pandemics seem to have originated in India as well. Many die as the disease spreads throughout the country and Sri Lanka in 1818. It reaches Southeast Asia and China by 1820 via several routes, and Japan by 1822. In 1821 British troops bring the disease to the Middle East, from where it spreads to Russia. Arab slave traders carry it to East Africa that same year. Large numbers take ill and thousands die as the disease takes root in endemic form in all the countries it reaches, laying the groundwork for more widespread and deadly pandemics later in the century.

1826–37

- Perhaps the worst cholera pandemic in history begins in 1826, and this one brings Europe and the Americas into play. Scattered reports put the death toll at 100,000 in Hungary, 25,000 in Ireland, and 15,000 in Mexico. The epidemic in the United States, where tens of thousands die, causes social tensions between the middle class and the poor. The poor, often immigrants living in crowded conditions with inadequate water and sewer lines, suffer the most. They are criticized in the press for their supposedly irresponsible and unhealthy behaviors. Returning pandemics in 1849, 1866, and 1873 evoke a more informed and sensible response, and they help pave the way for improvements in public health and water systems.

1829–32

- An influenza pandemic similar to the one of 1781–82 strikes some 50 years later. This one too apparently begins in China. Once again, mortality is fairly low.

1838

- At the initiative of the European powers and Turkey, an international Sanitary, Medicine and Quarantine Board is set up at Alexandria, Egypt. The goals are to prevent tropic diseases from being transported to Europe. Its mission is later expanded to cover the control of epidemic disease during the annual Muslim pilgrimage to Mecca. Similar boards are later established in Constantinople and Tangier.

1846–63

- Third great cholera pandemic occurs. By now, the disease is endemic in many regions, and it passes back and forth across the world. In Japan, several million die in 1858–59 and 1872. It becomes difficult to decide when a pandemic begins and ends. India continues to be a focal point.

1845–48

- In Ireland, a population exposed to severe hunger becomes easy prey for typhus and dysentery. Several hundred thousand die and hundreds of thousands more leave the country. Many emigrants die of disease on board ship or after arrival at their destinations.

1851

- The first International Sanitary Conference is held in Paris, largely in response to the first cholera pandemics. The delegates fail to agree on any practical measure, but they lay the groundwork for future global cooperation in matters of public health.

1854

- Florence Nightingale arrives in Scutari, Turkey, to tend to the sick during the Crimean War. Her sanitary reforms reduce the death rate in hospitals, launching Nightingale on a life-long struggle to improve sanitation in British hospitals.

1854

- During a London cholera epidemic, physician John Snow demonstrates that cholera spreads via drinking contaminated water. His discovery spurs construction of modern water and sewer systems around the world.

1861–65

- Disease kills over 400,000 Union and Confederate troops during the U.S. Civil War, as compared with 200,000 battle deaths.

1865–75

- Fourth great cholera pandemic of the century brings the disease to its widest distribution. In Mecca, one-third of the 90,000 pilgrims die in 1865. Nearly one-10th of the population of Martinique are wiped out that year and the next. Death tolls in Europe, India, and China are huge.

1866

- The British parliament passes the Contagious Diseases Act. The police now have the right to detain women in ports and army towns if suspected of prostitution and examine them for sexually transmitted diseases. If they are found infected, they are imprisoned in hospitals until free of signs of disease. After a campaign of opposition led by many women, the act was repealed in 1886.

1876

- The "germ theory" of disease begins to conquer the medical world and the public after German biologist Robert Koch demonstrates that a particular bacterium causes anthrax, a disease of cattle and sheep that can also infect humans.

Chronology

1881–96

- Fifth cholera pandemic strikes.

1882

- Robert Koch isolates and identifies the bacterium that causes tuberculosis, perhaps the most widespread infectious disease in the world at that time.
- First International Sanitary Convention is signed. The signatories agree to a series of prevention measures (including inspections and rat extermination) at ports and border crossings. They also agree to report on any cases of certain infectious diseases.

1885

- French biologist Louis Pasteur inoculated the first human patient against rabies. The boy, Joseph Meister, had been bitten by a rabid dog, which was until then considered a death sentence. Pasteur injected the boy with a weakened form of the virus taken from an infected animal. The patient's immune system was strengthened by fighting the injected virus, and he was able to fight off the more virulent strain passed along by the dog. The boy got better and lived a long, healthy life.

1889–90

- The worst influenza pandemic recorded up to this time breaks out somewhere in Central Asia or western Siberia in the spring of 1889. Due to the rapid spread of railroads and steamship lines all over the world, disease often spreads at unprecedented speed. By the end of the year it has reached all across Europe and the East Coast of North America. From there it spreads across North America and to South America within a month or two. All of North and Central Africa are affected in 1890. By early that year Southeast Asia and Australia have been hit as well. The death rate is higher than in the previous pandemics; subsequent waves, which strike in each of the next few years, are even more deadly.

1894

- French scientist Emile Roux announces a cure for diphtheria, a widespread and often fatal respiratory disease. He uses antitoxins extracted from the blood of animals infected with the disease.
- During an outbreak of bubonic plague in Hong Kong and South China, French biologist Alexandre Yersin and Japanese researcher Shibasaburo Kitasato jointly isolate the bacterium that causes the disease from human victims. Yersin also isolated the bacteria from rats, thus confirming the connection between the animal and human hosts.

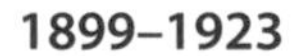

1899–1923

- Sixth cholera pandemic strikes much of the world, but causes few deaths in the developed countries of Europe and North America. It is particularly devastating in India. Annual death tolls typically run into the hundreds of thousands in this period.

1900

- The U.S. Army Yellow Fever Commission frees Cuba of malaria by eradicating mosquito breeding sites. The achievement makes possible the subsequent building of the Panama Canal, whose path had previously been blocked by mosquito-borne disease.

1902

- International Sanitary Bureau of the Americas is established at Washington, D.C., the world's first permanent international health organization. It later became the Americas Regional Office of the World Health Organization.

1916

- The United States is hit by its first large-scale polio epidemic, which kills some 7,000 patients and paralyzes another 20,000. From that point on, every summer brought a new epidemic, which grew more and more intense through the 1950s.

1918

- The first cases of what becomes the Great Influenza Pandemic appear among army recruits at Fort Riley, Kansas. The disease soon spreads across the country with troops being readied to ship overseas to the European front. In October 195,000 Americans die of the disease. By the end of the epidemic, total deaths in the United States reach about 600,000. In the meantime, troops apparently bring the virus to the trenches, where it spreads exponentially. Within months, every continent and country is affected. About one-third of mankind takes ill. The death toll has been estimated variously at from 25 to 100 million people. Unlike previous influenza epidemics, the worst mortality is among young adults; perhaps their healthy immune systems overreact to the virus, causing shock and rapid death.

1920

- The Health Organization of the League of Nations is founded.

1920s–1930s

- The deadliest strain of HIV virus jumps from chimpanzees to humans in West Central Africa, and begins its slow, quiet spread around the world.

Chronology

1928

- Alexander Fleming discovers penicillin. He notices that a common bread and fruit mold that entered his laboratory and was contaminating a sample jar was killing off staphylococcus bacteria.

1932

- The infamous "Tuskegee Experiment" begins, using 399 African-American men, mostly illiterate sharecroppers in Alabama, who are found to be infected with late-stage syphilis. The subjects are registered by the U.S. Public Health Service and observed to track the natural course of this devastating and fatal disease, lured by the false promise of free medical care. For 40 years the PHS never provides any of the subjects with appropriate treatment, even preventing them from getting penicillin via legitimate treatment programs. Over the years 40 of their wives become infected and 19 children are born with congenital syphilis. In 1972 the study is finally exposed. The resulting scandal causes changes in test protocols concerning informed consent, but it also undermines trust among many African Americans toward doctors and hospitals.

1938

- Howard Florey and Ernst Chain succeed in purifying penicillin, opening the way to its commercial use. Within a few years it becomes the most effective and famous of the new "miracle drugs."

1944

- The new antibiotic streptomycin, isolated from a fungus, cures a tuberculosis patient. The drug, and other similar medicines, ushers in a "golden era" in which a large number of infectious diseases are effectively eliminated in the developed world. Unfortunately, the era lasts a mere two decades as many bacteria begin to develop resistance.

1946

- The International Health Conference, held in New York by representatives of 61 countries, approves the constitution of the World Health Organization (WHO). The organization begins operations in 1948. That year the first World Health Assembly is held in Geneva, Switzerland.

1955

- The Salk polio vaccine is introduced to the general public, after a massive test among over 1 million schoolchildren that began two years before. The often fatal or paralytic disease, which had grown to serious epidemic proportions in the previous 40 years, was subsequently conquered in the developed world. By 2007, the disease stubbornly persisted in several poor countries in Asia and Africa, despite many years of intense vaccination programs.

- The World Health Organization launches a global malaria eradication program. In the first few years, cases do indeed plunge in many countries. But the effort proves too difficult to sustain, and malaria rates begin to rise once more by the late 1960s.

1957–58

- An influenza pandemic strikes, known as "Asian flu." More than one-third of the world's population is infected, but relatively few deaths are recorded, mostly among the ill, the aged, and the very young. It is the first flu pandemic since the dreaded "Spanish flu" of 1918, caused by a far more deadly strain of virus.

1959

- A blood sample is taken from an ill man in Kinshasa, Belgian Congo; decades later it is found to contain HIV virus particles. This is considered the first recorded case of AIDS in the world. HIV is later isolated from blood samples taken as early as 1959 in Africa and 1969 in the United States.

1962

- Rachel Carson's *Silent Spring*, an environmental manifesto, undermines support for the pesticide DDT. Although the book's condemnation was against widespread spraying of cropland, many nations eventually ban even the more limited, safer indoor spraying, which had been the strongest weapon against malaria and other mosquito-borne diseases in the previous 20 years.

1969

- Teenage boy dies in St. Louis with symptoms later identified as AIDS.

1975

- Doctors in Old Lyme, Connecticut, diagnose the first cases of Lyme disease, which eventually is found in rural and suburban areas across most of the United States.

1976

- Legionnaire's disease, a deadly new form of pneumonia, sickens many American Legion conventioneers in Philadelphia and kills several of them. The bacteria is eventually discovered lurking in a hotel's cooling system. The scare raises the specter of "sick buildings" and leads to a new focus on environmental causes of illness.

Chronology

1977

- The last case of naturally-occurring smallpox is recorded, as a massive 10-year global campaign to eliminate the disease comes to a successful end. In the subsequent 30 years not a single naturally occurring case of the disease is reported. Later revelations that Soviet laboratories had produced weaponized smallpox, and fears of its use in bioterror, keep the United States from destroying its remaining stocks of the virus.

1979

- Several dozen Russians die in a mysterious outbreak of anthrax in Sverdlovsk (today Yekaterinberg), Russia. Soviet authorities claimed a natural cause, but after the fall of the Soviet Union in 1991, officials admitted that the outbreak resulted from an accident in a massive Soviet biological warfare campaign, supposedly illegal under a 1973 U.S.-Soviet pact. Later analysis found that the toxin was a deadly combination of four different anthrax strains.

1981

- On June 5 the Centers for Disease Control and Prevention report that hundreds of gay men in New York and San Francisco are suffering from certain rare ailments associated with weakened immune systems. Over 200 die that year of what will later be named AIDS (Acquired Immune Deficiency Syndrome). Within two years the disease is recognized in countries around the world. By 2006, 25 million people around the world have died of AIDS, and 40 million more are infected with HIV. In the United States, a staggering total of over 550,000 AIDS deaths have been reported through the end of 2006.

1983

- Scientists at the Pasteur Institute isolate the virus that causes AIDS. It will eventually be names HIV (Human Immunodeficiency Virus). Cases of AIDS emerge in Europe and Africa that are transmitted through heterosexual sex.

1985

- FDA approves the first HIV antibody test, which enables the screening of donated blood to prevent the spread of AIDS via transfusion.

1986

- The first cases of "mad cow disease," or bovine spongiform encephalitis, are uncovered among cattle in Britain. Eventually some 200 people, most of them British, are diagnosed with the disease, which causes massive brain damage and death.

1988

- The Global Polio Eradication Initiative is launched by a coalition of U.S. and UN agencies. At that time, the disease was endemic in 125 countries and struck some 1,000 children every day. In the largest public health initiative in history, 20 million volunteers immunized 2 billion children. By 2006, polio was still endemic in six countries, with Nigeria and India accounting for most of the caseload, which had fallen to only six per day. The new target for complete global eradication is 2008.

1995

- A new class of anti-HIV drugs is introduced, known as protease inhibitors, which sharply reduce the death toll among those with access to drugs. By 2007, some 1 million AIDS patients in developing countries were receiving appropriate medication, and aid programs proliferated even in the poorer countries of Asia and Africa.
- Over 300 people die in a town in Zaire from Ebola hemorrhagic fever.

1997

- The first documented cases of avian influenza (bird flu) in humans occur in Hong Kong. The H5N1 virus sickened 18 people, of whom six died. The same strain was then raging through the city's poultry population, and all serious human cases involved direct human contact with infected birds. A few health care workers took ill as well, but with a mild form of the disease. The city immediately destroyed all 1.5 million birds within three days—possibly avoiding a pandemic.

2001

- U.S. and UN bodies jointly set up a global Measles Initiative. By 2005, it had exceeded its goal of cutting measles deaths in half by 2005, when some 345,000 deaths from the disease were recorded around the world—most of them children.
- Shortly after the terrorist attack in September that destroyed the World Trade Center in New York, a series of letters containing deadly anthrax spores were mailed to news media and to the offices of two U.S. senators, causing widespread concern. A total of 22 people were infected as a result, five of whom died. Massive investigations yielded no credible suspects.

2002

- The Global Fund to Fight AIDS, Tuberculosis, and Malaria is founded. It serves as a conduit for contributions from governments and other sources to fund a variety of local and regional programs fighting these three major epidemic diseases in the developing world.

Chronology

2002–04

- In November 2002 an epidemic of a new viral disease called SARS (Severe Acute Respiratory Syndrome) rapidly spreads from South China to several cities around the world, in part due to secrecy and delay within China. Extraordinary international efforts curb the epidemic within months, after 8,500 are infected and 800 die. The coronavirus that causes SARS is traced to wild civet cats. The last human cases appeared in January 2004.

2003

- The United States institutes PEPFAR, the President's Emergency Plan For AIDS Relief, pledging $15 billion to promote prevention and treatment for AIDS, malaria, and tuberculosis in developing countries. It is the largest single commitment of funds to fight the AIDS epidemic. An additional $30 billion was authorized in 2007.

2003

- Beginning in 2003, H5N1 avian influenza began spreading widely among wild and domesticated bird flocks in China, Hong Kong, and Southeast Asia. By 2005 and 2006 it was showing up, albeit in limited cases, in Europe and Africa as well. Human cases were diagnosed in 10 countries, stretching from East Asia to East Africa. By April 2007, 332 people had been found ill with the virus, of whom 204 died. Nearly all the cases appeared to be transmitted directly from birds to humans, although a handful of human-to-human transmissions may have occurred in Indonesia.

2005

- The WHO's World Health Assembly adopts new International Health Regulations after a drafting effort lasting 10 years. The regulations mandate international cooperation in preventing, monitoring, and controlling the spread of infectious disease, in particular across borders.

2006

- For the first time, the number of African AIDS patients receiving antiviral drug treatment surpasses 1 million. Still, the large majority of sufferers remain untreated.
- The U.S. Food and Drug Administration approves a vaccine against four strains of human papilloma virus, which is known to cause cervical cancer in women.
- Several large-scale studies in Africa show that male circumcision is an effective prevention measure against the spread of HIV during sex.

2007

- The World Health Organization approves the first vaccine against rotovirus. Nearly all children pick up rotovirus infections, which causes diarrhea, but most avoid serious disease. In poorer countries, however, some 600,000 children die each year. The WHO is planning a mass vaccination campaign.
- A leading nongovernmental organization and a major pharmaceutical company report the development of a new inexpensive combination antimalaria pill designed for children. Children make up most of the death toll from the disease.
- Revised International Health Regulations go into effect in June. They call for greater public openness and provide guidelines for international cooperation during health emergencies.

2008

- The H5N1 strain of avian influenza remains a potential global threat. Authorities in Indonesia and several other countries continue to report isolated cases among people and among domestic and wild birds. However, the feared breakout human pandemic has not occurred. Public health officials have become cautiously optimistic, thanks to increased supplies of vaccine and anti-viral drugs, new discoveries in basic research, and improved flu-response capability around the world.

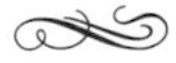

Glossary

antibiotic A drug that is used to kill or disable harmful bacteria in a human or animal host. Antibiotics are vital in the fight against infectious diseases such as tuberculosis, syphilis, cholera, and bubonic plague. At first the term was used only for drugs produced by microorganisms found in nature, such as bacteria or fungus, but it is now often used even for drugs manufactured synthetically from chemicals.

antibody A protein produced by an individual's immune system that recognizes foreign bodies, such as a bacteria or virus. The antibody typically attaches to the foreign body and allows other immune cells to kill it.

antiseptic A chemical used on external surfaces (such as skin) to prevent or stop the growth of harmful microorganisms. Antiseptic practices are methods used in health care settings to clean and disinfect all objects that might be contaminated with harmful organisms.

antitoxin An antibody produced by an organism (e.g., an animal) that can fight bacteria and other microbes within that organism. Antitoxins to some diseases can be extracted from an animal and used to create immunity in people to protect them from epidemic disease.

antiviral Any drug that kills a virus or prevents it from reproducing. Antivirals were first discovered in the 1960s, and are only now becoming widely used against diseases such as herpes, hepatitis, AIDS, and influenza.

avian influenza (bird flu) A viral disease found among domestic and wild birds around the world, similar to human influenza. Some strains of avian flu are very contagious and fatal to their hosts. Many strains can also infect humans.

bacteria A huge class of microscopic single-celled, plantlike organisms, that live everywhere on earth. Many bacteria are essential for human health, while others cause many of the worst epidemic diseases.

biodefense Any measures or products designed to protect people against biological weapons.

bioterrorism The deliberate use of disease-causing agents against civilians to provoke widespread terror in support of political aims.

carrier An individual who is infected by a disease agent, such as a bacteria, but does not show any symptoms. A carrier can unknowingly pass the agent on to others.

cell The smallest self-contained unit within all living organisms, including humans. The organs and tissues of the human body are composed mostly of cells. Many life forms, such as bacteria, have only one cell.

chronic Long-lasting or repeated; a chronic illness can last for years without killing the patient.

circumcision Surgical removal of the foreskin from a penis, for religious or health reasons. Recent studies show that circumcision helps prevent transmission of HIV/AIDS.

clinical Anything involved in the treatment of patients; clinical research deals directly with patients as opposed to theoretical or basic research, which may be done entirely in a laboratory.

contact tracing (or tracking) A method of fighting epidemics in which health care staff try to find every person who has come into contact with an infected individual. These people are examined and treated if necessary, and their own contacts may be tracked as well.

dehydration The loss of too much water from an individual, often due to diarrhea, leading to exhaustion and sometimes death. Diseases such as cholera often kill patients through dehydration.

diagnosis The job of finding out what disease a person has, or what microbe is infecting the individual. In epidemics, diagnosis may include finding out exactly what strain of virus or bacteria is involved.

dormant Inactive; an epidemic can enter a *dormant* phase when few people are infected, only to reemerge later. Bacteria or viruses can often remain *dormant* for a period inside the host, causing no symptoms.

endemic Always present in a country or region; an endemic microbe or disease can always be found somewhere in the area, residing in a natural "reservoir" of people, animals, or insects. An infectious disease is *endemic* in an area if it strikes a steady number of people every year; sometimes it can break out into an epidemic.

epidemic A sudden outbreak of a disease in a country or region, or a rapid increase in the number of new cases of a previously existing endemic disease.

epidemiology The study of epidemics; also used to refer to the sector of public health concerned with preventing and controlling epidemics and pandemics.

exposed In contact with a disease microbe or with someone already ill or infected; an exposed person is in danger of becoming ill, or may in turn pass the microbe on to another person.

fecal matter Human or animal solid waste. It can contain dangerous microbes that can cause disease if not properly disposed of. Traces of fecal matter in drinking water is a prime cause of cholera.

flu (influenza) A common infectious disease usually affecting the respiratory tract (lungs, throat, nose); many different flu viruses exist, some of which can be fatal. Many bird and animal species suffer from flu, and they can sometimes infect people.

generic drugs In most countries, drug companies can obtain patents giving them exclusive use of the drugs they develop; when the patents expire, other companies can manufacture "generic" (nonbrand name) versions of the same drugs, and sell them at lower prices.

genus One of the categories of living things that scientists use. Often living things are identified by their genus and species names, such as the deadly malaria parasite *Plasmodium falciparum*. The genus name is often abbreviated, as in *P. falciparum*.

health care delivery system The people and institutions that provide medical care to a population: doctors, nurses, clinics, hospitals, pharmacies, insurance companies, government agencies, etc.

hemorrhage A severe loss of blood either internally, through leakage from blood vessels, or externally from a wound. Some deadly viruses kill by causing hemorrhages.

host An organism (such as a person, animal, or plant) that is infected by a microbe or parasite. The host serves to feed and support the infectious organism, and it may be harmed or killed by it.

immune system The organs, cells, and proteins within the body that protect it from foreign agents such as bacteria, viruses, and parasites. People with weak immune systems, such as infants, the elderly, those suffering from certain diseases such as HIV/AIDS, or those treated with certain strong drugs, can easily get sick if exposed to dangerous microbes.

immunity A person's ability to resist a disease or any foreign agent such as a bacteria or virus. The body naturally develops immunity against many agents, while some vaccines and drugs can artificially stimulate or increase immunity.

immunization The process of stimulating a person's immunity to a disease agent, usually through a vaccine that contains a weakened form or part of the agent.

incidence The percentage or number of people who become infected by a disease agent in a given period: usually the percentage of a country's population to be infected during a given year. Compare prevalence.

incubation The development of an infectious disease from the time the pathogen enters the body until symptoms appear; the common cold may have an incubation period of one to three days; HIV can have an incubation period of many years.

infectious disease Any illness caused by an outside organism that enters (infects) the body. It can be caused by a bacteria, virus, fungus, parasite, or prion.

influenza *See* flu.

inoculation Injection into the body of a vaccine or other product in order to create or increase immunity to a disease; often a synonym for vaccination.

isolate 1) To discover the cause of a disease within tissue samples taken from an infected person; a researcher may isolate a known or a previously unknown virus from the blood of a patient. 2) To separate an infected person from healthy people to prevent contagion.

larva (e) An early stage in the life cycle of many insects. Larva can act as hosts for many parasites or other disease agents.

microbe Any living organism that is too small to be seen by people without the aid of a microscope, such as bacteria, viruses, parasites, and fungal cells.

microorganism Synonym for microbe.

morbidity 1) The harmful or painful symptoms of a disease. 2) The rate of illness in a country or population: most flu epidemics bring high morbidity but low mortality.

mortality Loss of life, especially as a result of disease or poor living conditions. Poor sanitation can cause high mortality rates among children.

negative In laboratory tests a negative result means that the individual being tested does *not* show evidence of having the disease in question. Thus, a negative result is good news for the individual.

outbreak The start of an epidemic or pandemic. Often refers to the moment when an endemic disease, a small local epidemic, or the release of a dangerous microbe suddenly causes a widespread epidemic.

organ A division of a plant or animal that can be regarded as a distinct body and can perform a particular function. The lung is the organ that controls breathing and respiration.

organism An individual plant or animal.

pandemic An epidemic of infectious disease that has spread to many countries, often to most of the world, and that infects a large number of people.

parasite In medicine, any small animal that lives within a host animal such as a human being and draws nutrition from it; parasites often cause diseases. Sometimes the term is used to refer only to single-celled animals and not to parasitic worms.

pathogen Any living body that causes disease, such as a bacteria, virus, worm, or parasite.

pathology 1) The abnormal and usually harmful conditions within an organism that result from disease, such as damaged cells or organs. 2) The study of diseases, their causes, and the changes they produce in the body. A pathology lab can diagnose disease by examining tissue samples from individuals.

placebo A substance that has no physical impact on the body. It is used as a control in tests of new drugs—some patients receive the drug, some the placebo, but neither is told which substance they are receiving.

pneumonia Any severe inflammation of the lungs that causes them to be partially filled with fluids and interferes with breathing. Pneumonia is typically caused by bacteria or viruses.

positive In laboratory tests a positive result means that the individual being tested shows evidence of having the disease in question. Thus, a positive result may be bad news for the patient.

present A patient "presents" symptoms of a disease when he or she shows visible or testable evidence of infection; the patient may incubate the disease for a long period before presenting its symptoms.

prevalence The number or percentage of a population that is infected with a disease or a pathogen at any one time. They may have acquired the disease that year or at any time in the past. Compare incidence.

preventive care Any treatment or regimen that will help prevent a person from becoming ill from a particular disease. It can include vaccination, antiseptic measures, better nutrition, and/or healthier living conditions or life styles.

prion A single protein particle that has taken an abnormal shape and can cause certain brain diseases such as mad cow disease.

protein One of the basic building blocks of all living cells. All living organisms are largely built up of the many different kinds of proteins; they also do most of the work of the cell.

protocol A standard guideline for treating a particular disease in an individual, or for responding to a potential epidemic.

public health The field that deals with protecting and improving the health of people in a community, country, or throughout the world. It usually covers preventive measures including vaccination, health-related environmental matters such as clean food, air, and water, and education for health and healthy life styles.

quarantine The practice of isolating an individual or a group who are or who may be infected with a contagious disease, so as to stop an epidemic from spreading. The term was originally used for ships who were required to wait for 40 days (*quarante* in French) before docking and unloading.

rehydration A method used in treating certain diseases such as cholera that *dehydrate* patients; the patient is given liquids enriched with electrolytes either by mouth or intravenously in order to restore body fluids to healthy levels.

reservoir In the study of epidemic disease, a reservoir or reservoir host is an animal in which disease organisms can safely live even when no humans are infected. Future human epidemics could spread from this reservoir.

resistance The ability of an individual to avoid getting ill even after being exposed to a disease pathogen. The immune system gives people different levels of resistance to many different organisms, which can be increased through vaccination or by a bout of the disease itself.

respiratory Relating to breathing. The respiratory system includes the lungs with their muscles and blood vessels, together with all the airways that lead from the mouth and nose down to the lungs. Respiratory diseases can affect any one of these organs.

sanitation The public function of keeping the environment clean, especially by removing waste.

secondary infection Certain diseases have the effect of lowering the body's overall resistance, so that various random microbes can take hold and cause "secondary" infections or diseases. For example, HIV/AIDS weakens the immune system and may allow diseases like tuberculosis to infect the patient as a secondary infection.

serum The watery fluid in blood that carries the blood cells. The term is often used to refer to serum taken from animals who have been exposed to a disease, which can contain valuable *antitoxins.*

species One of the categories of living things that scientists use; one or more species make up a *genus.* Human beings make up one species; many deadly microbes come in a variety of species, each one of which may affect the patient in different ways and may respond to treatment differently.

sterilization Eliminating all microbes from objects such as medical instruments, through the use of high temperatures or through the use of antiseptic substances.

strain The lowest level category used by scientists to classify living things. Many species (including disease microbes) come in a variety of slightly different strains; the different strains often act in very different ways.

surveillance In public health, surveillance involves keeping track of all cases of infectious diseases, in order to head off emerging epidemics. Modern surveillance includes close international cooperation, mandatory reporting, and daily Internet searches, among other techniques.

susceptibility The opposite of resistance; a person or population is susceptible to a disease if they lack immunity to it. Populations who have been isolated by geography or social circumstances tend to be highly susceptible to infectious diseases.

therapeutic Used to describe any substance or practice that will help an individual deal successfully with a disease.

toxin Poison; in medicine, this most often refers to a poisonous substance produced by a bacteria or by a poisonous animal.

transition In epidemiology, the process by which a microbe or a new strain of an old microbe passes from one host species to another, for example, from birds to humans. The microbe usually mutates in order to survive successfully in the new host.

transmission The passage of a microbe from one individual to another, either within or across species. For example, mosquitoes transmit malaria parasites between one human and another; flu can be transmitted by a simple sneeze.

vaccination Treatment with a vaccine—a substance made up of live or dead microbes, or parts of microbes—in order to stimulate the body to produce *antibodies* to that microbe. The antibodies will protect the vaccinated individual from future infections.

vector An organism that helps transmit a disease. Rats and fleas are vectors for bubonic plague; black flies are vectors for onchocerciasis.

viral Pertaining to or caused by a virus.

virus Any one of a huge collection of microscopic life forms that cannot live long or reproduce on their own but must infect host animals or plants. Viruses cause many of the worst human epidemic diseases, including HIV/AIDS, smallpox, polio, and influenza.

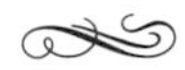

Index

Note: page numbers in **boldface** indicate major treatment of a subject. Page numbers followed by *f* indicate figures. Page numbers followed by *b* indicate bibliographic entries. Page numbers followed by *c* indicate chronology entries. Page numbers followed by *g* indicate glossary entries.

C

Index

Index

Index

Index

Index

T